CLINICAL PRACTICE IN PSYCHOSOCIAL NURSING: ASSESSMENT AND INTERVENTION

CLINICAL PRACTICE IN PSYCHOSOCIAL NURSING: ASSESSMENT AND INTERVENTION

EDITORS

DIANNE C. LONGO, R.N., M.N.

Instructor-Clinician II
University of Rochester
School of Nursing
Rochester, New York

REG ARTHUR WILLIAMS, R.N., M.N.

Assistant Professor
Department of Psychosocial Nursing
University of Washington
Seattle, Washington

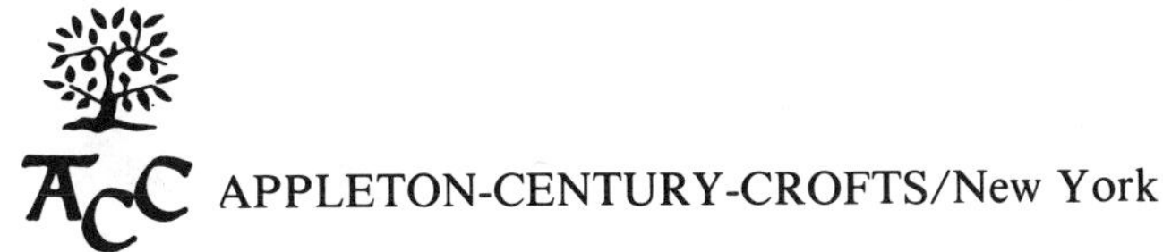

APPLETON-CENTURY-CROFTS/New York

78 79 80 81 82 / 10 9 8 7 6 5 4 3 2 1

Prentice-Hall International, Inc., London
Prentice-Hall of Australia, Pty. Ltd., Sydney
Prentice-Hall of India Private Limited, New Delhi
Prentice-Hall of Japan, Inc., Tokyo
Prentice-Hall of Southeast Asia (Pte.) Ltd., Singapore
Whitehall Books Ltd., Wellington, New Zealand

Library of Congress Cataloging in Publication Data

Main entry under title:

Clinical practice in pyschosocial nursing.

Includes index.
1. Psychiatric nursing. I. Longo, Diane C.
II. William, Reg Arthur. [DNLM: 1. Psychiatric nursing. WY160 C641]
RC440.C54 610.73′019 77-21502
ISBN 0-8385-1167-8

Text design: The Old Typosopher
Cover design: B. Andrew Mudryk

PRINTED IN THE UNITED STATES OF AMERICA

CONTRIBUTORS

KAREN SUE BABICH, R.N., M.S.
Doctoral Candidate in Education
University of Colorado
Boulder, Colorado;
Formerly Assistant Professor
University of Northern Colorado
School of Nursing
Greeley, Colorado

JOAN M. BAKER, R.N., M.S.
Assistant Professor
Department of Psychosocial Nursing
Alcoholism Nursing Program
University of Washington
Seattle, Washington

MARIE ANNETTE BROWN, R.N., M.N.
Clinic Supervisor, Planned Parenthood
Clinical Instructor
Department of Psychosocial Nursing
University of Washington
Seattle, Washington

MARY T. BUSH, R.N., M.N.
Assistant Professor
Department of Psychosocial Nursing
University of Washington
Seattle, Washington

ALICE COAD-DENTON, R.N., M.A.
Family and Psychosocial
Nurse Practitioner
Renton, Washington

DENISE CONLIN-FORT, R.N., M.S.N.
Doctoral Candidate
Clinical Psychology
Catholic University
Washington D.C.

LEONA L. EGGERT, R.N., M.A.
High School Nurse
Bellevue Public Schools, District 405
Bellevue, Washington;
Formerly Assistant Professor
Department of Psychosocial Nursing
University of Washington
Seattle, Washington

NADA J. ESTES, R.N., M.S.
Assistant Professor
Department of Psychosocial Nursing
Alcoholism Nursing Program
University of Washington
Seattle, Washington

HELEN HOPE GRAVES, R.N., M.S.
Assistant Professor
Department of Psychosocial Nursing
University of Washington
Seattle, Washington

M. EDITH HEINEMANN, R.N., M.A.
Professor
Department of Psychosocial Nursing
Alcoholism Nursing Program
University of Washington
Seattle, Washington

THOMAS H. HOLMES, M.D.
Professor
Psychiatry and Behavioral Sciences
School of Medicine
University of Washington
Seattle, Washington

LUCILLE KINDELY KELLEY, R.N., M.N.
Instructor
Department of Psychosocial Nursing
University of Washington
Seattle, Washington

MARGARET L. LARSON, R.N., M.N.
Assistant Professor
Department of Psychosocial Nursing
University of Washington
Seattle, Washington

DIANNE C. LONGO, R.N., M.N.
Instructor-Clinician II
University of Rochester
School of Nursing
Rochester, New York

P. M. MACELVEEN, R.N., Ph.D.
Assistant Professor
Department of Psychosocial Nursing
University of Washington
Seattle, Washington

L. (SISSY) MADDEN, R.N., M.N.
Educational Coordinator
and Family Counselor
Southwest Community Alcohol Center
Seattle, Washington

CAPT. R. H. RAHE, MC, USNR
Head
Stress Medicine Division
Naval Research Center
San Diego, California

MARI K. SIEMON, R.N., M.A.
Instructor
Department of Psychosocial Nursing
University of Washington
Seattle, Washington

ELAINE ADAMS THOMPSON, R.N., M.A.
Research Associate
Department of Psychosocial Nursing
University of Washington
Seattle, Washington

MARILYN PEDDICORD WHITLEY, R.N., M.A.
Instructor
Department of Psychosocial Nursing
University of Washington
Seattle, Washington

CINDY COOK WILLIAMS, R.N., A.C.S.W.
Social Worker
Veterans Administration Hospital
Seattle, Washington

REG ARTHUR WILLIAMS, R.N., M.N.
Assistant Professor
Department of Psychosocial Nursing
University of Washington
Seattle, Washington

CONTENTS

PREFACE

Providing psychosocial nursing care is an obvious and important focus of the nursing process. However, *how* one goes about delivering this aspect of care is not so obvious to most students and practitioners. This is particularly true because psychosocial concepts are complex and abstract and consequently difficult to translate into meaningful behavior at the bedside or in ambulatory care settings.

Partly for this reason, a few years ago we collected many of the teaching materials, organizing guidelines and references that we found helpful for students in operationalizing principles of psychosocial nursing. We had these materials printed in handbook format and sold to the students at cost, as a required adjunct to their basic textbook.

The handbook served the students well since they appreciated having a variety of resources under one cover. Without our being aware of it at the time, nursing students studying in other specialties, students from related disciplines, and practicing staff nurses working in nearby hospitals and clinics also purchased the text. The success of the original work, rudimentary as it was, supported us in our decision to expand both the format and the content and present it in a more formal way. The main purpose of this text is to present the assessment process in such a way that the reader can see more clearly the relationship between theory and practice. Hopefully this will enable the student to move with greater ease through levels of abstractions and to operate more successfully, with enhanced self-confidence in the actual clinical situation.

The reader might wonder how we decided which topics to include in the text. Some of the chapters were chosen as a direct result of recommendations from 200 undergraduate students. They identified the most helpful areas as suicide assessment, human sexuality, anxiety, and alcoholism. Group, family, social networks, and cultural systems move the focus of intervention from traditional dyadic interaction to alternative definitions of the "patient." The material on school-age children and adolescents was included so that generalists could benefit from the specialists' experience and gain an understanding of patients in these stages of development.

Throughout the book, the reader will notice the frequent mention and integration of physical health and physiological variables. Many of the authors used the medical-surgical setting as well as the mental health background to illustrate the assessment and intervention process. This is simply a reflection of each contributor's commitment to a holistic approach to patient care. Many of the authors maintain a considerable amount of interest in their former areas of expertise. Some of the contributors are presently practicing as medical nurse practitioners in addition to their roles as educators and psychosocial clinical nursing specialists.

We did not intend to explore every significant mental health issue in the text and recommend using it in conjunction with other basic psychiatric nursing books. Although this was written specifically for psychosocial nurses, we hope that the material will be helpful to other disciplines as well.

Many authors in the text used the term "she" when referring to the nurse. This was not intended to discount the many men in the field of nursing; it was used primarily for convenience and readability.

We would like to extend our thanks and appreciation to all the individuals who made contributions to this book. We would also like to thank Betty Mitsanaga, R.N., Ph.D., Chairperson, Department of Psychosocial Nursing, Oliver Osborne, R.N., Ph.D., and Helen Nakagawa, R.N., Ph.D., for their encouragement and support during the development of our text. We would like to acknowledge the many hours spent by Kathy Smith-DiJulio, R.N., M.A. serving as a reader for the manuscripts and Charles Bollinger for his encouragement and support.

Our appreciation is also extended to our typists, Shannon Peterson, Wendy Chinn, Bee Spanfelner, Kathy Arnold, Alice Hama, Deanna Rio, and Marty Streb. Their hours of typing outlines, rough drafts, and completed manuscripts made our efforts possible. Lastly, we thank a very important person in our lives, Cindy Williams, for her inspiration, concern, and support during the development and publication of this book.

D. C. L.
R. A. W.

CHAPTER

1

COMMUNICATIONS AND HUMAN BEHAVIOR

Dianne C. Longo

Most student nurses are required to complete a course in psychosocial nursing. Depending on the program followed, these courses can be variously labeled with names such as psychiatric nursing or mental health nursing. In these educational experiences it is expected that the nurse will master the basic communication skills involved in an interpersonal relationship. Before examining the specific verbal skills used within a therapeutic relationship (Chapter 2) it will be helpful to consider human behavior and communication from a larger perspective.

Only a few undergraduate nursing schools offer strong programs in cross-cultural nursing (Chapter 3). This lack in our nursing education has many implications, one of which has particular relevance for the communication that is necessary in the nurse–patient relationship. Involved as we are as participants in our culture, it is difficult for us to view our own values and assumptions objectively. One of these values concerns the fact that we are a noncontact people. North Americans, as compared with Arabs, for example, generally do not touch each other; we maintain large interpersonal distances when interacting. In place of physical contact we have substituted the use of words as a means to communicate; we place great value on verbal exchanges in communication rather than nonverbal exchanges (Hall 1959).

Similarly, it is characteristic of many students during their initial exposure to psychiatric mental health nursing or psychosocial nursing to assume that they are about to learn all the proper verbal responses to the questions they expect patients to ask them. They expect the emphasis to be placed on how to say the right thing at the right time, or at least how to say something innocuous in a tight situation. Being left stranded without the usual security that words provide can raise anxiety in students and practicing nurses alike.

The purpose of this chapter is to propose a construct or model to be used in the assessment of communication and for intervention in communication in the nurse–patient relationship. It is hoped that use of the construct will help nurses to think of communication in a broader perspective and that the construct will serve as a guide in evaluating verbal and nonverbal exchanges with patients.

The idea of communication is a complex conception, and the nurse–patient relationship is complex. No model can cover all aspects of such a complicated and critical interchange. However, this model has been found useful in helping nurses focus on those aspects of communication that our cultural biases prevent us from fully appreciating.

REVIEW OF COMMUNICATION PRINCIPLES

This section will briefly review the basic communication principles: content in communication, context in communication, and process in communication.

The content of communication is the most obvious aspect and it is the easiest to identify and assess. Content refers to the literal meaning that words or other symbols have for us. For example, in asking someone "Why do you say that?" the nurse is asking for content with respect to motivation and is expecting a reply such as "Well, I thought we had agreed to do it this way" or "Because I would feel foolish if I didn't say I was sorry." Similarly, by asking "How does that make you feel?" the nurse is asking for content with respect to an emotional experience and is expecting a reply such as "That makes me feel sad" (or happy or depressed or joyful). The content of the reply is important, and each of the words literally means quite a different thing, which in turn indicates a great deal about the responding individual.

The context involves the setting and the circumstances in which communication takes place. For example, if a patient responds to a nurse's first contact with him by commenting "I trust you implicitly, and I'm glad you came to talk to me," that is certainly not what he really means at all. The words need to be evaluated in light of the context. Implicit trust is not established within the context of an initial encounter. After considering the context, reformulation of the content could give a different meaning to the patient's words.

Process is the element of communication that involves the manner in which something is said or done. The most obvious example of process is the technique of indirect questioning. Instead of numerous questions to assess the patient's status (eg, Are you feeling fine? Are you relieved to be here? Are you sad to be away from your wife? Are you feeling bad?), the whole conversation can become more effective and less complex if the nurse simply asks "How are you doing here on your first day?" The manner in which statements, questions, and responses are formulated is very much part of process in interpersonal communication. The way the words are arranged in a statement or a question can influence the responding individual; this in itself can make it relatively easy or relatively difficult for the patient to reply in a productive manner.

THE CHANNEL CONSTRUCT

It might be said that the need we have to communicate and to establish a sense of relatedness to others is so important that we have evolved a fail-safe system for communication. The following model contains six channels or levels of communication that one can use to relay information to the outside world concerning an inner experience. The system, as seen in this model, is relatively fail-safe, inasmuch as when one channel fails or is dysfunctional (eg, verbal expression) another channel can take over (eg, the physiologic channel).

A construct is a framework or model for use in organizing information in a systematic manner. It is important to keep in mind that this is a model to be used for learning purposes. There is nothing sacred about its labels; there is no strict division between channels. For example, it does not really matter whether you label the act of crying as a physiologic activity or think of it as a behavior. What is important is that all channels have communicative value. The six channels of this construct are the following:

1. Physiologic channel
2. Fine motor channel (kinesic and proxemic)
3. Behavioral channel
4. Verbal channel: expression of behavior
5. Verbal channel: expression of thoughts, opinions, and ideas
6. Verbal channel: expression of feelings and emotions

The rationale for nursing assessment and intervention is drawn from knowledge and understanding of the basic physical and social sciences as well as from research and clinical data. Social anthropology has many implications for psychosocial nursing, and anthropologic concepts form a part of the basis for the model presented.

One of the most pervasive themes in social anthropology is the simple fact that human needs are universal; however, the processes through which these needs are met are certainly not simple. The essential elements of any culture remain constant (eg, kinship, law, religion), but the various forms (processes) that different cultures have evolved to deal with these elements can be vastly different from one another. For example, a marriage ceremony in one culture entails rituals that last three weeks; in another culture the marriage contract is unspoken and is treated in what we North Americans would consider a nonchalant manner.

There is a striking relationship between what is happening in a given culture (content) and how it is happening in that culture (process). One may observe similarity of content from one culture to another, but the process of one may vary dramatically from the process of the other. In this respect process may actually be the key to content.

The same principle holds true for human communicative efforts. There are many different outward ways to express the same inner experience. For example, given the same situational crisis to deal with we react in different ways, eg, at the death of a close friend each of us will handle grief in a different manner: on a given day one of us might be sitting alone and crying (one process), another might be spending the day reflecting on the friend's life (another process), and another might be involved in funeral arrangements (yet another process). Regardless of the different behaviors we are engaged in we are all involved in the same content: grief. Without an understanding of this relationship between content and process the analysis of behavior can be a more confusing project than it ought to be.

In addition to anthropologic concepts, traditional principles of communication and psychodynamics were used in the formulation of the channel construct. The focus is on process rather than content, and it is assumed that behavior is meaningful and that it has communicative value, that all parts of a person are involved in the communication process, that communication is inevitable: we cannot *not* communicate.

Physiologic Channel

The physiologic channel is that level involving observable or measurable changes in physiologic activity in response to or concurrently with emotional experience. We may express joy or sadness through tears, we may blush self-consciously when we feel embarrassment, we may turn red or white when we feel angry, we may experience pounding headaches when under stress.

Fine Motor Channel

The fine motor channel encompasses a variety of communicative processes. It involves body motion or body language—such things as eye contact, body position or posture, facial expression, gait, rate of speech, and quality of body movement. It also involves proxemic behavior, ie, a person's use of space, interpersonally or in relationship to inanimate objects.

Behavioral Channel

The behavioral channel involves activities that we usually consider goal-directed and purposeful, whether they are functional or dysfunctional in nature. Examples are innumerable: playing the piano, taking a walk, keeping an appointment, attending classes, reading a book, going to a movie. Behaviors that are usually considered dysfunctional include suicide gestures, using drugs or alcohol to excess, spending large sums of money one does not have, destroying property, rape, physical abuse, and extreme social withdrawal.

The first three channels presented (the physiologic, the fine motor, and the behavioral levels of communication) transmit what is usually referred to in the literature simply as nonverbal communication. However, many specialists in the field, most recently Spiegel and Machotka (1974), are strongly opposed to the use of that term. They contend that the label nonverbal reinforces the misleading notion that words are more important than other forms of communication in establishing the validity of one's inner experiences. We know that defense mechanisms play a large part in determining what is consciously experienced and therefore what can be expressed verbally; therefore, unless verbal expression is consistent with expression from the first three levels of communication it is usually wise to reserve judgment about the accuracy of what a patient verbalizes.

For example, if a patient were to say that he was not the least bit anxious and was not under any stress, but the nurse knew that he had recently begun to drink heavily, then the nurse would not accept his words alone as an accurate and complete picture of his inner experiences. People who feel secure and comfortable about themselves and their environment do not need the relief from anxiety or depression that one seeks in drinking large amounts of alcohol. Rather, the nurse may assume one of two things: either the patient is not in touch with (conscious of) his feelings of discomfort and therefore cannot be expected to express them in words or the patient is aware of his feelings but consciously chooses not to verbalize them. In either instance, although the nurse may respect the patient's statement, she will not assume that his words negate his behavior. This assessment process will be further discussed later in the chapter.

The first three channels are presented in the order of our ability to exert conscious control over them, ie, we have the least control over the physiologic channel. Normally we do not consciously control the rate of our heartbeat, the degree of vasodilatation or vasoconstriction, or the level of gastric secretions (at least not without biofeedback training or meditative effort). Our autonomic nervous system simply functions without our conscious control.

The kinesic and proxemic channel also operates for the most part without our awareness. Most people establish a predictable interpersonal distance in social situations, a distance that is culturally determined. Facial expressions can be consciously manipulated, but most people can differentiate the forced smile and the spontaneous one. Body posture also can be consciously controlled, but anyone who has tried to force or control his body's movements for any length of time is aware of the considerable strain involved and usually is relieved when he can drop the pretense and let his body act naturally.

Sometimes a person's rate of speech (rather than the content of the discussion) is the only indication that he is upset or very concerned about something at the moment. A person whose body position appears relaxed and whose facial expression appears serene may be speaking about something at so rapid a pace that a listener can hardly understand anything he is saying. The information being conveyed on the fine motor channel can override the information from the verbal channels in terms of significance. The patient may be trying to convince his listener verbally that he feels fine, but his rate of speech conveys the opposite content.

The behavior channel operates both consciously and unconsciously. Generally speaking, the greater the degree of emotional health a person has the more control he has over his behavior. The more emotionally mature a person is the better he understands the motivation for his behavior and the reasons he acts in certain ways. Another characteristic of the mature person is the ability to express feelings interpersonally, in words, in the appropriate setting.

On the other hand, people at the opposite end of the continuum "behave out" their emotions, rather than verbalizing them. (Behaving out is coined here as a general term. It is not necessarily synonymous with "acting out.") Behaving out can occur without the person being aware of why he is behaving the way he is and without his being aware of how his behavior patterns are reflective of and are related to his inner experience. Abusive behavior is one unfortunate example. If overcome for the moment by intense emotion, a person may strike out against those around him or inflict pain on himself (suicide or self-mutilating gestures) in an effort to release the accumulated tension that bottled-up feelings generate. This is usually done without the person realizing why he is hurting others or himself and without being aware of what else he could do to handle his feelings.

All of us have a very basic need to express our feelings. If we are inhibited in direct verbal expression, either because we have not learned to talk openly about ourselves or because our defense mechanisms prevent us from consciously expressing our feelings, then our emotions must be expressed in another manner; they must come out somehow. The channel for expression is frequently behavioral. Thus behavior, when viewed from this perspective, becomes more communicative than arbitrary in nature.

It is not surprising that generally, patients in need of mental health services are not sophisticated and open in verbalizing their feelings. Therefore the nurse's communication skills play a large role in helping patients to function more adequately in this area. There are levels of sophistication that patients move through in the process of acquiring the ability to verbalize their feelings. The three verbal channels that will be presented as part of our construct are discussed in the order of increasing sophistication, with verbal expression of behavior being the easiest to achieve and verbal expression of emotions being the most difficult.

There are many ways to assess content at this level of communication. This method of discriminating levels of sophistication can be used as a basic framework. How to help patients move specifically from one level to another will be discussed in later sections of this chapter.

Verbal Channels

Expressions of Behavior. The first verbal channel conveys verbalizations formulated in terms of activities or actions. This is the easiest channel for people to use when carrying on a conversation about themselves. For example, assume that a nurse is working with a male patient who has recently experienced a financial setback. If he were comfortable only at this level of communication the conversation might run something like this:

N: Mr. Smith, what was your reaction to the news about your investment?
P: Well, I got up that morning and went to work as usual. I couldn't stay the whole day, though. At noon I took a long walk in the park instead of eating lunch.
N: How were you feeling at the time?
P: That I could find another job if I had to and that I would have to switch stock brokers, that's for sure. I didn't know if I could tell my wife what had happened.

In this example the patient is describing his experience in terms of his behavior and the activities he engaged in, rather than in terms of his emotions or feelings. This form of response is not uncommon; it is the safest channel, and it is the one used most frequently in social and business interactions. Most people begin a therapeutic verbal encounter using this channel. Some need more help than others in moving to a more sophisticated and more functional level of emotional expression.

Expression of Thoughts, Opinions, and Ideas. The second verbal channel conveys thoughts, ideas, and opinions. Asking a patient "What do you think?" can mean at least two things: "What does logic tell you about this?" or "What is your stream of consciousness?" This level of communication is somewhat more difficult for people to attain; it requires that one commit himself to a position on an issue under discussion or share his inner thoughts with another. On this level, using the same example of the nurse and the patient who has recently experienced a financial setback, the dialogue between the nurse and patient will be somewhat different:

N: Mr. Smith, what was your reaction to the news about your investment?
P: Well, evidently the investment was not based on sound advice. I think, though, that my decision to invest was timely; there was a lot of evidence to suggest I could make a lot of money. However, in these situations one cannot always predict success.
N: How were you feeling at the time?
P: That my broker had been unwise in his judgments and that I had been equally unwise in committing that much capital to the investment. My wife agrees with my analysis of the situation. At this point we are both of the opinion that we have learned from this experience; these things, of course, happen to a lot of people.

In this example, the patient is describing his experience in terms of opinions and rational statements (as well as behavior) based on judgment and logical deductions, rather than in terms of emotions and feelings. This channel is used most frequently by people with strong intellectual defenses, ie, people whose principal defense mechanisms include rationalization, intellectualization, and denial. When someone uses this channel exclusively it takes time, patience, and trust to help him move to direct expression of feelings. At the same time, the ability to integrate experiences in a logical manner can be a strength the patient can certainly retain.

Expression of Feelings and Emotions. The third verbal channel conveys feelings and emotions. This level of communication is the most difficult to attain, but it is the most functional and the most necessary for emotional health. Unfortunately, many people are not taught the use of this channel by example, nor are they rewarded when they do use this channel to communicate with others. Direct expression of feelings in social situations, business situations, and many family situations is frequently seen as too threatening and is therefore not sanctioned. For many people the therapeutic encounter may be the only setting in which expressions of feelings are acceptable and in which the patient can be encouraged to continue verbalization at this level.

If we again use the example of the patient who has recently experienced a financial setback, and if we assume that the patient feels comfortable using this channel, the patient–nurse interaction will differ from the earlier two sets of dialogue:

N: Mr. Smith, what was your reaction to the news about your investment?
P: Well, I was naturally upset and also really shocked. I counted on this deal coming through so that my wife and I could buy a new home.
N: How were you feeling at the time?
P: I was furious with the broker who had made the suggestion, and I was really angry at myself for having agreed to go along. I was so anxious about telling my wife, and I really felt embarrassed when I did tell her. I was also afraid we wouldn't have enough money for the year, and I was devastated about myself as a provider for my family.

If we were to examine our own conversations, in both social and personal contexts, we would readily find examples of the use of each of the verbal channels described. There might be some instances when even within the context of a very trusting relationship we would find it difficult to express some of our true feelings. Most often we would probably find our channel usage mixed: part behavior, part thoughts, part feelings. However, if we kept track of our own levels of verbalization over a long enough period of time, certain patterns would emerge.

One of the most valuable experiences nurses can have is the opportunity to learn about themselves in this area. It is important to establish a sense of one's own strengths and limitations. It is very difficult to help a patient verbalize uncomfortable feelings if one has not experienced the positive effects of this exercise for oneself.

Channel Congruence

Congruence is important in this discussion of the various channels of communication. Congruence as used here simply means consistency. If we say that a person is congruent for all levels of channel usage we mean that the pieces of information coming from all levels have similar content.

The channel construct is presented below with a congruent example of expression of anger:

1. Physiologic channel: Face flushed, neck veins distended, hypertension.
2. Fine motor channel: Wavering eye contact, fists clenched, speech pressured.
3. Behavioral channel: Slamming of doors, hurried pacing, fists pounding table.
4. Verbal channel (expression of behavior) "I feel like breaking every dish in the house."
5. Verbal channel (expression of thoughts, opinions, and ideas): "What you said was totally unfair, and I do not agree with any of it."
6. Verbal channel (expression of feelings and emotions): "I am really furious about this issue. I feel awkward and uncomfortable."

As was mentioned earlier, because of the strength of defense mechanisms some emotions are blocked; one is not conscious of them, and they cannot be expressed verbally. However, people usually communicate these experiences indirectly through other channels. Here is an example of an incongruent channel outline of someone expressing anxiety behaviorally rather than verbally:

1. Physiologic channel:	Diaphoresis, rapid breathing, difficulty in hearing what is being said.
2. Fine motor channel:	Locking and unlocking fingers, frequent position changes, tense posture.
3. Behavioral channel:	Walking up and down corridor, bumping into chairs, dropping papers, misplacing important items.
4. Verbal channel (expression of behavior):	"I think I'll go for a ride; it's such a nice day."
5. Verbal channel (expression of thoughts, opinions, and ideas):	"That idea is just fine with me. No, it doesn't bother me at all to take the exam again."
6. Verbal channel (expression of feelings and emotions):	"Oh, I'm very relaxed, and I feel comfortable. No, I'm not worried about my grade being so low."

Obviously the person in this example is neither comfortable nor relaxed. There are many indications of anxiety, and the verbal responses do not totally reflect the person's actual experience.

ASSESSMENT AND INTERVENTION

A full assessment of the communication assets and limitations of a patient can be made quickly and simply with the channel construct in mind. Gathering data in this way also helps one to focus on possible goals for the nurse–patient relationship, and the data can easily be applied to a problem-solving model. It also allows the nurse to monitor changes in the patient's progress in interpersonal relationships more systematically and concretely.

The following outline may be helpful:

1. Examine each channel as information becomes available, eg, in the nurse–patient relationship and from history, physical examination, presenting complaints, and past and present behavior patterns. Note which channels are used and which are unused.
2. Do not close the assessment process until all channels have been reviewed.
3. Consider all pieces of information gathered as having equal communication value.
4. Review data for congruence.

5. If the content from one channel is inconsistent with that from another, closely examine those channels that operate outside of the patient's conscious control, and contrast this information with information from channels that are subject to conscious control.
6. Consider the medical-psychiatric diagnosis, as well as its implications for the communicative process and its indications of defense mechanisms you might expect to encounter. In addition, look at symptoms that would influence baseline functioning.
7. Review the context of the situation.
8. Reformulate content in light of context and process.

The remainder of this chapter will focus on assessment and intervention as presented within the context of clinical situations and examples. Further remarks about each channel are included. Intervention specific to each channel will then be suggested and discussed.

Physiologic Channel

When significant emotions are repeatedly blocked from adequate expression and a chronic state of physiologic readiness ensues, organic changes and tissue destruction will follow. This chain of events can result in a full-blown psychosomatic syndrome (Alexander 1950). Psychosomatic diseases, which include such syndromes as essential hypertension, peptic ulcer, ulcerative colitis, and bronchial asthma, represent the end point of years of complex psychodynamic and physiologic responses. Working with these patients requires close collaboration with and supervision from the medical team. For that reason specific interventions are not discussed here.

There are also patients who present with exclusively physical symptoms in whom there have been no concomitant organic changes and no pathophysiology has been found. Examples are hypochondriacal neurotic and hysterical neurotic patients, conversion types. The nurse should be aware that approaches to these patients are presented in most nursing texts, and the reader is referred to that literature for more specific information.

The focus of this section is not to review assessment and nursing intervention for patients with these clear-cut syndromes; it is to suggest another perspective when working with patients. MacKinnon (1971) reminds us that "everyone has a psychosomatic aspect of his emotional life" (p 363). Every person will at one time or another use the physiologic channel to express feelings that have been blocked from other channels. Loosely speaking, this is what is referred to as somatization. It must be emphasized that for the nurse to react to a patient's physical complaints as if they are "only in his mind" is not only inappropriate but also dangerous. Somatic complaints are complaints of real distress, and they should be treated as such. The patient who has transitory episodes of diarrhea during a crisis in his hospitalization or during the confrontive stages of psychotherapy is actually having diarrhea; it is not just a symptom "in his mind."

The nurse's intervention in such instances should include three aspects of care: (1) neutral statements that acknowledge the patient's physical or emotional distress, (2) administration of physical treatment if appropriate (eg, medication), and (3) collaborative effort with the patient to connect the stressful event with the communicative aspects of the physiologic channel.

Assuming that the physical symptoms are not organically based, the following interventions are suggested:

1. Help the patient identify when and under what circumstances these symptoms appeared.
2. Help the patient identify thoughts, feelings, and behavior that are connected with these situations.
3. Collaborate with the patient in identifying alternative responses the patient can utilize in the situation if it happens again (eg, use of other channels of expression).
4. Support the patient while new responses are being tried.
5. Observe for change in frequency of physiologic response.
6. Confirm changes with the patient and together evaluate the approach taken.

CLINICAL EXAMPLE

Mrs. Green is a 52-year-old woman who was admitted to the hospital with a diagnosis of depression. She and her husband have grown apart in recent years, and her youngest son has just begun to attend college away from home. Her husband visits in the evening. After every visit Mrs. Green requests p.r.n. medication for headache. Her requests for medication are made only at these times.

In exploring such a situation with a patient the nurse should react in a calm but direct manner. It is frequently useful to share observations with the patient if he cannot make these connections himself. Questions or statements that are usually effective include:

When did the pain begin?
What were you doing at the time? Whom were you with?
What was being discussed?
What were you thinking of while you were involved in the conversation or activity?

AND THEN

This is what I think could be happening . . . . What are your impressions?
I think there could be a relationship between these events and your pain, but you may have another opinion.
I have no doubt that your pain is real and that your body is uncomfortable, but I am also interested in how it happens. There may be some things we can do together that can prevent the pain.

With patients who can nondefensively acknowledge the connection between physiologic pain and stressful events the nurse can usually point out that when our feelings are blocked from direct expression sometimes our bodies feel the discomfort for us. At that point the nurse can encourage the patient to keep track of the thoughts and feelings he experiences but does not directly express during stressful periods. It can further be suggested that these feelings be expressed to the nurse so that patterns can be examined more clearly and alternatives can be chosen in cooperation with the patient. The long-term goal of the intervention is to help the patient move to more functional channels of communication (eg, verbal expression), as well as to utilize the channels as indicators of distress when working with the patient.

CLINICAL EXAMPLE

A 16-year-old girl who had been admitted to an inpatient service for obsessive-compulsive symptoms had repeatedly stated to the staff that she just couldn't wait to go home. As the day for discharge drew near, the patient began to experience stomach cramps and vomiting. She had not displayed these symptoms before. With exploration the nurse and the patient discovered that the young girl was in reality extremely concerned about rejoining her family. The relationship between her physical symptoms and her imminent discharge was discussed, and the patient was able to relate more directly and consciously experience her feelings of fear and anxiety about leaving. Although her discharge date had to be postponed, the additional time in the hospital was well spent. Together the nurse and the patient explored ways the patient could relate to her family that would decrease the anxiety the discharge had precipitated. The patient began to learn to use verbal and behavioral channels for expression rather than physiologic ones.

The nurse does not simply have to "wait and see" if the patient will use the physiologic channel for communication. Physiologic symptoms occur with surprising frequency in many patients in commonly stressful situations. These incidents can almost be anticipated. Interaction with family members is frequently a cause of anxiety, as is the first day back at work or the first weekend visit home. More obvious situational crises can also precipitate this response. The mechanisms cited in these examples are capable of bringing out the psychosomatic side of every patient.

Fine Motor Channel

Because gestures, facial expressions, and one's use of space operate at an unconscious or preconscious level they are important communicative variables. There are many clinical examples that illustrate the importance of the fine motor channel. One situation in which nurses operationalize theories about interpersonal distance and its relationship to gender is in the seclusion or restraint of a patient. In situations where staff members approach a male patient who is out of control in order to restrain him it is becoming standard practice that both female and male staff members participate in the physical act of restraint. The same is true for a female patient who is out of control. This is done in order to decrease the likelihood that the patient will misinterpret the physical proximity and will view the seclusion activity as a potential homosexual or heterosexual assault.

Kinzel (1969) found data to support the contention that this practice is based on sound principle. In a body buffer zone experiment with male prisoners who had histories of repeated and apparently unprovoked assaults on other prisoners he found that their personal space zones (especially if the subjects were approached from the back) were physically four times greater than those of other prisoners. During the experiment the assaultive inmates consistently misperceived the distances between themselves and other people to be four times less than they actually were. They reacted instantaneously and automatically to the perceived invasion of their personal space zones by physically pushing people away in order to handle their anxiety in such situations.

Horowitz (1964) found that schizophrenic patients (in contrast to other psychiatric patients) also have exaggerated needs to protect larger personal space zones around their bodies. They prefer that both nurses and other patients maintain larger interpersonal distances. The patients in Horowitz's study also exhibited too much anxiety with face-to-face positioning for conversation; they preferred a side-by-side arrangement.

Theoretically, the difference between the spatial organizations found in Horowitz's study is understandable if we consider Freud's observation (1927) that "the ego is first and foremost a body ego: it is not merely a surface entity, but is itself the projection of a surface." Bender (1952) and Schilder (1950) also regard an internal conception of spatial organization to be a part of functional body image. Since we know that patients with schizophrenic symptoms have disturbances of ego and body image, it is not surprising that the issue of personal space as an extension of body integrity would be important to these patients. Consequently it is recommended that the nurse pay close attention to the personal space zone needs of these patients, particularly when the patient is actively psychotic. The general rule is to allow the patient to control the interpersonal distance between himself and the nurse. The nurse should not comment on this process; she may comment on interpersonal distances later when the patient has stabilized and is no longer acutely psychotic and when she thinks that some trust has been established in the relationship.

In later experiences the same patient may develop a tendency to the opposite extreme, ie, he may invade the personal space zones of others without realizing that he is encroaching. He may not understand the need of other patients or family members to maintain normative distances.

The nurse can raise these behaviors to the verbal level by commenting on them during an interaction. She can help the patient explore the meaning of his behavior, and she can make suggestions to the patient as to what a normative distance is. She can model for the patient: position the patient far enough away so that she feels comfortable. This helps the patient practice the subtle differences in distance through controlled behavior so that more satisfying interpersonal relationships can result.

There are also various clinical examples of the role body language can play in communicating important information to the nurse. Again, the recommended intervention is to raise this behavior to the verbal level. The nurse must take the initiative in this, because these movements are not initially conscious.

CLINICAL EXAMPLE

In a family therapy session an adolescent girl was presented to the therapists as being depressed and unable to function on her own. The mother and daughter sat side by side, and the father chose a chair opposite them. During the discussion the identified patient wouldn't speak, even when directly asked to do so. Whenever a question or remark was directed to her she would automatically turn her head to look at her mother, at which time her mother would automatically reply for her. This happened so quickly and so smoothly that it took a few minutes for the therapists to become aware of the pattern. Finally, when a therapist commented on this pattern and expressed curiosity about it, the mother replied almost with relief and without hesitation: "Well, yes, you know sometimes I almost feel like my daughter's ventriloquist." The remark characterized the mother-child relationship better than any comment from the therapist.

CLINICAL EXAMPLE

In another family therapy session a psychiatrist was meeting with a couple to discuss how they might better handle anger in their marital relationship. The wife began to get somewhat angry during the encounter, and the husband immediately moved his chair so close to hers that he was practically pushing her away in his effort to decrease the distance between them. When the therapist pointed this out the patient first denied any communicative value of his behavior; then he said, "I only did it so we could share the ashtray." However, this was a concrete example of the couple's underlying conflict. The husband was physically expressing his fear that expression and acknowledgment of angry feelings would be sure to separate the couple permanently. Later he agreed that the therapist's statement made more sense to him, and he agreed to give it more thought.

Behavioral Channel

What does it mean when people behave in any given way? If we consider not only the behavior itself but also what it implies we may come closer to an understanding of why behavior is an important area for assessment.

Ask yourself about your own behaviors and coping mechanisms.* What behaviors do you engage in when you are upset, happy, relieved, fearful, or suspicious or when you feel overpowered or in control? What would it imply to your friends if you left school in the middle of the semester, or got married next weekend, or gave away all your belongings? Of course people would wonder why. What were the reasons? What were the circumstances? They would probably think you had good reasons for your behavior, but they would still be curious.

With patients it is likewise helpful to assume that either on a conscious level or on an unconscious level the behavior makes sense and that people do not behave in a vacuum. Behaviors are related to thoughts and feelings, and nurses should be curious about their relationships.

Unless a patient is self-referred and openly seeks counseling, it is safe to assume that there has been a change in behavior that has attracted the attention of family, friends, or authorities. Even the self-referred patient will usually describe behavior changes rather than feelings that are distressing.

It is not just behaviors in themselves but also changes in behaviors that are indicative of underlying problem areas. The following are common examples:

The housewife who cannot sleep, does not prepare meals for her children, and stops eating.

The businessman who fails to meet contract agreements, starts drinking heavily, and starts taking time off from work.

The adolescent who stops participating in class, hands in assignments late, and refuses to eat any meals with the family.

CLINICAL EXAMPLE

Mrs. Blue was a psychotic patient who was in remission. She had been maintained in the community for 3 years with the help of a supportive nurse-patient relationship. She came into the clinic infrequently, preferring to use the telephone for contact. One day she called and asked for an appointment to see the nurse in the clinic. When she came for the appointment she looked tired and complained that she was "just depressed" and felt really sick. She could not state why she felt that way and could not clearly describe any new problem areas: "Everything was the same."

The nurse was aware that Mrs. Blue's mother had died 2 months earlier; they had discussed this a number of times in previous interactions. Mrs.

**Coping mechanisms are usually thought of as conscious actions that help us deal with stress and are usually described in behavioral terms. Defense mechanisms are unconscious mental mechanisms that block anxiety and psychic pain from our awareness. Coping mechanisms are directly observable; defense mechanisms can only be inferred from observation.*

Blue denied any interest in discussing this further. When asked what she had been doing lately, she replied, "I can't do anything for myself anymore. I wake up early in the morning with thoughts about killing myself. My husband just bothers me all the time; sometimes I get so angry with him I think about killing him. I gave away some jewelry to my daughter and told my son he could have my mother's china I have stored in the basement."

Mrs. Blue was clearly describing behaviors that not ony were unusual for her but were indicative of disequilibrium. The nurse knew the patient's relationships with family members were basically ambivalent. Considering this in conjunction with the grieving process, some anger was to be expected. However, in this instance the patient's anger fluctuated both inward and outward in suicidal and homicidal ideation, rather than toward her mother who had died.

In addition to other behavioral changes the patient had given away her personal belongings, a behavior that the nurse found particularly disturbing. Implicit in these actions was this underlying message: "I might not be around to give these to you later." In other words, the patient was actively preparing for suicide. The patient later described vivid homicidal fantasies that seemed possible for her to execute and which may have been successful. She was hospitalized on the day the interview took place.

Mrs. Blue had not come to the clinic consciously seeking admission to the hospital; she only knew that she was doing things and thinking about doing things that were frightening to her. The nurse assessed the patient with regard to the implications of her behavioral changes, as well as with regard to what the patient conveyed verbally. It is interesting that this patient verbally resisted hospitalization; however, she actively and cooperatively engaged in the admission procedure itself and then appeared relieved to have been placed in the hospital.

In the inpatient setting the nurse finds patients who are not able to use verbal channels to communicate. By utilizing the communicative value of her own behavior the nurse can then begin the relationship at that level. Taking a walk with a patient, playing cards with him, and accompanying him to some other activity are behaviors that begin the relationship on a concrete level and help establish a sense of relatedness for the patient. Most patients will gradually begin to talk to the nurse on their own if this approach is consistently carried out.

When patients are better able to use words to communicate the nurse can direct the conversation to the level of verbally expressing behavior. This is the safest verbal channel to begin with, and the nurse can then proceed with some assurance that she is not pushing the patient too fast.

When the relationship is better established the nurse can help the patient examine behaviors he would like to alter. Substituting functional behaviors for nonfunctional ones demands time, patience, and persistence. The nurse must be realistic about what can be accomplished immediately if she has only a short time to work with a patient. Short-term and long-term goals are helpful in delineating the intervening steps that can help make behavioral changes attainable.

Patients should always be encouraged to express their thoughts and feelings. Sometimes the questions intended to achieve this are not sufficiently structured for the patient to see how specific behaviors can be altered. If it becomes clear that attempts at these communication skills are only confusing the issue, the nurse can be more specific. For example:

> "It seems that whenever you get angry you go in your room and start pounding on the wall. What else could you do?"
> "There may have been a time when you didn't do that. What did you do to get out your feelings then?"
> "Everyone gets angry and everyone has to find a way to deal with this in a productive way. What do your friends do when they get mad?"
> "If you were to put your behavior into words when you pound the wall, what would you say?"
> "Let's make an agreement about what else you can do if you get this angry and feel like pounding on the wall again."

The changing of behavior patterns is difficult for anyone. In the process it is better to emphasize the successes rather than the failures. During this time it is critical for the nurse to acknowledge this difficulty openly with the patient, lending her support and attention while change is being attempted and verbally pointing out progress to the patient as change occurs.

Verbal Channels

In this section the three verbal channels will be presented in an interrelated manner. In general there are two main goals at this level of intervention. The first is to phrase questions and elicit responses in such a way that the difficulty of each level is acknowledged. The second is to assist the patient to connect all channels of communication by words within appropriate contexts, one of which is the nurse–patient relationship.

If the nurse knows the patient well she probably will already have assessed the degree to which the patient is comfortable discussing behaviors, thoughts, and feelings. In the example that follows the patient was unknown to the nurse. However, the nurse was quickly able to determine the patient's best level of functioning by changing levels until the patient appeared comfortable. In this example the nurse started with the most difficult level. She could also have started in the reverse order. The fine motor channel was used for validation.

N: How do you *feel* about being here?
P: I don't know. (Eyes downcast, posture uncomfortable.)
N: Well, what do you *think* about coming to the clinic?
P: It's OK. (Eyes scanning room, looking out window.)
N: What would you like to *do* right now?
P: Leave! (Anxious smile but good eye contact.)

N: It was difficult for you to come here. (Behavioral response indicated this; nurse is also relating feelings to behavior.)
P: You're not kidding! (As above).
N: Most people who come to the clinic for the first time feel nervous. Is that true for you too?
P: Yes, I really didn't know what to expect.
N: Well, since you're here and we have some time, what would you like to do?

In this example the patient was clearly more comfortable discussing behavior, and the nurse reacted to this by staying on that level for the last half of the conversation. She also understood the implications of behavior, and she verbalized what was implied so that the patient might validate it ("It was difficult for you to come here").

When helping the patient move toward more direct verbalization of feelings, the nurse should begin with questions that ask for a description of behavior or thoughts. Then she should move on to verbalizing what she sees as the feelings the patient is implying. Finally, she should verbalize possible connections between thought, feelings, and behavior for the patient to validate. For example:

N: Mr. Smith, we were discussing your thoughts about getting a divorce the last time we talked. Have you thought more about that?
P: Yes, I've been thinking about it, but I haven't called my lawyer.
N: Actually doing something is different from thinking about it.
P: That's really true; anyway, I haven't had the time.
N: You haven't made any calls then?
P: No, but I came close once.
N: What did you do?
P: I dialed the number, but the line was busy. I never called back.
N: What were your thoughts when you discovered the line was busy?
P: I was a little relieved, to tell you the truth. I don't know, I just can't decide right now. I think I should give it more time.
N: You said you were a little relieved when the call didn't get through. What else were you thinking or feeling?
P: Well, actually I was hoping the office was closed or something. I just keep thinking that this isn't really serious; my wife and I have always patched up our problems. God, we've been married for 26 years. Why does she want a divorce?
N: You must be feeling pretty confused about all this and really unable to decide what to do.
P: I am; I really am confused. I mean, I just don't understand this. I feel so miserable I can't stand it.
N: It looks like you have a lot of feelings that are making this a very uncomfortable time. Although it can be very painful to talk about these feelings, it will help you feel less overwhelmed if you do.
P: Sometimes it does help. But a grown man can't go around crying about his problems, can he?

When talking with patients it is helpful to explore systematically each major issue the patient brings up. Explore is a term frequently used in psychosocial nursing. It means looking at an issue with a patient from every possible perspective. This is easiest to do if an attempt is made to recapture significant events the patient is discussing in one's own mind and then ask the following questions: Is there a clear picture of what the patient was doing, thinking, and feeling during this event? If not, what area is unclear? In this way the nurse can understand the patient's experience, as much as possible, from at least these three significant perspectives.

This method of putting the pieces of the puzzle together also helps the patient to reconstruct the event in a new way or to experience a present interaction in a new way. In social relationships others are not usually interested in this systematic search for the total experience. Relating patterns of behavior to thoughts and to feelings is a different kind of experience for the patient. Since each patient is unique, it is also a different therapeutic experience for the nurse as well.

In closing this section on verbal interventions it seems appropriate to comment on the two most widely advertised clichés in psychiatry and mental health counseling, namely, the questions "How do you feel about that?" and "Why?"

The first question includes several variants: "What are your feelings?" "How does that make you feel?" and "Tell me how you're feeling," to name a few. In initial encounters with patients it is easy for nurses (as well as other mental health professionals) to use these phrases too frequently. Of course it makes sense to question patients about their feelings, but many patients do not respond well to such a direct and immediate style in their first few encounters with a nurse. The best response that many patients can produce may be a blank stare, a long uncomfortable silence, or an "I don't know." It is helpful to remember that spontaneous direct expression of feelings in an interventive situation is a measure of mental health, not emotional impairment. It is not true that most patients can automatically begin at this level and then quickly progress to analyzing and answering the question "Why?"

As the nurse develops a greater appreciation for the complexity of psychodynamics and the role of defense mechanisms it becomes clearer that the patient who is not in contact with large parts of his emotional life cannot be expected to know why without some exploration first. People who do understand the relationship between what they do, how their bodies respond, how they think, and how they feel can usually put together the why of their experience for themselves.

To repeatedly ask a patient "How do you feel?" or "Why?" when it is apparent that no answer will be forthcoming is to put the patient in a position to fail. To realize that you don't know the answers about something as intimate and private as your own self is distressing enough. To have to admit this to another person over and over again in the same interaction makes for an unnecessarily confusing and uncomfortable experience.

One might assume that immediate use of these phrases should remain within the psychoanalytic framework. In an analytic relationship the patient will have been assessed for his ability to handle such a stressful encounter. Analysis is thought to be best suited for people who can begin treatment from an articulate, introspective, intelligent position.

With patients who would not be good psychoanalytic candidates (the majority of patients), other interventions are usually more successful in helping the patient toward more direct expression of feeling and attainment of more functional problem-solving abilities.

SUMMARY

Interpersonal communication is an essential element in nursing practice. Communication, however, is a complex and diverse dimension of mental health care. Communicative efforts involve content, context, and process. The manner in which people communicate is influenced by physiologic, cultural, psychodynamic, and behavioral variables. A six-channel construct has been presented in order to guide the nurse to an appreciation and an understanding of some major dimensions of the communicative process in dyadic interaction. Suggested interventions have been presented to demonstrate these principles in the clinical setting. Interventions have been described that relate to each channel in the construct.

References

Alexander F: Psychosomatic Medicine. New York, Norton, 1950

Bender L: Child Psychiatric Techniques. Springfield, Ill, Thomas, 1952

Birdwhistle R L: Kinesics and Context: Essays on Body Motion Communication. Philadelphia, University of Pennsylvania Press, 1970

Freud S: Ego & Id. London, Hogarth, 1927

Hall E T: The anthropology of manners. Sci Am 192:85–9, 1955

——— The Silent Language. New York, Doubleday, 1959

——— Man's spatial relations. In Goldston I (ed): Man's Image in Medicine and Anthropology. New York, International Universities Press, 1963, pp 422–45

——— The Hidden Dimension. New York, Doubleday, 1966

Horowitz M J, Duff D F, Stratton L O: The body buffer zone: an exploration of person spaces. Arch Gen Psychiatry 11:651–6, 1964

Kinzel A F: Body buffer zone in violent persons. In Proceedings of the American Psychiatric Association Annual Meeting. 1969, pp 209–10

MacKinnon R A, Michels R: The Psychiatric Interview in Clinical Practice. Philadelphia, Saunders, 1971, p 363

Montagu A: Touching: The Human Significance of the Skin. New York, Harper & Row, 1971

Rogers C R: On Becoming a Person. Boston, Houghton Mifflin, 1961

Ruesch J, Kees W: Non-Verbal Communication. Berkeley, University of California Press, 1956

Schilder P: Image and Appearance of the Human Body. New York, International Universities Press, 1950

Spiegel J P, Machotka P: Messages of the Body. New York, Free Press, 1974

CHAPTER

2

THERAPEUTIC SUPERFICIALITY AND INTIMACY

Alice Coad-Denton

Any sharing of behaviors, thoughts, and feelings occurs within one of many possible interactional frameworks that determines how superficial or intimate a relationship is or will become. Initially, most social and therapeutic interactions begin at a superficial level and progress toward interpersonal closeness and sharing. Within the framework of social interaction, such as that experienced with friends and acquaintances, the involved individuals mutually determine the pace of progression and the degree of personal involvement. This involvement may remain superficial or may develop into an intimate friendship.

However, in the development of psychosocial relationships, a major focus is the establishment of therapeutic intimacy. The nurse guides the development of this therapeutic intimacy, and she needs to know the variables that comprise a therapeutic relationship. In order to facilitate the development of therapeutic interactions the nurse must understand how an intimate therapeutic relationship differs from an intimate social relationship. Once this understanding is achieved, the nurse must utilize nursing interventions to promote and maintain therapeutic intimacy.

SOCIAL AND THERAPEUTIC RELATIONSHIPS

The progression from superficiality to intimacy in both social and therapeutic relationships has distinct components that may be considered to constitute a continuum. Superficiality, or the dynamics of a newly initiated social relationship, occupies one end of the continuum. The interpersonal dynamics of these superficial interactions are characterized by limited self-disclosure, discussion of general or nonpersonal topics, and minimal knowledge and understanding of the participants. There is no interdependence between the participants, and they do not seek to fulfill their needs within the relationship. Rarely are personal goals, perceptions, and needs shared. Typically such interaction occurs in large social gatherings, in time-limited relationships, and on initial meetings of new social contacts.

In contrast with this style of superficial interacting are the interpersonal interactions at the opposite end of the continuum that reflect a sense of interpersonal closeness or intimacy in social relationships. Intimacy implies an awareness of psychologic interdependence among two or more individuals. It is a vital component in the development of close, meaningful relationships. The mutual acceptance of one another by the participants leads to feelings of security and safety and to assurance that the other individual will always respond in an accepting, nonevaluative manner. The process of achieving this acceptance is characterized by mutual disclosure of perceptions, needs, desires or wishes, behaviors, and feelings. This personal sharing promotes a feeling of a close and satisfying relationship and contributes to an atmosphere of generalized support, acceptance, and trust. This is reflected in a sense of interdependence that is characterized by mutual abilities to meet needs and understand one another. In this sense intimacy is characterized by mutual self-actualization and not by the promotion of dependence. Recognition that the behaviors, thoughts, and feelings of one person can influence these factors in the other person is assumed in the definition of self-actualization. Within the range of social relationships the individuals involved in intimate relationships are very close friends, family members, and housemates.

The realm of social intercourse is familiar to all. But this realm does not completely transfer into the framework of therapeutic interaction. In a therapeutic relationship the sense of progress from superficiality to intimacy emerges in a different manner. While social superficiality and intimacy are characterized by the degree of sharing of behaviors, thoughts, and feelings, therapeutic superficiality and intimacy are not characterized by such mutuality. The sense of intimacy and closeness in a therapeutic relationship derives from the content and expression of feelings the patient shares with the nurse and from utilization of the nursing process. Within the scope of therapeutic interactions the nursing process supports the patient as he explores his areas of need, solves his problems, and acquires or confirms his skills in coping and solving problems. The nurse's support is not necessarily passive; rather, the supportive process is an active contributing component of care.

The nurse responds to the patient's actions and his shared thoughts and feelings. The patient is not asked to respond to the nurse's personal needs. Thus the style of interdependence that characterizes social relationships does not characterize therapeutic relationships. The interdependence in therapeutic intimacy occurs because the nurse fosters the development of a supporting, accepting atmosphere. This type of atmosphere has a quality of openness, and the patient is free to be himself, with no need to hide his actions or feelings. He can risk self-disclosure without fearing repercussions. The patient begins to develop confidence and trust in the ability and expertise of the nurse and in the emerging therapeutic relationship.

The feeling of closeness emerges in a therapeutic interaction as the patient and nurse focus on the content and feelings that the patient shares with the nurse. The patient's part in this interactive process is to provide meaningful content, ie, the patient shares his behaviors, thoughts, and feelings as they relate to his problems or situation. The nurse's role is to help facilitate the patient's production of meaningful content and to support the patient's problem-solving skills. This process is frequently complex and difficult. To the novice it is often an area that appears to have no landmarks and no structure to suggest where the nurse and patient are on the superficiality–intimacy continuum scale or in what manner the relationship needs to progress. But the landmarks or components on the continuum do exist in all relationships. They include the following: self-disclosure, the focus of the interaction, the pertinence of any topic to the goal of the interaction, the past-present-future time reference, the utilization of feelings, the sense of involvement, and acknowledgment of the dignity and autonomy of the individual. In Table 2.1 social superficiality and therapeutic intimacy are contrasted.

In the therapeutic relationship both the nurse and the patient must understand that there are none of the expectations of mutual self-disclosure that characterizes social relationships; the nurse does not discuss her personal problems with the patient. At first this is difficult for both the patient and the nurse. Prior to learning how to use communicative skills therapeutically the nurse relied on social skills to achieve feelings of closeness and intimacy. For most people this is a comfortable and predictable manner of interacting that has been learned from infancy. However, within the therapeutic setting it is necessary to learn new skills in order to develop an effective relationship. These skills include not only verbal skills but also the use of factors that contribute to the development of therapeutic intimacy. Most therapeutic relationships begin at the superficial end of the continuum and progress in sophistication and intimacy. It is during the beginning phase that the nurse's knowledge of the factors that contribute to intimacy is crucial to facilitation of a sense of therapeutic closeness. When closeness is achieved, these skills are necessary to maintain it.

Table 2.1. SOCIAL SUPERFICIALITY AND THERAPEUTIC INTIMACY CONTRASTED

COMPONENTS OF RELATIONSHIP	SOCIAL (SUPERFICIAL)	THERAPEUTIC (INTIMATE)
Mutual self-disclosure	Variable	Patient: self-disclosure; nurse: self-disclosure in terms of response to patient only
Focus of conversation	Unknown to participants	Known to nurse and patient
Pertinence of topic	Social, business, generalized, impersonal	Personal and relevant to nurse and patient
Relationship of experiences to topic	Sense of uninvolvement and use of indirect knowledge	Sense of involvement and use of direct knowledge
Time orientation	Past and future	Present
Use of feelings	Sharing of feelings discouraged	Sharing of feelings encouraged by nurse
Recognition of individual worth	Not acknowledged	Fully acknowledged

ASSESSMENT

The major areas requiring assessment during the development of therapeutic intimacy are those components of any relationship that were mentioned earlier: (1) the focus of the interaction; (2) the pertinence of any topic to the goal; (3) the time orientation; (4) the relationship of one's experiences to the topic and to one's cognitions; (5) the use of and expression of behaviors, thoughts, and feelings; and (6) the recognition of individual worth and autonomy. The assessment of the development of the therapeutic process is facilitated by an assessment of the progression of each of these variables toward intimacy. In utilizing these variables as a basis for assessment the nurse should recognize that the progression of the variables can also be taught to both patient and nurse. In Table 2.2 the variables contributing to therapeutic intimacy are delineated. These will be discussed in detail as part of the assessment process. For a smooth progression toward therapeutic intimacy all of the variables must simultaneously be at the same point on the continuum. The dashed line indicates this. Note that the dotted line passes through past and future orientations to time; at this point the nurse will recognize the need to encourage the patient to focus on a present time orientation so that all the variables will be congruent in their placement on the continuum. A brief example is provided by the following dialogue:

Table 2.2. CONTINUUM OF THERAPEUTIC INTIMACY

THERAPEUTIC INTIMACY DEPENDS ON:	Superficiality ———				——→ Intimacy
Focus of conversation	Focuses on people or events not personally known to nurse and patient	Focuses on people or events known to either nurse or patient	Focuses on people or events known to both patient and nurse	Focuses on patient's concerns and self-disclosures or on nurse's concerns re patient	Focuses on mutually shared aspects and concerns of therapeutic relationship
Pertinence of topic	Topic is not pertinent or important to nurse or patient		Topic is important to nurse or patient		Topic is of concern and importance to both nurse and patient
Time orientation	Past or future orientation that does not clarify or relate to present time			Focus on present time; any discussion of people or events that helps to clarify the present	
Relationship of experiences to topic	Abstractions and vague reports of events or interactions; no supportive, illustrative examples; sense of uninvolvement			Sense of involvement in interaction or event; supported with specific, concrete examples and observations; recognition that distortion occurs with indirect knowledge	
Use of feelings	Sharing of feelings is avoided and is considered disruptive and meaningless; indirect reflection of feelings is common: generalizations, judgments, intellectualizations about events and people			Sharing of feelings is considered beneficial; feelings are considered natural and acceptable by nurse and patient; initially, feelings are shared from patient to nurse, but as therapeutic relationship develops the nurse shares feelings re present time and therapeutic relationship	
Recognition of individual worth and autonomy	Lack of acknowledgment of individual worth and autonomy; patient or nurse may strive to convince the other to be like him/her; to do as he/she does			Fundamental integrity and worth of individual is acknowledged; respect for personal autonomy. This concept is valued by nurse and patient.	

Dash line indicates that all variables are not simultaneously at the same point on the continuum. Dotted line indicates that all variables are simultaneously at the same point on the continuum.

N: I understand you are not working now.
P: Yes, actually I have been out of work six times. The first time was in 1950. . . . The second time was in 1952. . . .
N: Tell me about right now, about the job you just left.

Focus of Interaction

The focus of the interaction of conversation varies with the degree of trust in the relationship and the level of superficiality. At the beginning of a therapeutic relationship the depth of personal sharing by the patient is frequently minimal. The superficiality is reflected in the choice of topics, which usually involve events or people not personally known to the nurse and patient. Such topics might include recent actions of governmental agencies, events reported by the news media, or life styles of well-known persons. As progress is made beyond the superficial level the patient begins to focus on events and people known to both himself and the nurse (see Table 2.2). Within the hospital setting this might include the admission procedures, the patient's family, the attending physician and nurses, and the patient's behavior and activities. Gradually the focus becomes the mutual sharing of the concerns of the nurse and the patient about the therapeutic relationship. The last stage involves the mutually shared aspects of their own relationship.

In Table 2.2 the dotted line indicates congruity of all the variables at the intimacy end of the continuum. When this occurs the therapeutic process is well established. The following dialogue is indicative of this:

N: I would like to talk about your asking me for a date this morning.
P: Well, I am getting to like you a lot, and I thought that after I went home we could get together sometime. I've told you how lonely I get and you seemed to want to help me. Besides, I like seeing you every day.
N: Yes, I think I understand your feelings, but I do not think my dating you after your discharge from the hospital will change what makes you lonely. I'd like to talk about how I understand your suggestion of dating, and then let's talk about how you might possibly solve some of the problems your loneliness causes.

The important thing here is the focus on mutual concerns about the therapeutic process and the relationship. The nurse does not offer to share the concerns and problems of her personal life. Since the emphasis is to be for the nurse to focus on the patient's needs and offer effective interventions, the sharing of her personal concerns would be detrimental. This would suggest friendship and might lead to the expectation that the nurse would be asking him for help with her problems. In the foregoing example, instead of discussing the possibility of a social relationship the nurse focused on the underlying problem that the patient was indicating by his request for a date. The problem, loneliness, is a concern that the nurse and the patient can work on together.

Pertinence of Topic

The second variable is the pertinence of any selected topic of conversation. Frequently at the beginning of any therapeutic interaction the lack of pertinence and importance of the topics of conversation is evident. There are many possible reasons for this: The patient probably is accustomed to beginning all interaction as though it is occurring in the social realm. Until trust is established the patient may feel that any self-disclosure is problematic. The nurse must help the patient recognize the necessity of discussing significant topics. Progress on the continuum toward intimacy occurs as the topics become increasingly related to the patient's problems and concerns. In the middle area of the continuum this assignment of value and significance to the topics selected may be done by the nurse or the patient. When intimacy finally occurs for this variable the nurse and the patient should concur on the importance and pertinence of any topic to the therapeutic process. Topics should reflect the issues that must be explored, integrated, and resolved in the therapeutic process. For example:

N: Yesterday you were telling me about the problems you are having with your diabetes. Perhaps it would be helpful to explore those problems further.	Topic: Diabetes.
P: Well, when I became a diabetic my family blamed me because they said I had always eaten too many sweets.	Focus: Family's reaction (blaming and accusatory).

In this example the nurse and the patient can discuss how the patient has dealt with his family's reaction, which is the focus of the interaction. This would include exploration of his behaviors, thoughts, and feelings about his family's reaction to his diabetes.

As was stated earlier, an indicator of increasing intimacy is the negotiation of what topics are pertinent and important. At times, because of her knowledge, expertise, or experience the nurse's opinion of what is important may override the patient's opinion. Often, however, there will be the option of the patient choosing which aspects of a topic area he would like to discuss initially. An example of this would be a young man who has difficulty in defining heterosexual relationships. It would be pertinent for the nurse to explore aspects of his relationships with women. This might include his relationships with his mother, female siblings, other women, female peers, and female nurse-therapist. The patient should then choose the aspects he wants to explore initially.

Time Orientation

Whenever a past or future orientation, unrelated to the present, is utilized in order to avoid having to deal with the present, superficiality tends to be perpetuated. It is not uncommon for therapeutic relationships to begin from such an orientation, and of course the patient finds this orientation easy to maintain. On the other end of the continuum (the intimate relationship) the focus is on the current needs, problems, and feelings, and the major time focus is the present. This orientation to the present enables the individual to develop competence in relying on his own faculties and sense of expressiveness, although events from the past or events anticipated in the future may contribute to an understanding of current thoughts, feelings, and behaviors and may aid in resolution of present problems. The patient's ability to achieve a sense of actualization and autonomy is dependent on his ability to achieve a meaningful sense of time and to be comfortable in the present.

Relationship of Experiences to Topic

Individuals must be able to relate their experiences to the topic areas being explored in the therapeutic process. Thoughts and feelings reveal the sense of involvement that an individual experiences, and they provide content for mutual therapeutic focusing. These experiences are personal and are experienced singularly until they are expressed and shared, through either behaviors or verbal sharing.

At the superficial end of the continuum the patient may exhibit a pervasive sense of uninvolvement and a lack of interest in development of a closer relationship. The patient may neither like nor accept the nurse-therapist, and no warmth toward others is conveyed. Events and interactions may be related in an uninterested manner, and descriptions are frequently vague.

As the relationship becomes increasingly therapeutic a sense of involvement is experienced by the nurse and the patient. This involvement emerges within the guidelines established by the focus of interaction, the topic of discussion, and the orientation to present time. Specific examples and observations encourage the development of depth and intimacy. These specific examples presented to support the thoughts and feelings of the patient contribute to clarity and help to prevent distortion. Without this specific verbal experience it is difficult to relate experiences and cognition. Lack of clarity and the use of abstractions make it difficult for the nurse to help the patient resolve problems and explore his concerns. For example:

N: You mentioned that you found it difficult to keep your job as a gardener. What were some of your experiences with this?	Topic: Occupation.
P: Well, it seems that I am defeated before I start. I remember the last time the boss got angry and fired me. I didn't know what to say. What if that happens to me next time and I don't know what to say again?	Experience: Termination from last job. Relationship to topic: Clear, not abstract. There is a sense of patient involvement in the interaction.

Use of Feelings

As the nurse helps the patient to focus on the relationship of experience and cognition, the use and expression of feelings become important. For the most part, one's feelings constitute a personal and private experience. Thus in a superficial relationship any discussion of feelings is avoided. Indeed, in many social situations a discussion of feelings would be meaningless or even disruptive. Feelings are revealed in many ways during the therapeutic process, and the nurse should be attuned to the cues that are offered and to the variety of ways that feelings are expressed, both verbally and behaviorally.

Feelings can be related indirectly through behaviors, through verbal descriptions of behaviors, and through the sharing of thoughts. In many instances patients as well as nurses have to learn to recognize their feelings. Within a therapeutic relationship the sharing of feelings is essential to the development of intimacy and increased knowledge of oneself. The recognition of one's feelings appears to be a learned phenomenon. Most patients initially need help in recognizing their feelings or in refining their processes of recognition. Recognition alone is not enough; once feelings are recognized they need to be expressed as directly as possible. Recognition of feelings is not any easy process; it is an area that frequently is not utilized effectively in the therapeutic relationship. Instead, indirect experience of feelings is often utilized as the basis for intervention. This may include generalizations, judgments, and intellectualizations about events and people.

Direct Use of Feelings. The direct use of the patient's feelings depends on the nurse's ability to recognize those feelings in her patient and use direct examples to which the patient can relate. The nurse may recognize feelings of frustration and initiate a discussion of alternative behavior. This is indicated in the following example:

N: As you talked about your experience with your boss you sounded frustrated.
P: I never thought of that; but, as I think about it, you're right.

N: When you feel frustrated, as with your boss, what do you do?
P: Not much. I think I had better learn what to do; maybe I'll be able to handle it better next time.
N: There are ways to deal with your feelings of frustration and the bind you get into with them. We need to start by exploring what you do and how you feel when you are frustrated.

Indirect Use of Feelings. For the novice it may be easier to use an indirect approach to utilize the patient's feelings in the therapeutic process. Generalizations and intellectualizations carry less risk of inaccurate perception of feelings and behavior:

N: A lot of people feel frustrated when they are fired, because they think they have worked hard. Sometimes people are totally surprised when they are fired.
P: You think a lot of people feel that way? I don't know if I do, but I'd like to learn how they solved the problem.

Many patients as well as nurses experience difficulty in sharing their feelings. This may be because of the newness of the experience, because of the difficulty of accepting and using feelings constructively, or because an intimate and personal aspect of one's being is being revealed to another. The capacity to experience feelings is vital to man. Without feelings we would not be capable of responding to others.

Feelings that reflect negative emotional states—anger, hate, fear, and distrust, for example—are often the most difficult to recognize. Additionally, because of the inadequacy of conventional terms, the expression of these feelings is problematic. Nonetheless, they arise in many situations, and the nurse needs to convey to the patient the normalcy of these feelings. In fact, it is crucial for the nurse and the patient to recognize in these feelings their universal aspect and to utilize them constructively. The constructive expression of negative feelings in a therapeutic relationship is vital to the continued productivity of that relationship. For example:

N: Whenever I make a suggestion you tell me that you like my suggestion and then give me several reasons why it won't work for you. I am irritated that you always say "Yes, but . . . ."
P: I didn't mean to make you angry. I suppose you always want me to follow every one of your suggestions or stop seeing you.
N: No, I don't think it would be helpful to discontinue our relationship. I do think it would be helpful to discuss your response to my feelings of irritation and how we are going to resolve this situation.
P: You have a good point. Whenever I've been mad at someone, I haven't wanted to see them again.

The manner in which the patient expresses such feelings determines their usefulness in the assessment of behavior. There are various ways of expressing and using these negative feelings. One person's expression of despair might be quiet contemplation of suicide, whereas another might attempt a specific suicidal plan. Another might share his feelings with friends or health professionals and utilize various aspects of the social network. The feeling motivating the behavior in each instance is the same, but the behavior varies. The behavior alternatives can be learned, and they can be incorporated into anticipatory guidance for mental health. The nurse can aid in the proper utilization of feelings by helping the patient understand how to control and understand his feelings as they relate to his actions.

Initially in the therapeutic process the patient shares his feelings with the nurse for a variety of reasons. When a patient is experiencing difficulty in solving his problems it is important for the nurse to understand how he is perceiving the situation and to understand the personal feelings accompanying the situation. When the patient introduces his feelings into the therapeutic exchange he signals a move from superficiality toward greater self-revelation. It is necessary that the patient share his feelings about events and interactions that pertain to the problem. This permits the patient to examine his feelings as they relate to his behavior. Since the nurse generally does not share in the events of the patient's life, her responses should focus on the events and feelings in the nurse–patient relationship. Since this relationship is known to the patient and the nurse, it is possible to explore the components that contribute to the nurse's feelings and to the therapeutic process.

As the patient begins to share his feelings and behavior and a sense of involvement in the therapeutic process emerges, the fundamental integrity and worth of the individual must be acknowledged. The nurse must establish that she perceives the individual as being equal with others. She must also convey her belief that the patient has the potential to utilize his strengths to change himself and develop. This is an essential part of the nursing process, regardless of the setting. It is from this premise that the nurse is able to accept individuals with minimal judgment.

Recognition of Individual Worth and Autonomy

In initial social interactions a failure to acknowledge an individual's worth and uniqueness is not uncommon. Unfortunately this attitude is often maintained throughout a relationship. Its result can frequently be recognized in the individual who attempts to convince another to like him or to do as he does. At times this may be viewed as competitiveness or as the dynamic of one-upmanship. When a person has to strive to convince another of his individual worth, the process prevents acknowledgment of that individual as he is underneath his distorted competitive presentation.

This prevents the development of closeness and makes the sharing of feelings and behaviors difficult. This often occurs as the initial stage in the development of therapeutic relationships. Patients employ this approach because they do not know another or because they find any kind of involvement difficult. If therapeutic relationships are to develop beyond the superficial level it is necessary to value and openly acknowledge the individual's inherent integrity and worth. The nurse can do this through her actions, by her promptness for appointments, by realistic praise, by support and encouragement. This also conveys respect for personal autonomy, the ability to develop and change. On the intimacy end of the continuum these concepts are valued by both the nurse and the patient. With autonomy, the patient is liberated from adherence to rigid parental values, social pressures, and expectations. Instead, values and principles are adopted such that the patient learns behavior appropriate to his life style and situation.

Summary

Ideally, if all of the aspects of the therapeutic relationship discussed here are utilized the nurse–patient relationship should rapidly progress toward therapeutic intimacy. It is on the intimacy end of the continuum that much of the progress of therapeutic interaction is achieved. However, this progress is frequently slow and can take several weeks or months to achieve. The nurse's ability to assess the development of each of these aspects, as well as their congruent occurrence on the continuum, is important in facilitation of an effective therapeutic interaction.

Relating effectively to others is important to the fulfillment of the individual. The therapeutic nursing process is important in helping the individual to achieve and maintain this ability to relate. Today rapid facilitation of the therapeutic process is important in order to reduce patient costs and help him strengthen his coping skills as quickly as possible.

The importance of building effective and meaningful relationships with patients cannot be overemphasized. By utilizing the superficiality–intimacy continuum the nurse ensures that the important aspects of the therapeutic process are initiated and that placement of the variables on the continuum is congruent with the progress in the development of intimacy.

INTERVENTION

As progress is made toward a greater degree of sharing and a sense of intimacy, more sophisticated communication skills are required, as well as more knowledge about the process of communication. It is important to determine the advancement of each skill along the continuum so that the nurse can utilize each effectively in the development of an intimate therapeutic relationship. These skills may be utilized in a variety of ways, but they must remain goal-directed. The skills presented may be viewed on a continuum that ranges from the basic skills that build trust to those that are more sophisticated and that need the framework of an established relationship for their effective utilization. These skills are adapted from Brammer (1973), and Table 2.3 relates them to the discussion that follows.

Table 2.3. INTERVENTION SKILLS: PROMOTION OF THERAPEUTIC EFFECTIVENESS*

LISTENING AND INTERVENTION SKILLS TO PROMOTE THERAPEUTIC EFFECTIVENESS	Superficiality ———————→			Intimacy
Listening	Attending	Paraphrasing	Clarifying	Checking perception
Guiding	Indirect Guiding	Direct Guiding	Centralizing	Inquiring
Reflecting	Content		Feelings	Congruence of expression and behavior
Consulting	Guiding			Suggesting
Summarizing	Content		Feelings	Process
Interpreting	Questioning		Explaining	Fantasizing
Confronting	Repeating		Describing and expressing	Feedback and opinion

**Adapted from Brammer: The Helping Relationship Process and Skills, Englewood Cliffs, Prentice-Hall, 1973.*

Listening

Active listening is important in the development of effective communication skills. The following discussion concerns the four aspects of listening that reflect increased sophistication and closeness between individuals.

Attending. The first aspect, or the initial listening behavior, is attending. Basic attending involves listening to or heeding what is being said. It is not the hollow action of nodding or agreeing without listening. Rather, it is an action in which an individual gives close attention to what is said and what is behaviorally expressed, both in individual nurse–patient interactions and in the larger milieu.

Attending is enhanced when the nurse is comfortable in the use of the skills that convey interest. These include eye contact, a comfortable posture and position, and natural actions that reflect the nurse's receptiveness and warmth. This skill also tends to reduce the nurse's anxiety, because it is difficult to remain anxious and listen carefully at the same time.

In an interview situation skilled attending can have a major effect on the interaction because it helps the nurse to focus on the patient and to create an atmosphere of interest and trust. In time, as a relationship progresses, this interest is always maintained and conveyed in additional ways.

Paraphrasing. The next component of listening is paraphrasing. This means an overt responsive activity on the part of the nurse. It is easier to attend to what another shares than to paraphrase what is shared. Paraphrasing, because of the responses required from the nurse, is an activity that compels the nurse to continually focus on and attend to the patient. Paraphrasing enables the nurse to test her understanding of what the patient says by summarizing what she thinks is he saying. Frequently this involves making the patient's statements more concise; at times it means elaborating so that the nurse conveys to the patient that she fully understands what he is saying. Paraphrasing has many purposes, one of which is to reflect back to the patient how someone else is understanding him. This enables him to assess his ability to communicate.

A special aspect of listening and paraphrasing is that it enables the patient to feel that another person is helping to bear his feelings, and often his sense of psychic pain. The act of paraphrasing demonstrates involvement with the patient and helps to reduce emotional distance in the therapeutic process. Examples of paraphrasing are the following:

P: I am all tired out and I just can't cope anymore.
N: You're saying that you don't have the energy to keep going.
P: Sometimes I don't understand what is going on, and I just want out.
N: You're confused about what is happening, and at times you think of leaving the situation completely.
P: I know my children are lonely and unhappy, but what can I do? I can't see them as often as I like because of my work.
N: Your children's welfare concerns you, and your job schedule complicates your relationship with them.

Clarifying. The next aspect of listening is clarifying, which diminishes emotional distance and begins the approach to emotional closeness. The process indicates the nurse's increased awareness and understanding of the patient's problems, feelings, and needs, and it contributes to a sense of therapeutic intimacy. The following is an example of clarifying:

P: I am all wrung out, and I just can't cope with what is happening to me.
N: You're feeling exhausted, and you're thinking the situation is really hopeless for you. What does that mean to you?

Clarifying goes beyond paraphrasing and begins to explore the meaning behind what the patient is sharing with the nurse. It is a way of asking the patient to give a more succinct account of what he has left vague. However, in the early phases of development of the therapeutic relationship any interpretation or explanation of behaviors, meanings, and situations is to be avoided.

Checking Perception. Checking perceptions is the most sophisticated and complex skill involved in active listening. It is utilized as the therapeutic process approaches intimacy, because the nurse is reflecting her perception of the patient's behaviors, thoughts, and feelings. Essentially, the nurse is sharing her view of how she perceives and hears the patient. Usually this is done at the completion of a discussion of a thought or an aspect of a problem. When perceptions are shared, the patient is asked to verify or give feedback. When perceptions are confirmed as accurate the patient also experiences an increased sense of understanding. If patients do not think they are being understood or do not sense the nurse's interest in them, feelings of therapeutic intimacy will not develop. Consider this example:

P: Sometimes I think I know what to do and sometimes I don't. It's really a mess. How did this all happen?
N: Let me tell you what I see from our discussion. I'm impressed with the amount of work it has been for you to talk with me about this. I also get the feeling from listening to you that you're still confused and perhaps feeling pressured to make a choice. What do you think of what I've said?

When the nurse actively listens to the patient she is also role modeling for the patient and teaching him new listening and communicating skills. Active listening is a skill that all individuals can learn, and it provides them with a strong foundation for effective interaction. As the patient becomes increasingly involved in the therapeutic process and learns this skill he also becomes responsible for actively listening to the nurse. To achieve an understanding of himself and facilitate his personal growth and development he needs to master the attending, paraphrasing, clarifying, and perception-checking skills that have been described.

Guiding

In the early stages of the development of an effective therapeutic relationship the guiding and encouraging skills should be well utilized. Guidance aids the patient in choosing a direction or an area that he would like to pursue or that it is necessary for him to pursue. It may involve direct questions or the use of questions and statements to keep the interaction in productive channels. Guidance is involved in all aspects of listening and understanding skills, but it can also be considered a discrete entity.

Indirect Guiding. During the superficial stage of the interaction indirect guidance is frequently utilized. Indirect guidance consists in general statements, questions, or expectant looks and pauses. It involves such questions as the following: "Tell me more about that." "How do you feel about that situation?" "What problems brought you to the clinic?" These give the nurse additional information needed for understanding the patient and for continued work with him. Early in the relationship this helps the patient to assume responsibility for the primary content of the discussion, and it helps to establish the role of the nurse as the helping partner.

If indirect guidance is kept general, open-ended, and vague, patients frequently are eager for the opportunity to share and elaborate on their feelings, situations, and behaviors. A patient sometimes intuitively understands the process of developing therapeutic closeness. In other patients such an approach may provoke anxiety, thus forcing the nurse to take the primary responsibility for introducing issues and concerns. These patients require additional support in understanding how to be active in the therapeutic process.

Indirect guidance can be approached by structuring the situation for the patient and by not moving too rapidly toward therapeutic intimacy. The structuring of the situation occurs with the nurse's understanding of the patient's dilemma: he wants to discuss his problems but he does not know what is expected of him. First, the nurse can explain this to the patient and gently encourage and guide him as he begins to discuss his problems. Second, the nurse can assess the progress of each variable on the continuum as it contributes to therapeutic intimacy, and she can be responsible for helping the patient address all the variables at the same place on the continuum. Third, the nurse can use her initial contact skills in all of the listening skills. The more sophisticated skills (those farther on the continuum) may be threatening to the patient during initial encounters. As the patient and nurse move to diminish their emotional distance the need for more specific information and a definite focus emerges.

Direct Guiding. Questions and suggestions to direct the interaction are next utilized. Initially this is to establish a basis for future understanding of behavior and feelings. As the patient and nurse understand the details and ramifications of the content that emerges with direct guidance, other skills that increase therapeutic closeness can be utilized. Direct guidance helps patients to explore behaviors, thoughts, and feelings directly. Direct guidance is not general, open-ended, or vague in character; rather, specificity is sought. The following questions are examples of direct guidance: "What do you do when you are angry?" "How did you think your suicide would affect your wife?" "How did you feel when you left work?"

Centralizing. After the initial problem is assessed, centralization can be employed to further explore any issue, feeling, or action that the nurse and the patient think they would find beneficial. The nurse, using her knowledge and expertise, helps the patient to focus on the central issues of his problem. Once again, this demonstrates how the nurse and the patient share responsibility for developing therapeutic closeness. The patient provides the content and decides to trust and risk, while the nurse provides the expertise and knowledge that enable the patient to determine the priorities of his concerns. Centralization may be at the nurse's discretion, or it may be negotiated with the patient. When active listening occurs and the patient's autonomy and dignity are acknowledged through this process, the patient frequently enjoys deciding with the nurse what issues are important and where the focus is to be. In addition, this facilitates the development of therapeutic closeness. Consider this example of centralization:

N: During our last visits together you have told me about your relationships with several different men, and it seems that in each of these relationships you became very unhappy. I think it is important for us to discuss the reasons that you select men who will make you unhappy. There are several places we could start, but I think it is important for us to explore what happens with you when you select men who cannot return your feelings of love and concern. We also need to discuss your relationship with your father, brothers, and male colleagues. Where would you like to start?

Inquiring. Inquiring occurs when the nurse and the patient have developed some degree of closeness. It is part of the process of helping the patient to understand his problems, behaviors, thoughts, and feelings. It differs from other skills in that the focus is on increasing the patient's understanding, not the understanding of the nurse. The nurse helps the patient to examine and investigate the multiple aspects of his problem and its ramifications for him in daily life, as well as potential resolutions of his problem. As the nurse develops her therapeutic skills and integrates her nursing knowledge and expertise, her inquiries often prove the catalyst that helps the patient recognize crucial dynamics and develop appropriate insights.

The process of inquiring includes questioning, and statements that encourage exploration of a problem, so that the patient gains increased understanding. The nurse and patient are achieving the beginning of therapeutic intimacy and interdependence at this point. The patient is involved in the process of self-disclosure as well as in seeking insights. The nurse's utilization of listening and understanding skills and knowledge is influencing the development of therapeutic closeness. For example:

P: I have such a hard time staying on a diet, but I hate being overweight. My wife fixes marvelous meals and always serves snacks in the evening. I just can't say no when I should. I don't want to hurt her feelings.

N: Tell me what you think would happen if you did say *No* to your wife.

Reflecting

Reflecting involves integration of feelings and content obtained by the nurse through the use of the above skills and reflection of these back to the patient. In general, the components that are reflected are content and feelings and the nurse's perception of the congruity between the patient's verbal expressions and behaviors. In practice it can often be difficult for the novice to separate these elements and to share the information with the patient.

Content. The mirroring of content and behavior back to the patient differs from paraphrasing. The nurse shares her empathy and also presents the patient with a comprehensive picture of what she sees at that moment. This can also mirror back to the patient confusing or contradictory elements. Since reflection presents a synthesis of what the nurse perceives, her feedback often provides the patient with new ways of considering his behaviors, thoughts, and feelings. In order to be fully utilized, reflection of content requires knowledge of the patient and understanding of his sphere of reality. For example:

N: Mr. Piper, we've talked about your relationship with your wife and your problems at work. It seems that you separate them in your mind, but I see some similarities there that I think need discussing.

Feelings. Reflection of feelings requires an understanding of the content expressed by the patient and knowledge of how behaviors relate to feelings. The nurse must employ her expertise to recognize feeling tones and cues. Increasing therapeutic intimacy occurs because she responds to and shares with the patient the feelings she perceives to be behind his behavior or his description of a situation. This is done in order to help the patient become aware of his feelings or to elicit clarification of feelings. However, clear and accurate perception of feelings that are behind behavior is often difficult.

It can be difficult for individuals to recognize their feelings, although feelings are an essential part of being human. Reflection often helps individuals to integrate or reintegrate their feelings into their awareness. This can be a personal and intimate experience, and it occurs as superficiality diminishes. The following is an example of reflection of feelings:

N: Mrs. Gray, we've discussed your concerns about your two children. It seems they are both a joy to you and a source of frustration as well. I say this because I've noticed that you can talk about them easily when it's been a good week and you've had a good time together. But sometimes it seems difficult for you to talk openly about the arguments you also have. I wonder if this isn't related to some feeling of guilt on your part. I could be wrong, but a lot of people have the idea that you're just not supposed to feel angry and fight with children, and then they feel guilty when this happens. Do you think this might be true for you?

Congruence of Expression and Behavior. The full sense of therapeutic intimacy occurs for this skill when the nurse is able to share with the patient that she perceives congruence of the patient's words and behaviors or body language. The nurse is responding to the total experience offered by the patient; this includes the physiologic aspect as well as the psychologic aspect. A guideline in this area is to include all the reflective components: content, feelings, and description of what she perceives as occurring. An example: "You tell me that you do not care that your wife left you, but when we discuss her leaving you clench your fists and tighten your jaw. It seems that you are upset."

Consulting

During the course of the patient's hospitalization and follow-up on an outpatient basis there inevitably are times that the nurse will be asked for her suggestions and guidance in areas with which she is not familiar or in which she has no expertise. On the other hand, the nurse usually has a certain store of life experience that she may utilize in giving advice on a wide range of topics.

Guiding. Once the nurse begins to understand the scope of the problem and the patient's subjective assessment of his situation, pertinent information and guidance can be helpful to the patient. By recognizing the patient's needs and abilities, and by accurate referral by the nurse, the patient and nurse begin to appreciate what they can accomplish together. Referrals for specific advice on family planning, credit consolidation loans, development of assertive skills, and weight reduction programs are appropriate in helping patients alleviate some of the myriad human problems. Often such guidance is so helpful to the patient that a decrease in tension can easily occur.

Suggesting. Suggestion involves the presentation to the patient of ideas or tactics for his consideration of their use in resolution of his problem. Often the nurse will make recommendations for the patient's consideration, but the nurse does not make the final decision. At times this makes associations more meaningful and provides impetus for further exploration. It occurs with therapeutic intimacy because it involves sharing of the patient's problems by the patient and the nurse. It is frequently more effective than advice because of the patient's involvement in adapting the recommendations or suggestions to his life. For example:

N: I think there are several solutions to consider as you decide whether to keep your baby. I'd like to share them with you, and then we can discuss whichever ones you like. One possibility is an abortion, another is giving the baby up for adoption, and another is keeping the baby and remaining at home or moving to your own apartment. Take a few minutes to think about each of these and how it would fit in with your life. Then we can discuss them.

Summarizing

Summarizing includes the same components that constitute reflecting. The goal of summarizing is to give a feeling of movement and accomplishment to the therapeutic process. It can occur at any point during a discussion or in the process of problem resolution. Summarization is utilized to synthesize the topics under discussion.

Content. The first few minutes of any interaction with a patient can be used to summarize the last interaction. This has a twofold purpose: First, it enables the patient to maintain a perspective on the areas discussed and on his progress in these areas. Second, by beginning with the stated content the patient is able to see how the nurse synthesizes the content of a previous interview or interaction.

The patient can share in the responsibility of summarizing at the end of interviews and interactions. Alternatively, the nurse and patient can discuss their individual summarizations. As this occurs the mutuality of their work together is enhanced. The following is an example of content summarization:

N: In our talk yesterday you told me about your daily activities and how difficult it was for you to care for your children before you came to the hospital.
P: I think that sounds right. When I take time to think about our talks, it helps me to see how things happened and how hard it was for me to do much of anything.

Feelings. As the patient departs from objective content and begins to elaborate on subjective content, or thoughts and feelings, a sense of therapeutic intimacy begins to emerge. This may be facilitated by mutual summarization of this aspect. The same process of summarizing occurs. Feelings are summarized, change or lack of change is noted, and the patient's increased sharing of feelings is discussed. For example:

N: Today, I think we covered a very difficult area. It is hard to understand anger and often difficult to handle our angry feelings. For the first time I heard you make direct references to your anger about your friends and discuss what you are going to do about the situation.

Process. When intimacy is established, the most sophisticated aspect of summarizing is utilized. The nurse can summarize the dynamics of the nurse–patient interaction and relate them to the feelings and content of the interaction. This permits all the dynamics and content to be related and establishes the premise from which further exploration will be necessary. This is educational for the patient because he can learn from the nurse's skills and observations, as well as increase his understanding of interpersonal and intrapersonal dynamics. For example:

N: Today I felt as though you put me in your wife's shoes. I would like to share with you how I felt and what I saw happen. Perhaps this will contribute to your perspective on your relationship with your wife.

The nurse–patient interaction is in many ways analogous to a jigsaw puzzle. At times it is difficult to visualize how the pieces fit together and to see that each small completed section is a component of the entire puzzle. It is beneficial to continually relate the complete portions to the picture of the completed puzzle. Similarly, the summarizing process keeps the interactions goal-directed and in perspective for the nurse and the patient.

Interpreting

Interpreting skills are used by advanced practitioners. Interpretation is best suited for work with patients who are in long-term treatment, who are capable of testing reality, and who are introspective, intelligent, and well motivated. Patients are given interpretations by the practitioner when therapeutic intimacy is firmly established. Interpretive skills, although not used by beginning practitioners, are included here so that the nurse can identify them and contrast them with other skills. Unfortunately, many interpretations are made without the practitioner being aware that this skill is being employed and without being aware of the demands interpretation makes on the patient. Consequently many patients are subjected to ill-timed interpretations (usually too early rather than too late) that serve only to demonstrate the beginning practitioner's intellectual understanding of the patient's psychodynamics rather than a high level of accurate empathy and sound clinical judgment.

Interpretation of the patient's behaviors, thoughts, and feelings is a process of sharing explanations and definitions of those feelings and behaviors with the patient. The art of interpreting provides the nurse with a vehicle for helping the patient bring to his awareness the circumstances, beliefs, judgments, and feelings that motivate his behavior. Skill, integrity, and empathy are required in interpreting the patient's behaviors and feelings.

It is important for the nurse to share her interpretations in such a way that the patient feels he can respond to them, negotiate their meaning and accuracy, or indicate that he is not ready for the interpretation. There is potential for tremendous impact on the patient inherent in interpretation. In order for it to be meaningful it must relate to the aspects of the interaction that are occurring in present time. The value of this intervention is measured by how it contributes to patient change and development. Patients may develop or enhance insight by learning to utilize this skill.

All behaviors are meaningful, as are the thoughts and feelings that accompany them. The nurse's interpretation of events and behaviors is an integral part of her influence on the patient's thoughts, feelings, and behaviors. Often the nurse will make interpretations of behaviors or events but not share them with the patient. These are for the nurse's personal reference and can be validated or negated as the therapeutic process continues. Learning when to share an interpretation is an advanced skill. The following is an example of interpretation:

N: You told me about your father's suicide and how you felt because you failed to prevent it, as well as how you felt about working very hard to care for your mother after his death. I wonder if your great concern and caring for your suicidal friend is related to that incident. By working very hard to prevent your friend from commiting suicide it sounds as though you are alleviating the guilt you feel about your father's suicide. Will you share with me some of your thoughts on what I just said?

Questioning. The interpretation can be presented as a question. Questions have a tentative quality, and they can permit validation of a suggestion or a hunch to occur. For example: "Do you think you are having problems preparing for your examination because you have done poorly on other major examinations?" This process minimizes the risk, and it enables the patient to explore the problem in a broader context.

Explaining. The explanations that occur farther on the continuum reflect the nurse's orientation to the therapeutic process. The framework in which she understands behavior is shared. As the patient accepts or rejects these interpretations of behaviors he learns more about the nurse's knowledge and orientation, and he also obtains increased knowledge of himself. For example:

N: It appears that you suddenly dislike anyone who criticizes you and find ways to avoid them after that. I think this is a problem of not knowing what to do after you are criticized; perhaps we can look at this more clearly.

Fantasizing. Fantasizing is the most sophisticated aspect of interpretation, and it is utilized when therapeutic intimacy is established. It includes the aspects of interpretation, but the major focus is on the nurse's frame of reference. This is a part of the therapeutic process that enables the nurse to share her comprehension and application of knowledge about the patient. Fantasies permit the nurse free play with her imagination, in which she creates mental images that are modified by what she perceives the patient's needs to be; the process is analogous to daydreaming. Through the sharing of fantasy the nurse is also modeling ways in which fantasy can be used. For example: "Let me just pretend for a minute about what I think you might do in a situation, based on what you have told me about yourself. You suddenly receive a gift of $1 million, tax-free. You decide that you have two basic choices: The first is that you can continue your job as an engineer and keep the money in the bank earning interest to supplement your income. The second is to spend the money and have everything done for you, to be taken care of with no responsibilities. In this fantasy I think you would choose to be indulged and taken care of. What do you think?" With time and effort many patients learn to use this effectively. Ultimately, this is part of the goal of teaching the patient how to formulate his own interpretations of the interrelatedness of behaviors, thoughts, and feelings.

Confronting

Confronting skills are complex, and they are utilized when therapeutic intimacy is fully developed. Success with confrontation skills depends on the establishment of trust, honesty, warmth, and sincere caring, as well as nurse–patient investment in the development of therapeutic intimacy. When employing confronting skills the nurse must keep her responses constructive for that particular patient. As she keeps her feedback within the framework of the established therapeutic goals, she must always be aware that her feedback affects the patient's thoughts and feelings.

Repeating. The patient often experiences a sense of risk or vulnerability during confrontation. The least threatening and most superficial risk is that of repeating feelings previously expressed by the patient or the nurse for emphasis or elaboration. Feelings are personal experiences, but when they have been openly shared no further intrusion is made by repeating what has already been said. The accuracy in the repetition is important, just as the nurse must be able to accurately recognize the feelings originally expressed. Self-awareness is an important adjunctive skill in this area. Often the nurse recognizes the patient's feelings by her own responses to them. An example of this might be the desire not to be near someone who is very depressed. Another manifestation of such awareness might be the development of a stomachache when in the presence of someone who is anxious. Based on her own feelings and on what she perceives of the patient's feelings the nurse might draw conclusions such as these: "I understand that you feel quite sad about the death of your dog. You seem to be feeling very anxious right now." "Often when people describe those feelings they are feeling bored and frustrated."

Describing and Expressing. Descriptions of feelings are the next degree of confrontation on the continuum. Description is based on the nurse's knowledge and expertise in the area of feelings and in the area of the resultant dynamics or benefits of sharing feelings at a particular moment. The description of her feelings that the nurse shares with the patient helps to contribute to the mutual process of investment in the therapeutic process. The nurse is no longer a stranger when her feelings are shared. The feelings that are shared are those involving her interaction with the patient, not those of her personal life. The benefits of sharing and developing a sense of intimacy are facilitiated at this stage by the linking of feelings with content or behavior. This reinforces the process and the importance of sharing feelings. It also helps the patient to differentiate between thoughts, feelings, and actions. Some examples: "When you pace the floor, I find myself feeling anxious." "I experience a warm feeling when I see you working so hard not to be anxious during exams."

Feedback and Opinion. As the nurse shares her feelings, often in a modeling role, the patient is encouraged to share his thoughts and feelings. Before this can be utilized effectively the sense of therapeutic intimacy should be well established, and the variables contributing to therapeutic intimacy should be congruent on the continuum. At this point the nurse shares with the patient her reaction to him and how she is affected by him. The nurse helps to contribute to the patient's definition of himself by offering her opinion about his feelings and behaviors. Needless to say, this is a level of skilled interaction that must be supported by a strong therapeutic relationship. The nurse must be able to recognize that the patient is ready for feedback. One way to assess readiness is when the patient asks for feedback: "Tell me what you think about my plans." Some patients have difficulty with this, and they need to have openings provided. In these instances the nurse can ask the patient if he would like her thoughts or feelings on an issue.

With this skill, as with other skills, it is helpful for the nurse to link the feedback about her feelings to specific patient behaviors or events in order to contribute meaning to the observation. Effectiveness is enhanced when she is able to discuss what she thinks the observation means and relate it to other facts and data about the patient. Feedback must be kept in this sphere in order to prevent the interjection of personal biases, prejudices, or problems. Care must be taken, because this personal extension by the nurse can have tremendous impact on the patient.

Informational feedback exercises provide information on the perception of behaviors, the consequences of actions, and the nurse's reactions to behaviors; care must be taken not to give the impression of attacking the patient. When utilized appropriately, with recognition of the possible consequences and the vulnerability involved, feedback helps to promote therapeutic intimacy. This can be reflected in the process of increased self-exploration and subsequent behavioral changes.

Nursing interventions must be based on an assessment of where the nurse–patient relationship is on the therapeutic superficiality–intimacy continuum. By employing active intervention skills the nurse is able to promote therapeutic intimacy and subsequent acquisition of self-knowledge, alteration of behaviors and feelings, and resolution of problems.

The paradigm of intervention, accompanied by the discussion, shows increasingly sophisticated intervention skills may be utilized as therapeutic intimacy emerges. Utilization of intervention skills reflects the increasing sophistication that is facilitated by the emerging intimacy that is necessary for the maintenance of therapeutic intimacy.

SUMMARY

The characteristics of intimacy and superficiality in social and therapeutic interactions have been discussed: the focus and topic of the interview, the pertinent patient experience, the time orientation of the patient, the uses of feelings, and the recognition that each individual is unique and has inherent worth.

The nurse's utilization of intervention skills aids in the development of therapeutic intimacy. By appropriately utilizing these skills at various stages of emerging therapeutic intimacy she is able to help patients resolve their problems efficiently and understand their thoughts and feelings.

Reference

Brammer LM: The Helping Relationship Process and Skills. Englewood Cliffs, Prentice-Hall, 1973

CHAPTER

3

CULTURAL VARIATION

Mary T. Bush
Karen Sue Babich

The idea that ethnicity is an important factor to be considered in providing quality nursing care is more often manifested in rhetoric than in action. Some isolated facts regarding the characteristics of cultures occasionally are taught (eg, the importance of the extended family in the Chicano culture), but usually little effort is made to place the facts in the context of the overall beliefs of that culture or to understand the dynamics of a minority culture as they are influenced by the economic, political, and social forces of the majority culture. Thus viewing individual behaviors out of context often leads to the interpretation that the different behaviors of nonwhites in our majority white culture are pathologic and require psychiatric intervention. It is not necessary that the nurse be an expert in other cultures, but she should have an awareness of her own racial identity and values, an understanding of the roles social systems play in influencing behavior, and a willingness to learn from the client from another culture.

The first two chapters in this book presented information about communication and therapeutic relationships. Before moving into more specific concepts, skills, and interventions the nurse should consider the impact that cultural variation can have on her practice. Therefore the overall goal in this chapter is to provide the nurse with an understanding of the importance of cultural diversity, a framework for assessment of needs, and some general principles for intervention that can be utilized to provide safe and senstive psychosocial care for ethnic people of color.*

**The term ethnic people of color is preferred because it avoids connotations of inferiority that are associated with the term minority groups (Rich 1971, p. 230). While there is some disagreement on the scientific accuracy of this term (there being no standard differences in skin tones), the term itself addresses the real psychologic issue. Objections may be raised because of the use of the word color, with its connotations of discriminatory practices; on the other hand, acceptance of the term may be based on association of the word color with a sense of racial pride (Branch 1975, p. ix).*

HEALTH CARE DELIVERY AND ETHNIC PEOPLE OF COLOR

The Bureau of the Census in 1970 estimated the population of the United States to be approximately 200 million, 87.64 percent white and 12.36 percent nonwhite (Fig. 3.1). There is general agreement that these data underestimate the numbers of nonwhite persons; more accurately, the figures appear to be black Americans 12 percent, Spanish-speaking Americans 5.9 percent, and native Americans 0.64 percent (Shyrock and Siegel 1973). The racial composition of each major ethnic group is outlined in Figure 3.2.

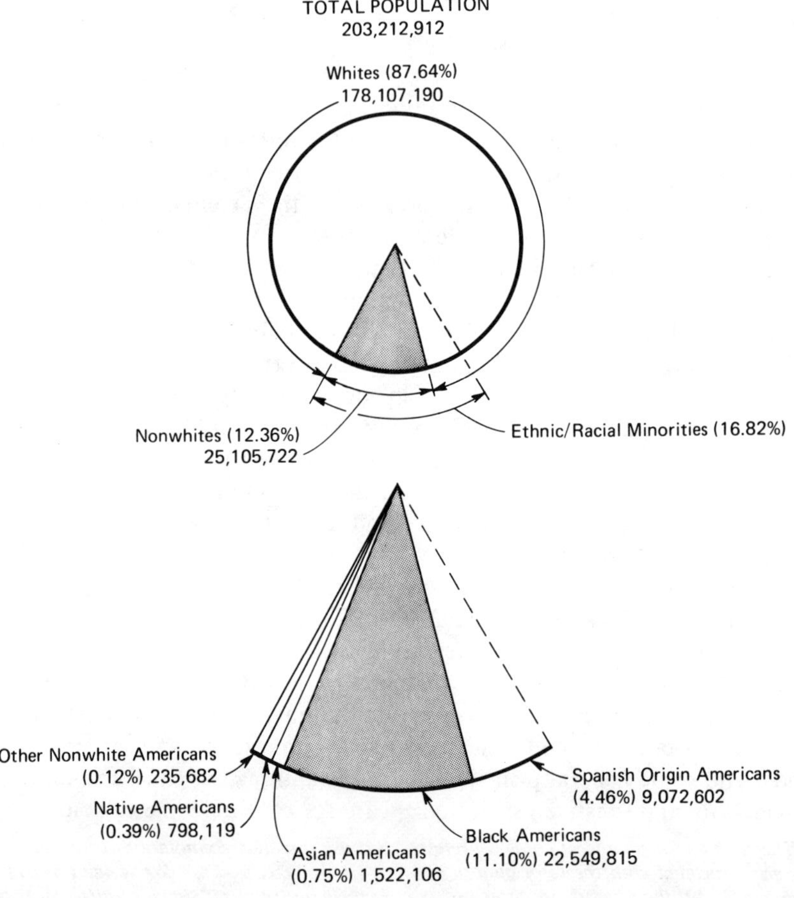

FIG. 3.1. Ethnic/racial minorities, United States population, 1970 census. (Minority Health Chart Book, USPHS/DHEW, Washington, DC, US Government Printing Office.)

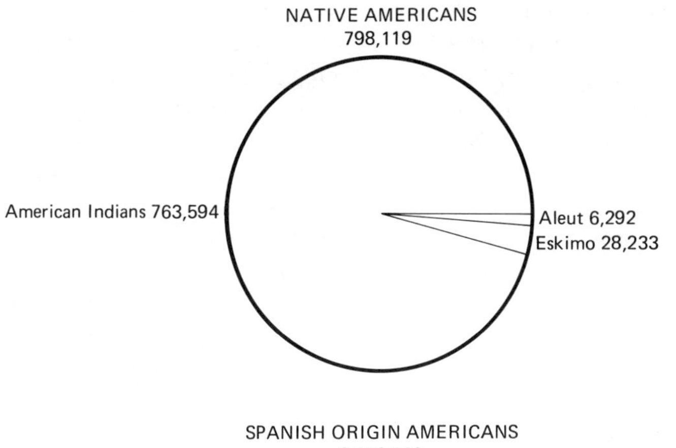

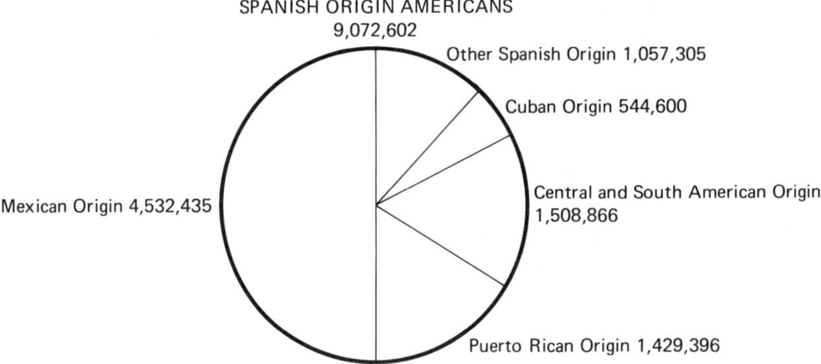

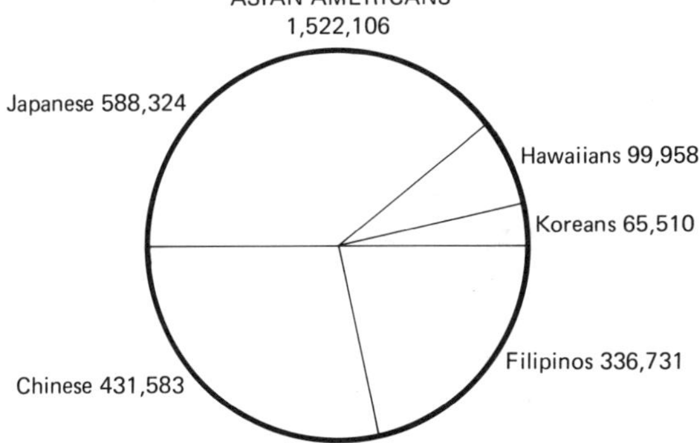

FIG. 3.2. Minority population composition, 1970 United States census. (Minority Health Chart Book, USPHS/DHEW, Washington, DC, US Government Printing Office.)

One might question such concern over an issue that involves only one-eighth of our total population. But in view of the fact that it is the nonwhite populations that historically have been systematically oppressed, the emphasis becomes more understandable. Discrimination on the basis of color is a violation of the principles this country has long espoused, if not practiced. From a socioeconomic viewpoint the issue involves underutilization of an enormous amount of human potential. Of major concern to the health care provider are the statistics (Fig. 3.3) showing that nonwhite persons have higher rates of chronic conditions requiring medical treatment and shorter life expectancy than whites. The Life Tables of the U.S. Department of Health, Education, and Welfare (1970) show that life spans are 7.6 years shorter for nonwhite males than for white males and 8.1 years shorter for nonwhite females than for white females.

Despite the statistics demonstrating that health needs are great among ethnic people of color there is a lack of content directed at the problem in nursing school curricula. Most schools of nursing do not include information and experiences that would prepare graduates to provide appropriate and sensitive care for minority groups with unique cultural patterns (Branch and Paxton 1976, p. xi). This deficiency in nursing education (as well as in most other forms of education) can be attributed to a lack of awareness and to the blind assumption that equality has been achieved as well as proclaimed.

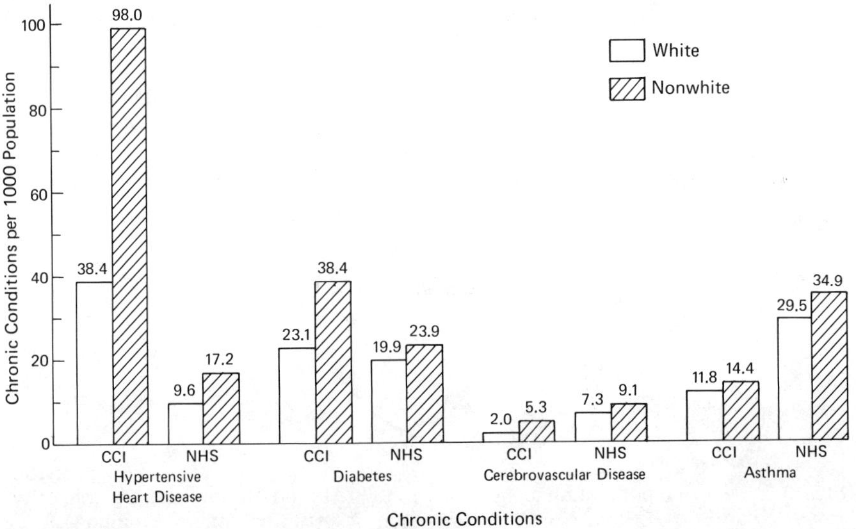

FIG. 3.3. Prevalence of selected chronic conditions. (Minority Health Chart Book, USPHS/DHEW, Washington, DC, US Government Printing Office.)

This lack of awareness derives from the fact that when one's background or frame of reference is all white and the people one associates with are all white (ie, when all one has ever seen has been white) there is nothing to lead one to suspect that there is an absence of color in one's world. One's difficulties in acknowledging differences and focusing on these differences to improve health care are most often related to a reluctance to deal with reality. The notion that we are basically all alike (as derived tortuously from doctrines of equality) not only discounts the unique attributes of each culture but also encourages a whitewash approach that does not provide any impetus for whites to examine the value sets within their culture.

Adherence to what might be called the great Clorox melting pot theory of delivery of health services results in ineffective interventions and unsafe nursing practice. A most striking example is that not until recently has information on the assessment of cyanosis in black skin been included in nursing and medical texts. While the loss of lives because of lack of information in this area may be appalling, equally appalling is the fact that over a period of many years either no one noticed this gap in information or anyone who did was unheeded. Another example can be drawn from the numerous studies that show underrepresentation in the use of mental health facilities by Mexican-Americans living in the Southwest United States. Gaitz and Scott (1974) have hypothesized that some of the reasons for this involve cultural differences from the majority of the population: cultural attitudes toward illness, their unique family structure, and their resistance to obtaining professional help in formal and impersonal Anglo-American institutions (pp. 104–105). However, they refer to a study conducted at the East Los Angeles Mental Health Service in which it was found that Mexican-American patients responded at least as well as Anglo-American patients when they were offered professional treatment in an atmosphere of cultural familiarity and acceptance (p. 105).

The responses of ethnic people of color to majority-culture psychosocial nursing care can lead to frustration for both practitioner and client, as well as to unsafe and unsuccessful intervention. In a paper presented to the American Public Health Association conference in New Orleans in June 1974 Rosemary Wood described quite vividly the positive influence that understanding and utilization of cultural factors in psychotherapeutic interventions can have. Her success in working with an institutionalized native American Kickapoo woman was attributed to focusing on content and process that were culturally relevant. The key to communication with the patient was to encourage her to speak and sing in her native language. An interpreter from the woman's hometown was engaged, and it was arranged to involve the family in treatment. As a result, dramatic positive changes occurred in the patient, who had been described for 10 years as dangerous, impossible to understand, and mentally retarded (Wood 1974).

CURRENT KNOWLEDGE BASE

Lack of awareness and denial of differences are not the only factors that account for our inability to provide safe and sensitive care to ethnic persons of color. There is also a dearth of accurate information in the many volumes of research done on the various ethnic groups; the groups studied have had little or no input into the analyses of the findings, and thus the research has generally served to perpetuate myths and stereotypes of the ethnic groups of color being studied by white researchers. Some examples from the literature on research concerning mental health and ethnic groups will illustrate this point.

First are the studies that fall in the category that might be termed mental health and the poor. In these studies the researchers tend to associate ethnic people of color with poverty so often that these disparate elements tend to become synonymous to the researchers. Not only is this an overgeneralization that denies the individuality and cultural richness of ethnic groups, but also it leads to misconceptions, as in the Hollingshead and Redlich study (1958). These researchers found a higher incidence of psychosis and treatment failure among lower socioeconomic groups, but they failed to acknowledge middle-class models of diagnosis, treatment, and communication as important variables influencing their findings; several challenges of their findings have appeared (eg, Miller and Mischler 1959). A review of Miller and Mischler would be worthwhile for many nurses.

Williams (1971) has suggested that the Moynihan report (1965) is a prime example of how research on specific ethnic groups can be both inaccurate and destructive to social planning and change. In addition to viewing black behaviors as pathologic, rather than as survival responses to white racism, Moynihan also suggested that there has been a general disintegration of the black family resulting in a matriarchal family structure that is not in accordance with what he terms the American way. Wilkinson (1970), in discussing this issue, suggested that if black researchers were to view the white middle class and note the frequency with which the male is out of the home and the woman is assuming conventional male tasks a similar diagnosis of matriarchal family structure could be made. He further speculated that the marked emphasis placed on matriarchy in the black community may in reality be the outcome of the white man's fears that his own patriarchal system is slipping away (p.

1090). While racism is the basic issue, a feminist is sure to note that in both cases the message implied is that a matriarchal family structure is inherently inferior.

The American Indians are other ethnic groups that have been extensively studied by social scientists, and the findings have been detrimentally generalized. Suicide and alcoholism are widely viewed as symptoms of severe personal mental health problems among native Americans rather than as the results of white social and political policies. Ignoring a person's environment while diligently searching for the characteristics of the person's problem creates a situation in which the victim of a social ill comes to be seen as the creator of the social ill. Ryan (1971) has labeled this process "blaming the victim," a process he delineates thus (p. 8):

> First, identify a social problem. Second, study those affected by the problem and discover in what ways they are different from the rest of us as a consequence of deprivation and injustice. Third, define the differences as the cause of the social problem itself. . . . The formula for action becomes extraordinarily simple: change the victim.

In an excellent article in *Psychology Today* Caplan and Nelson (1974) pointed out that focusing the blame on the person rather than on the system tends to justify the actions that these professionals advise under the guise of help for those the professionals have categorized as having problems. This maintains the status quo. However, it is also counterproductive to place all the blame on the system; what is needed in research is to establish a healthy balance between the person and the system, with a reasoned appreciation of the relationship between knowledge and the social, political, and economic consequences of its use (p. 104).

More recently, research and writings in professional nursing journals and textbooks have begun to present a more accurate picture of the relationships among the cultural environment, the person, and the health care delivery system. The emphasis is on how the information can be used to improve the quality of care, rather than on how to change the patient to fit our system of health care.

One project (Models for Introducing Cultural Diversity in Nursing Curricula) under the auspices of the Western Interstate Commission for Higher Education has as its goal "to develop models for the inclusion of multicultural course materials in nursing through a systematic approach for defining, teaching, and evaluating content which prepares students and practicing nurses to work with ethnic groups of color" (Branch 1974, p. 1).

Besides establishing a climate favorable for the development of cultural pluralism in nursing, much useful information has already emerged from this project: a study of the ideal characteristics of persons providing health services among ethnic people of color, a tool for the critique of culturally relevant references, and papers related to various aspects of culture, including white identity. Most important, however, is that nursing educators, nursing students, and practicing nurses participating in this project are developing cultural course materials that are validated by experts (ethnic health professionals and consumers).

It is hoped this and other efforts not only will add to our body of nursing knowledge but also will be the foundation from which we practice. Heightened awareness of one's own cultural value set and appreciation of beliefs that differ from one's own have the potential for contributing to safe and sensitive health care for consumers of all colors.

PSYCHOSOCIAL ASSESSMENT AND ETHNIC PEOPLE OF COLOR

Assessment is a vital step in the nursing process. It consists of the gathering of data that will aid in identifying a person's specific problem or need, as well as in recognizing the person's strengths. Too often in nursing the assessment is made by a practitioner from the majority culture who may lack either sensitivity or information on cultural variation.

A common problem in nursing is the incorrect application of norms from the majority culture to measure phenomena that occur in a bicultural setting. Ruffin (1973), a nurse psychotherapist, cited examples based on her experience in supervising group therapists. In many instances she found that the white therapist, either in an effort to prove that all people are alike or in an effort to prove that the therapist is an expert on another race, often avoids dealing with the basic racial issue the client presents. Instead, an attempt is made to provide interventions that will persuade ethnic persons of color to accept some white middle-class value. What the therapist should be doing is exploring the client's own racial experience (pp. 175–178).

While it is not possible for the white therapist to experience societal and cultural factors in the same way that they are experienced by an ethnic person of color, it is possible to increase one's understanding of some of the dynamics involved in cultural variation. Since educational materials usually do not provide the reader with the quality of feeling involved in an experience, it is suggested that such personal works as *The Autobiography of Malcolm X* (Haley 1964), *The Teachings of Don Juan* (Castaneda 1974), and *Bury My Heart at Wounded Knee* (Brown 1970) be used for this purpose.

Ethnoscience: A Method for Exploring Values

Anthropology is a discipline from which psychosocial nursing can borrow several concepts to improve assessment skills in relation to ethnic people of color. Anthropologists employ the holistic approach in their study of man; this can be adapted to include biologic, social, cultural, and personality factors as influences on illness and well-being (Osborne 1969). Anthropologists have traditionally explored cultures from the viewpoint of the participant observer in an effort to avoid bias in their conclusions. Of course, no discipline is totally free of bias, and care must be taken in utilizing any data; nurses, also, must constantly strive for validity and sensitivity. Specifically, in adopting the anthropologic approach the holistic concept must not exclude individuality or the enrichment that comes with diversity.

Anthropologists have developed ethnoscience as a method of exploring cultures. Originally the method was used in the study of kinship systems, color categories, and taxonomy to better understand diverse cultures through language organization. More recently ethnoscience has been applied to cultural groups within American society in an attempt to explore experiences, perceptions, or cognitive sets as expressed through the symbols of words. An example of this latter use of ethnoscience is Spradley's work (1970) with urban nomads, where the experiences and terminology of skid-row inhabitants of Seattle were explored and classified in an orderly manner. It is interesting that his work had an influence on city programs to provide services to these urban nomads; better understanding of the language and life style of this group of people led to attempts at more perceptive methods of delivering care.

Another example of the ethnoscience approach to understanding cultures within our society is the research of Bush and associates (1975); they examined the conception of mental health as understood by black central-city residents and as understood by psychiatric professionals. A basic finding that emerged from this research was that professionals use abstract, specialized, and intellectual terminology when speaking of mental health that often results in vagueness and ambiguity. On the other hand, black people living in the inner city use concrete, down-to-earth terms focusing on social and economic concerns. This produces a clear contrast between the illness-oriented professionals and the black residents concerned with wellness. For example, the psychiatrists in the study focused on interpersonal factors and intrapsychic dynamics in defining mental health, frequently using professional terminology such as defense mechanisms and developmental tasks. The black inner-city residents, on the other hand, utilized terms such as making it, beating the system, and survival as they relate to socioeconomic well-being (pp. 136–138). One wonders that the two groups ever succeed in communicating in a community health care setting.

The ethnoscience method involves several specific steps that relate to the assessment process nurses utilize. The first step in this method is learning which questions to ask, questions that are culturally relevant and meaningful. This is done by listening to members of the culture being examined; in essence, one is trained or taught by those in the culture. For example, a subject in the studies of Bush and associates changed the initial query of the researchers from "What does the term mental health bring to mind?" to "What does feeling good mean?" To that person the words feeling good defined a meaningful concept, and the nurse adopted this query in researching the definition of mental health.

The second step is to organize the data shared with the interviewer in a meaningful way. It is important to note that the organizing is done by those in the culture being explored, not by scientists at some location far removed from the culture. Thus the subject mentioned previously organized her thoughts about the concept of feeling good as shown in Table 3.1. In Table 3.1 T_1 to T_4 are levels of the subject's taxonomy; they indicate progress from broad concepts (T_1) to more specific ones (T_4). The subject developed this taxonomy by first stating that feeling good encompassed praying and having kids and friends. The subject then went on to elaborate what praying provides: luck, money, and physical health. All terms associated with feeling good were thus related to each other in a way that was meaningful to this subject.

The final step in the ethnoscience method involves verification by the subject of the data that have been gathered and their taxonomic arrangement. The ethnoscientist would ask, in relation to the taxonomy of Table 3.1, "Is talking a part of having friends as we have diagrammed?" The subject would then either verify the taxonomy or reorganize the data more appropriately. By this process cultural accuracy and sensitivity can be considerably enhanced.

Essentially, what ethnoscience can teach psychosocial nurses is that we are always learners and that we should explore cultures that are different from our own from the vantage point of the learner. Members of the cultures we are exploring and serving are the experts, the teachers. This is a reversal of the nurse–teacher/patient–learner roles we have been taught.The most obvious advantage of this approach is that our concepts of the culture being explored will be more accurate; they will not be based on prevalent stereotypes but rather on personal understanding. It is to be hoped that if our concepts and understanding are more accurate our assessments will be more accurate and therefore our treatment plans more effective. A less obvious but still important advantage is that the

Table 3.1. ONE PATIENT'S TAXONOMIC DEFINITION OF FEELING GOOD*

T_1†	T_2	T_3	T_4
Praying	Luck		
	Money	Strength Work Welfare	
	Physical health	Working problems out	Food Clothes Shelter Education
Having Kids	Luck		
	Giving help	Needed Important, worth-while Happy Proud	
	Getting help	Strength Secure (present) Secure (future)	
Friends	Talking	Strength Get help Give help	
	Getting out	Strength Free	

**From Bush, Ullom, Osborne: The meaning of mental health: a report of two ethnoscientific studies. Nurs Res 24:133, March–April 1975, by permission of The American Journal of Nursing Company, ©1975.*

†*T_1–T_4 refer to taxonomic levels.*

client–therapist inferiority–superiority distancing, which seems especially inevitable when a majority-culture nurse deals with an ethnic person of color, can be diminished.

Along with this learner approach to assessment the psychosocial nurse needs some direction in the areas that are important in assessing cultural diversity. Peter Koshi (1975) has developed a scale that may be used to assess cultural variables.

Koshi Scale: A Method of Assessing Cultural Variables

Just as it would be a mistake to assume that every nurse supports the Equal Rights Amendment, so it would be a mistake to assume that every member of a given group of ethnic people of color fits into the same category. To lock someone into a slot because of the color of his skin would deny his individuality and perpetuate stereotyping. While there may be a body of traditional beliefs in each culture, adherence to these beliefs varies between generations, families, and individuals. In the white culture, for example, one's adherence to the Protestant ethic of hard work and maintenance of the proper social image may be similar to that of one's peers but different from that of other family members, or vice versa.

In order to avoid stereotyping on the group level, Koshi (1975) has developed a scale to measure eight variables that affect one's perception and response in relation to one's cultural identity (Fig. 3.4). The nurse may use this framework to gain an awareness of the cultural factors influencing her client. The scale allows for assessment of each variable to be made along a continuum. The continuum does not suggest a good–bad value set but only provides valid data to the psychosocial nurse on the frame of reference of her particular client, in essence, the way in which he views his world, his problems, and the alternatives available in dealing

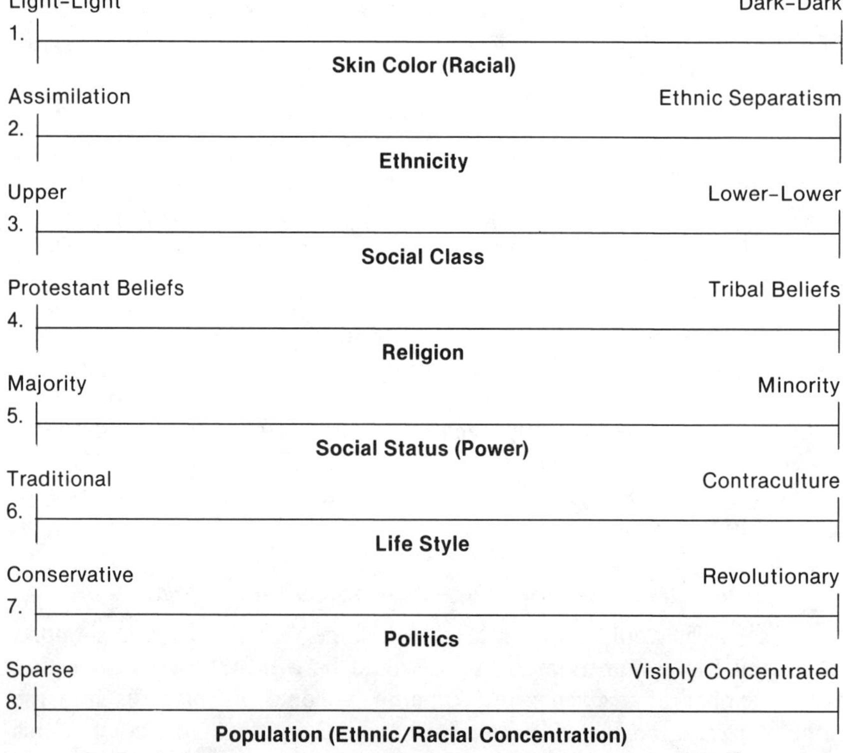

FIG. 3.4. Eight continua of cultural variables affecting practitioner and patient perception and responses. (Adapted from Koshi: J Nurs Educ 15:14–21, 1976)

with those problems. Such information is important to the nurse if she is to work collaboratively with the client in solving problems.

The process used to assess these cultural variables depends on the nurse's own style of interviewing, on the degree of comfort established, and on the level of awareness of racial prejudices. It is imperative to remember that the nurse is a learner and that the scale is a tool that can be used for focusing on relevant information. Each item can be discussed separately with the client, or the scale may be used as a general guide for discussion and observation. The scale itself is not offensive, but it can elicit defensive responses if the nurse uses it without sensitivity. Asking questions as if one were a newspaper reporter or as if one were doing market research does not induce sharing. But if genuine interest and caring are involved the client will be aware of it, and mutual exchange and learning about the client's cultural orientation can occur.

It may be helpful for the nurse to practice using this scale by assessing herself on each of the cultural variables. The significance of skin color may not be readily apparent to whites, but from one's readings (eg, *The Autobiography of Malcolm X*) the role it has played historically will become clearer. Instead of skin color the nurse may try assessing hair color. If she has blond hair does she automatically get labeled as a dumb blond? How does that affect her interactions with others? Religious beliefs are usually closely tied to ethnic practices. For example, for the Irish the wake is generally an essential part of grieving for the loss of a loved one. But it is possible to be Irish and not Catholic, to be Catholic and not observe a wake as part of the funeral service, or to be Protestant and observe wakes. The point to be made is that variations of the same sort exist among all groups of ethnic people of color. One must not assume; one must explore.

When the nurse has an accurate understanding of the client's cultural orientation she may then proceed to assessment of problem areas with greater empathy and accuracy. The following case study illustrates the use of Koshi's scale:

CLINICAL EXAMPLE

Mrs. Martinez, a 33-year-old client with light skin color and brown hair (continuum 1) attended two day treatment sessions at a large urban community mental health center, but then she did not return for several days. The nurse had observed that Mrs. Martinez usually remained silent during group activities, although her speech was clear and easily understood when she did participate. The nurse had been uneasy with the client and had noticed the client's considerable reluctance to take medications. She decided to make a home visit to further assess the situation.

Mrs. Martinez lived in a small house in a community where there were many Chicano families and small ethnic shops (continuum 8). The nurse was politely received by Mrs. Martinez, although conversation was quite tense at first. The nurse commented on the interesting shops she had seen, and gradually Mrs. Martinez began to talk with more ease about herself and her family, sharing bits of information about their culture. After some time she explained that she was in a dilemma about attending day treatment because her husband and parents disapproved of her participation in a program outside of her own community. They thought that a visit to a curandera would be more beneficial than "taking pills" (continua 4 and 6). The nurse left after promising to contact Mrs. Martinez the next day.

On returning to the community mental health center the nurse consulted with a Chicano staff member. He suggested arranging another home visit at a time when Mr. Martinez could be present, and he volunteered to accompany the nurse, as this might make Mr. Martinez more receptive to the visit. The plan at that point was to explore the community resources available in Mrs. Martinez's neighborhood and share this information with the family, thus providing alternatives that might prove more viable than the day-treatment program should Mrs. Martinez choose not to return.

Familiarity with Norms

Another consideration in assessment is the nurse's familiarity with the range of norms of a given cultural group; she must be able to recognize deviation from these norms. A brief but persuasive example concerns depression in black Americans. Until quite recently there was a prevalent belief that older blacks were seldom depressed. According to Carter (1974), depression is rarely diagnosed in elderly blacks because the data one would ordinarily use to formulate such a diagnosis can be misleading to the clinician who is ignorant of the black culture (p. 95). Carter believes that neurotic depression in the black community is frequently masked by somatic complaints and a facade of psychologic well-being, because racism has forced blacks to deny their natural impulses and feelings (p. 99). Probably not many majority-culture therapists are familiar with such thoughts as are expressed in these lines by the poet P.L. Dunbar (1970, p. 60):

We wear the mask that grins and lies
It hides our cheeks and shades our eyes
And with torn and bleeding hearts we smile.
Why should the world be overwise
Nay let them only see us while we wear the mask.

P.L. Dunbar, "We Wear the Mask"

It is hoped that through the psychosocial nurse's increased personal awareness, learner attitude, and appreciation of cultural diversity there will be less need for masks, for nurse or client.

PSYCHOSOCIAL INTERVENTIONS AND ETHNIC PEOPLE OF COLOR

In this book various frameworks for assessment are presented, and the psychosocial nurse can see that the intervention used depends on the assessment made. In psychosocial nursing any intervention actually begins at the time of assessment. That is, the process of talking with a client and helping him identify the issues that are causing him concern can be thought of as assessment, but at the same time the process is also intervention because of the therapeutic relationship that is being established. It is often frustrating to the nurse that interventions are not a series of standard tasks she can perform for the client to make him feel better. Instead, the focus is on what alternatives can be offered to remedy the problem, and in this area the client is the ultimate decision-maker. For an alternative to be acted on by the client it obviously must make sense and be perceived as feasible by him. The psychosocial nurse's role, then, is to establish a meaningful relationship, help the client solve problems, and locate resources.

The therapeutic process used with all clients is to employ a variety of assessment tools to help identify the problem and aid the client in solving the problem. Should the process be any different for an ethnic person of color? Obviously not, and yet nurses often approach the task of working with ethnic people of color in a state of bafflement, wondering "What am I supposed to do?" Perhaps the major problem is that the nurse often sees the ethnic client not as an individual person in distress but as an extension of the entire ethnic group, which can lead to the vague notion that the intervention must solve this nation's entire racial problem. Stereotyping and generalizing in this manner not only renders the nurse ineffective but also denies the individuality of the ethnic person of color. Utilization of the assessment tools described in this chapter, while maintaining a high sensitivity to the problem of racism, should avoid most of this stereotyping and still allow the nurse to be aware of cultural variables.

Language and Cultural Barriers

A discussion of intervention must include comment regarding the constraints of language and cultural norms. It is impossible to deliver services effectively to clients if there is no common ground for communication. This fact is quite obvious; yet many health care units in ethnic communities across the country are staffed with professionals from the white middle-class culture (Bullough and Bullough 1972, p. 174). The obvious solution to this dilemma is to employ bilingual professionals, and it is hoped that in the near future this can be achieved. However, at this time the need for bilingual, bicultural nurses greatly exceeds the supply; thus one must search for alternatives. One alternative is for the nurse to learn the language and nuances of communication of her clients; another is to utilize the services of a translator. A fairly common practice in hospitals is to use ethnic people of color who are on the housekeeping staff as translators. There is reason to question the reliability of this practice, because the translator usually lacks knowledge of medicine, and the advice given in the translation may not be exactly what the nurse was trying to convey. If no alternative exists the nurse must use sign language. Teaching aids for health communication are also available in many areas of the country.*

Even in working with clients who speak English there may be cultural barriers that require consultation or utilization of other resource people. The following situation exemplifies this:

CLINICAL EXAMPLE

In a group supervision session a student described the difficulty she was having in establishing a therapeutic relationship with an older Filipino man; he was aloof and reserved in spite of the student's efforts to put him at ease. She stated: "Manuel seems to avoid me. He is polite about it, but I feel he doesn't trust me." The student had spent considerable time sitting next to the client in silence. Another student in the group, a Filipina, shed some light on the dynamics in operation by sharing information on the norms of her culture. She mentioned that it was considered disrespectful to address an older person by his first name, that direct eye contact between an older man and a young woman usually implied either seduction or anger, and that personal space was quite extended outside of close family situations. She also stated that an open sharing of problems in this setting with the student would be almost impossible from the standpoint of this man's cultural norms.

The importance of having cultural diversity among health professionals is well illustrated by this example. In this case the Filipina nursing classmate served as a valuable resource person. In assessing such a situation based on new knowledge regarding a client's cultural norms the student will realize the need to increase her awareness of cultural variables in her efforts to establish a therapeutic relationship. She also might review Koshi's scale with her client. If the stalemate continues in this case, despite her sincere and open approach, she might seek the assistance of her classmate or the staff team in locating a resource person with whom the Filipino man could share his concerns. Such alternatives are much more therapeutic for the client than if the student continues her original efforts and either labels her client's behavior as resistance or comes to feel that she is a personal failure.

**A Spanish-language aid pamphlet may be obtained from the Public Inquiries Branch, Office of Communications and Public Affairs, Health Services and Mental Health Administration, Room 5-B-29, 5600 Fishers Lane, Rockville, Md. 20852.*

Cultural Therapies

In planning interventions the psychosocial nurse might need to consult with or utilize the services of a folk healer. Many cultures have folk healers; in our dominant white culture we could even consider mental health professionals as our folk healers. Whatever their titles, they all provide the same service: to help people with their problems. The success of the treatment used, whether it be transactional analysis, behavior modification, or the Navaho squaw dance, depends largely on the amount of faith the client and therapist have in that approach.

Curanderismo. Kiev (1968), in a study comparing curanderismo (Mexican-American folk healer treatment) and psychotherapy, concluded that neither approach was of more value than the other; the choice depended solely on the basic philosophic beliefs of the people utilizing the two treatments (p. 183). In psychotherapy the emphasis is on insight and personal change within the person, which reflects faith in personal and social progress through change and hard work (the Protestant ethic). The Mexican-American believes that the source of anxiety lies within the environment, not the self; thus the change that must occur to restore balance requires the intervention of a curandero (folk healer), who holds both mystic and religious powers (pp. 175–189).

In the Mexican-American culture two common forms of illness are sustos and mal ojo. Sustos, or spirit loss, usually is the result of the death of a loved one or the result of a frightening experience. The person experiences symptoms of anxiety (tachycardia, dyspnea, fear of illness or death) and depression (insomnia, anorexia, loss of interest). In interpreting the psychodynamics of this illness, Kiev (1968, p. 122) stated:

> The idea of death associated with "sustos" may contain elements of anxiety about punishment for death wishes against others, as well as anxiety about one's own excitement. This is reasonable in a culture where impulses must be controlled at all costs and where hostility to authority is strongly dampened by the strict patriarchal hierarchy.

Mal ojo, the evil eye, is accompanied by such physical symptoms as fever, excessive crying, vomiting, and listlessness, usually in a child. The parents believe that their child has been struck down with this illness because someone has given the child a compliment or made an affectionate overture, without touching the child. To afford protection against mal ojo a child will often wear a bracelet, necklace, or cluster of pink coral. These ritualistic steps help to relieve the parents' anxiety and guilt about the child's illness by projecting the cause of the disease onto someone outside the family who has upset the normal balance of interpersonal relationships in the family (pp. 106–107).

Navajo Squaw Dance. To the Navajo, everything originates in thought, and the power of thought is real, for good or evil. Good thoughts will maintain health and happiness; bad thoughts cause disharmony and illness in the mind and body. Consequently the Navajo has difficulty understanding the white man's separation of healing forces from the worship of life-giving forces, or the separation of medicine and religion. Therefore, to deal with his psychologic problems a Navajo may go for prayers or for a cermony conducted by a medicine man; the ceremony best known for its psychologic efficacy is the "enemy way" or squaw dance. Enemy Way kills the ghost of the haunting slain enemy; in other words, during the Enemy Way the Navajo healer overcomes the subconsious memories that torment the mind. According to Carl Gorman (1975, p. 13), director of native healing sciences at the Navajo Medical School:

> The white psychiatrist will try to probe the individual subconscious. The Navajo [medicine man] recognizes a pattern, uses a story of the Holy People to illustrate the same type of problem, tells how the Holy Person was cured and proceeds to follow the same ritual and treatment. Identification with the Holy Person is made [by the "patient"], and like the Holy Person in the myth the patient is cured.

All too often the merit of any treatment is judged on whether it is "scientific" rather than on whether the client gets better. Since mental illness occurs in a social setting and therefore is socially defined, the treatment of the disease must occur within the context of the person's cultural belief system. Only a few brief examples of cultural belief systems have been given, but it is hoped that the nurse will be stimulated to explore the richness and variety of cultures that exist within our society.

SUMMARY

Ethnic people of color comprise 18 percent of our population. All people have the right to receive accurate, safe, and effective mental health care. This can be accomplished only if the nurse is open to cultural variations. When working with ethnic groups different from her own she must be willing to give up the traditional authoritarian teacher role of the nurse and assume the role of a learner. In this way nursing as a profession will be enriched, but more specifically psychosocial nursing will become effective for our entire population.

All too often conscientious majority-culture nurses delivering services to ethnic people of color become overwhelmed and discouraged by the challenge cultural diversity presents and by racism in its many forms. The goals of this chapter have been to encourage personal awareness and sensitivity in the nurse and to provide concrete principles and tools that can be translated into practice. We firmly believe that feelings of frustration and futility can be replaced by feelings of excitement and anticipation of personal enrichment and professional gratification.

References

Branch M: Models for Introducing Cultural Diversity in Nursing Curricula. Western Interstate Commission for Higher Education, 1974 (project funded by W.K. Kellogg Foundation, 1974–1977)

——— Nursing Faculty Development to Meet Minority Group Needs (Final Report). Western Interstate Commission for Higher Education, August 1975

——— Paxton P: Providing Safe Nursing Care for Ethnic People of Color. New York, Appleton, 1976

Brown D: Bury My Heart at Wounded Knee. New York, Holt, Rinehart, Winston, 1970

Bullough B, Bullough V: Poverty, Ethnic Identity, and Health Care. New York, Appleton, 1972

Bush M, Ullom J, Osborne O: The meaning of mental health: A report of two ethnoscientific studies. Nurs Res 24:130–138, March-April 1975

Caplan N, Nelson S: Who's to blame? Psychology Today 8: 99–104, 1974

Carter J: Recognizing psychiatric symptoms in black Americans. Geriatrics 29:95–99, 1974

Castaneda C: The Teachings of Don Juan: A Yaqui Way of Knowledge. New York, Touchstone, Simon & Schuster, 1974

Dunbar P L: We wear the mask. In Kearns F E (ed): Black Identity, a Thematic Reader. New York, Holt, Rinehart, Winston, 1970, p. 60

Gaitz C, Scott J: Mental health of Mexican-Americans: Do ethnic factors make a difference? Geriatrics 29:103–110, 1974

Gorman C: Navajo theory of disease and healing practices. Unpublished paper presented at the First Navajo Nation Health Symposium, Tsaile, Ariz, July 1975

Haley A: The Autobiography of Malcolm X. New York, Grove, 1964

Hollingshead A, Redlich F: Social Class and Mental Illness. New York, Wiley, 1958

Kiev A: Curanderismo. New York, Free Press, 1968

Koshi P: Achieving a culturally diverse nursing curriculum. Original paper present at Region I Workship, WICHE, Models for Introducing Cultural Diversity in Nursing Curricula, Warm Springs, Ore, June 1975; revised paper published J Nurs Educ 15:14–21, March 1976

Life Tables, Vital Statistics of the United States 1970, Vol 2. Rockville, Md, U.S. Department of Health, Education, and Welfare, 1970, pp 5–31

Miller A, Mischler T: Social class, mental illness and American psychiatry: An expository review. Milbank Memorial Fund Quarterly 37:174–199, 1959

Minority Health Chart Book. Washington DC, USPHS/DHEW, US Government Printing Office, 1974

Moynihan D P: The negro family: Case for national action. Washington DC, US Department of Labor, Office of Policy Planning and Research, US Government Printing Office, March 1965

Osborne O: Anthropology and nursing: Some common traditions and interests. Nurs Res 18:251, May-June 1969

Rich A L: Some problems in interracial communication: An interracial group case study. Central States Speech Journal 22:228–235, 1971
Ruffin J E: Racism as countertransference in psychotherapy groups. Perspect Psychiatr Care 11:172, October 1973
Ryan W: Blaming the Victim. New York, Pantheon, 1971
Shyrock M, Siegel W: The methods and materials of demography. Washington DC, US Government Printing Office, 1973, pp 252–281
Spradley J P: You Owe Yourself a Drunk: An Ethnography of Urban Nomads. Boston, Little, Brown, 1970
Wilkinson C B: The destructiveness of myths. Am J Psychiatry 126:1087–1092, 1970
Williams R L: Abuses and misuses in testing black children. Counseling Psychologist 2:62, 1971
Wood R: Cross-cultural psychiatric nursing—psychotherapy with an American Indian. Unpublished paper presented at the APHA 102nd Annual Meeting, New Orleans, La, October 1974

CHAPTER

4

LIFE CHANGE, HUMAN ADAPTATION, AND ONSET OF ILLNESS

Cindy Cook Williams
Thomas H. Holmes

Many changes occur in one's personal environment during the course of one's life. Some of these changes may be desired and welcome, such as marriage or a vacation. However, others can be both undesirable and uncontrollable. We would avoid such events as the death of a loved one or bankruptcy if it were possible. Many of these experiences cause dramatic changes in one's life style. With repeated change, an individual's physiologic adaptive mechanisms can be activated to cope with the circumstances. Research has documented that life changes with their adaptive responses are often correlated with the onset of illness. In order to assess the type and degree of life change one experiences, the Schedule of Recent Experience (SRE) was developed (Appendix). The questionnaire itself can be a valuable clinical assessment tool for pscyhosocial nurses and other mental health professionals.

The first section of this chapter will discuss the historical development of the relationship among life change, human adaptation, and onset of illness. Research that documents this relationship will be cited, and the development of the SRE will be detailed. The second section will describe the use of the SRE as a psychosocial clinical assessment tool. Several cases will be discussed, with examples of how the questionnaire was used in client assessment and treatment.

HISTORICAL PERSPECTIVE

Why is it that a person frequently exposed to an infectious organism becomes ill at one time of exposure but not at another? Why does one individual catch the flu, while another person similarly exposed does not?

If the body's resistance is lowered one may be predisposed to becoming ill. One causative factor in lowered body resistance is prolonged physiologic adaptation to the environmental changes one experiences. Although common sense dictates that people who have to cope with great emotional burdens are likely to become sick, it is only during this century that researchers have scientifically documented this phenomenon (Holmes and Masuda 1972).

Dr. Adolf Meyer, a pioneer in psychobiology* during the early 1900s, noted that people often became sick near those times when their environments changed. Examples included changes in jobs, births and deaths in the family, entrance into school, and changes in habitat. From these observations Meyer developed a life chart. This device organized medical data into biographic form and demonstrated the interrelationship of biologic, psychologic, and sociologic processes in the health status of man (Lief 1948, Holmes and Rahe 1967).

A neurologist at Cornell Medical Center, Dr. Harold G. Wolff, began conducting research on the onset of illness using Meyer's concepts. These studies concluded that an individual's health is closely linked to the psychophysiologic demands placed on him by his environment. Wolff (1960) emphasized that an individual's usual coping mechanisms may prove inadequate if the environmental burden becomes too great or the frustration too prolonged. More primitive behaviors are often called forth to supplement these initial coping skills. Behavior patterns involving cardiovascular, respiratory, alimentary, glandular, urinary, sexual, and vasomotor activity are common. However, these adaptive arrangements cannot persist indefinitely. Over a prolonged period of time untoward effects on the bodily tissues can occur, and illness can be the unfortunate result.

Hinkle, one of Wolff's followers, found similar results when studying telephone company workers over a 20-year period. Illness often occurred when people perceived their lives as being over-demanding, unsatisfying, and full of conflict. These individuals generally felt unable to adapt to their life situations, and the by-product frequently was illness. It was found that illness patterns were established in early adulthood and generally remained the same for the next 20 years. Employees who were frequently ill when first beginning their jobs continued the same pattern throughout their entire employment. The reverse situation was also true. Hinkle determined that illness was not randomly distributed in the population: 30 percent of the people had 70 percent of the illnesses. Individuals with multiple illnesses often suffered the involvement of many body systems. The system most frequently involved was that governing

**Psychobiology is the study of psychosocial phenomena in relation to biologic processes.*

thought, feeling, and behavior—man's psychosocial and emotional system (Hinkle et al 1958).

Graham investigated the relationship between specific attitudes and the occurrence of disease. As an example, he found a high correlation between urticaria (hives) and a particular emotional attitude toward life circumstances. Nearly all his study participants with hives expressed intense resentment and saw themselves as victims of unjust treatment that they could do nothing about. This resentment generally was felt toward a significant person in their lives or an event of major importance. It was concluded that extreme dilatation of both the arterioles and minute vessels in the skin occurred partially as a result of the individual's emotional response to various life situations. The skin's physiologic response, it might be noted, was identical to that seen following actual trauma to the skin (Graham 1950).

Holmes, one of Wolff's colleagues, conducted further research on the relationship among life situations, emotions, and nasal disease (Holmes et al 1950). A group of patients who had recovered from colds and nasal infections were measured for their freedom of breathing, blood flow, swelling, and amount of secretion in the nose. Those events preceding the illness were then discussed with each patient, eg, a new job, a marriage in the family, a visit by a mother-in-law. Following the discussion of these life events the above measurements were repeated. Biopsies of nasal tissue confirmed that tissue damage was caused by talking about psychologically charged events.

DEVELOPMENT OF SOCIAL READJUSTMENT RATING SCALE

The rate of change in one's life, rather than the specific type of change, was found to be a particularly significant factor in the natural history of disease. Beginning in 1949 a study was conducted in which more than 5000 patients were asked to report those life events that occurred before the onset of their illnesses. A wide variety of circumstances were reported. The most common events cited by the study participants were compiled into a list (Table 4.1). It was found that many of the items were representative of the American way of life, such as marriage, education, occupation, and economics. Many of these events were socially desirable, and they supported the value system of achievement, materialism, self-reliance, and success. However, some of these life events were socially undesirable and unwanted. Examples included personal injury, sexual difficulties, and a jail term. All these life events did have one thing in common: their occurrence usually evoked some degree of coping or adaptation by the individual; they caused change from the existing steady state (Holmes and Rahe 1967).

Table 4.1. SOCIAL READJUSTMENT RATING SCALE

NO.	LIFE EVENT ITEM	MEAN VALUE
1.	Death of spouse	100
2.	Divorce	73
3.	Marital separation from mate	65
4.	Detention in jail or other institution	63
5.	Death of a close family member	63
6.	Major personal injury or illness	53
7.	Marriage	50
8.	Being fired from work	47
9.	Marital reconciliation with mate	45
10.	Retirement from work	45
11.	Major change in health or behavior of a family member	44
12.	Pregnancy	40
13.	Sexual difficulties	39
14.	Gaining a new family member (eg, through birth, adoption, oldster moving in)	39
15.	Major business readjustment (eg, merger, reorganization, bankruptcy)	39
16.	Major change in financial state (eg, a lot worse off or a lot better off than usual)	38
17.	Death of close friend	37
18.	Changing to different line of work	36
19.	Major change in number of arguments with spouse (eg, either a lot more or a lot less than usual regarding child-rearing, personal habits, etc.)	35
20.	Taking on mortgage greater than $10,000 (eg, purchasing a home, business)	31
21.	Foreclosure on mortgage or loan	30
22.	Major change in responsibilities at work (eg, promotion, demotion, lateral transfer)	29
23.	Son or daughter leaving home (eg, marriage, attending college)	29
24.	In-law troubles	29
25.	Outstanding personal achievement	28
26.	Wife beginning or ceasing work outside the home	26
27.	Beginning or ceasing formal schooling	26
28.	Major change in living conditions (eg, building new home, remodeling, deterioration of home or neighborhood)	25
29.	Revision of personal habits (dress, manners, associations, etc)	24
30.	Trouble with boss	23
31.	Major change in working hours or conditions	20
32.	Change in residence	20
33.	Changing to new school	20
34.	Major change in usual type and/or amount of recreation	19
35.	Major change in church activities (eg, a lot more or a lot less than usual)	19
36.	Major change in social activities (eg, clubs, dancing, movies, visiting)	18
37.	Taking on mortgage or loan less than $10,000 (eg, purchasing a car, TV, freezer)	17
38.	Major change in sleeping habits (a lot more or a lot less sleep, or change in part of day when asleep)	16
39.	Major change in number of family get-togethers (eg, a lot more or a lot less than usual)	15
40.	Major change in eating habits (a lot more or a lot less food intake, or very different meal hours or surroundings)	15
41.	Vacation	13
42.	Christmas	12
43.	Minor violation of law (eg, traffic tickets, jaywalking, disturbing the peace)	11

Using the list of life event items, a series of studies established that a cluster of life events was significantly associated with the onset of illness. Within 2 years preceding tuberculosis, skin disease, coronary occlusion, and hernias a cluster of life events was found. One health change, pregnancy, had its onset in a setting of increased environmental change (Rahe et al 1964). Through these studies it was concluded that life events can be necessary to the occurrence of disease but that they are not sufficient alone to cause the illness.

Different types of life events were found to have varying significances for different people. Some have greater impact on a given person than others. The death of one's spouse, as an example, cannot be compared to changing one's type of recreation. Thus, the process of assigning a magnitude score to each life event item began. The method used to quantify the impact of each life event was originally used in psychophysics.* Stevens and Galanter (1957) found that man can reliably rate his experiences in relation to a perceived physical phenomenon, such as the brightness of light, number of objects, or intensity of sound. It was later assumed that man could also make similar quantitative judgments about psychosocial phenomena. For purposes of comparison one life event item, marriage, was chosen as the psychosocial phenomenon to be examined; it was given an arbitrary numerical value of 500. The next step was to ask 394 individuals to rate each life event item based on the impact it had in comparison with marriage. The respondents compared the amount, severity, and duration of change the average individual would experience for each event (Holmes and Rahe 1967).

There was considerable agreement among the respondents as to which life events required major adaptation and which were not as significant. Table 4.1 illustrates the rank order for all 43 life event items. The completed list was then designated as the Social Readjustment Rating Scale (SRRS). Each life event score was divided by 10; thus marriage was assigned a value of 50 rather than 500. The life event item requiring the greatest amount of social adjustment was death of a spouse. Other items with significant impact included divorce, marital separation, jail term, death of a close family member, and personal injury or illness. Minor violation of the law was listed as evoking the least degree of adjustment; this was assigned a value of 11. Other low-adjustment items were changing one's eating habits, taking a vacation, and observing Christmas.

The ranking of the 43 life event items remained primarily the same when rated by persons of varying ages, sexes, races, and income levels. Replication of the scaling method using college students was conducted (Ruch and Holmes 1971). The college students and the original 394 respondents assigned essentially the same rank order to the events.

**Psychophysics is the study of the psychologic perception of the quality and quantity, the intensity and magnitude, of physical phenomena.*

The same outcome was also found in Pasley's work (1969) with students in the seventh, ninth, and eleventh grades. Literate individuals from other countries also gave similar ratings of most life events. High correlations were found between the American population and the populations of Spain, Japan, Denmark, French-speaking Western Europe, Sweden, and Malaysia.

Comparison of the Japanese and American samples revealed interesting findings. Death of a spouse was rated at the top of the list in both cultures. A jail term was considered by the Japanese to be in 2nd place on the list of items requiring the most adaptation; Americans, on the other hand, rated it 6th. Differences in ranking minor violation of the law were also noted. The Japanese rated the event in 28th place, whereas Americans placed it last at 43rd (Masuda and Holmes 1967). To account for these differences Holmes and Masuda (1972, p 72) concluded that "the cultures have different views of ethical conduct. Americans emphasize internal Christian moral values, placing guilt above humiliation as a guide to ethical conduct. The Japanese rank humiliation and the opinions of others as chief guides." Differences in family structure were also evident between the two cultures. Americans, as a primarily isolated grouping of parents with children, rated the addition of a new family member as the 13th item. Japanese families, on the other hand, often are part of a larger extended family circle. They rated the same life event item as 23rd, considering it to require much less adaptation than American families.

The scaling method of the SRRS has an interesting property. The magnitudes of life event items are directly proportional to the change associated with each. The following example was cited (Holmes and Holmes 1975, p 49): "Death of one's spouse (100 LCU) requires, in the long run, twice as much readjustment as getting married (50), four times as much as a change in living conditions (25), and nearly ten times as much as minor violations of the law (11)."

SCHEDULE OF RECENT EXPERIENCE

Using the life event items and their proportional magnitudes (Appendix B), the Schedule of Recent Experience (SRE) was developed. It is a self-administered questionnaire that assesses the occurrence of life events during specific periods of time. There are two sections of the questionnaire that must be completed by each participant. The first part includes questions about each individual's personal history, involving such factors as age, sex, marital status, birth order, and population of birthplace. The second section assesses the life event items experienced. The occurrence of these events in the following four time periods is determined: (1) 0–6 months ago, (2) 6–12 months ago, (3) 1–2 years ago, and (4) 2–3 years ago. The first 13 questions ask each participant to indicate whether or not a given event was experienced in each of the four time periods. Questions 13 through 42, on the other hand, require that one indicate how many times an event occurred in the four time periods.

After the individual carefully reads the instructions and answers both sections of the questionnaire the scores can be tabulated using the SRE mean value sheet (Table 4.2). Each value point assigned to a life event item is called a life change unit (LCU). Divorce, as an example, is given a score of 73 LCU. To determine the total magnitude of change experienced in a given time period the LCU scores for all reported life event items must be added. If items 13 through 42 on the SRE are reported more than once in the same time period their scores are doubled, tripled, or quadrupled accordingly. An individual might report the following items in a 1-year period:

One marriage	50 LCU
Five changes in residence	100 LCU
One vacation	13 LCU
One change in sleeping habits	16 LCU
One change in financial state	38 LCU
Two changes in working hours	40 LCU

The total LCU score experienced during this 1-year time period is 257.

It has been found that the higher the LCU score the more likely it is that a change in health will occur. In a study by Rahe and Holmes (unpublished) the SRE was administered to 200 resident physicians at the University of Washington. The participants were also asked to list the major health changes they experienced during the previous 10 years. The relationship between life change and health change was then analyzed. The 88 physicians who answered the SRE reported a total of 98 diseases. The major categories of health changes were: (1) infectious, (2) musculoskeletal, (3) allergic, and (4) psychosomatic. The LCU scores for each year were then totaled for each participant. It was determined that 89 of the health changes (93 percent) occurred 2 years after a cluster of life changes totaling 150 LCU or more. The odds of this happening by chance are less than 1 in 1000. A cluster of events totaling 150 LCU or more was then defined as a life crisis (Holmes and Masuda 1973). Three categories specify the degree of life crisis experienced. A score of 150–199 LCU in 1 year represents a mild life crisis, 200–299 LCU indicates a moderate life crisis, and 300 LCU or more indicates a major life crisis (Table 4.3).

Table 4.2. MEAN VALUE SCORES FOR QUESTIONS ON SRE

NO.	SRE QUESTION	MEAN VALUE
1.	Trouble with boss	23
2.	Change in sleeping habits	16
3.	Change in eating habits	15
4.	Revision of personal habits	24
5.	Change in recreation	19
6.	Change in social activities	18
7.	Change in church activities	19
8.	Change in number of family get-togethers	15
9.	Change in financial state	38
10.	Trouble with in-laws	29
11.	Change in number of arguments with spouse	35
12.	Sex difficulties	39
13.	Personal injury or illness	53
14.	Death of close family member	63
15.	Death of spouse	100
16.	Death of close friend	37
17.	Gain of new family member	39
18.	Change in health of family member	44
19.	Change in residence	20
20.	Jail term	63
21.	Minor violation of law	11
22.	Business readjustment	39
23.	Marriage	50
24.	Divorce	73
25.	Marital separation	65
26.	Outstanding personal achievement	28
27.	Son or daughter leaving home	29
28.	Retirement	45
29.	Change in work hours or conditions	20
30.	Change in responsibilities at work	29
31.	Fired at work	47
32.	Change in living conditions	25
33.	Wife begins or stops work	26
34.	Mortgage over $10,000	31
35.	Mortgage or loan less than $10,000	17
36.	Foreclosure of mortgage or loan	30
37.	Vacation	13
38.	Change of school	20
39.	Change to different line of work	36
40.	Begin or end school	26
41.	Marital reconciliation	45
42.	Pregnancy	40

Table 4.3. LIFE CRISIS CATEGORIES AND LCU SCORES*

CATEGORY OF LIFE CRISIS	LCU SCORE
No life crisis	0–149
Mild life crisis	150–199
Moderate life crisis	200–299
Major life crisis	300 or more

**The LCU score includes those life event items experienced during a 1-year period.*

Research has also revealed that the risk of illness increases as more life change is experienced. Holmes (1970) predicted the odds of becoming sick based on the amount of life change experienced. Of his study participants reporting under 150 LCU 33 percent experienced an associated health change during the next 2 years. The odds increased to 53 percent for those individuals with scores of 150–299 LCU. Of those participants with scores over 300 LCU 80 percent reported significant health changes. Based on this study it appears that an individual who experiences a major life crisis has an 8 out of 10 chance of becoming sick in the next 2 years. Those individuals with mild to moderate life crises, on the other hand, have a 5 out of 10 chance of experiencing a related health change.

Since the development of the SRRS and SRE many other studies have been conducted that support the life change–illness onset concept. Rahe (1968) found similar results when he studied 2500 officers and enlisted men in the U.S. Navy. In a study by Tollefson (1972) a correlation was found between bone fractures and increased life change. Even pregnancy was found to occur in a setting of increased environmental change. Women who had prenatal medical problems experienced major life crises during pregnancy and during the year prior to conception; many delivered prematurely (Williams et al 1975). Using a modified version of the SRRS Bramwell et al (1975) studied the life event scores of 82 college varsity football players. Those individuals suffering major time loss due to injuries had significantly higher life change scores than noninjured players. Holmes and Holmes (1970) conducted a study on minor health changes and life events. The health changes studied were colds, cuts, bruises, stomachaches, headaches, and backaches; none required medical care or sick leave from work. It was found that the minor health changes occurred on days of greater-than-average life changes. Another project determined that the greater the life change the greater the vulnerability to disease and the more serious the illness that can develop (Wyler et al 1971).

The relationship of life events to the onset of depression has been the focus of several studies. Paykel et al (1969) compared depressed patients with a cross section of the general population. The depressives were found to experience nearly three times as many life change items as the general population. They reported significantly more arguments with spouses, marital separations, deaths or serious illnesses in the family, beginnings of new types of work, and personal physical illnesses. Many of these events involve losses and socially undesirable experiences. Another study found that depressives experience more life change items than newly hospitalized schizophrenics (Jacobs et al 1974).

Within the past 10 years the concepts of life change and illness onset have received much attention in the popular press. Toffler's *Future Shock*

(1970) addressed the implications of the accelerating change in our society; the interrelationship of life change, human adaptation, and illness onset was discussed extensively in his Chapter 15. Several widely read magazines have brought these concepts to the layman. Examples include Wolfe's article (1972) in *Family Circle*, an excerpt in *Time* entitled "The Hazards of Change" (1971), and Lamott's article (1975) in *Today's Health*. Even hospitals and health insurance companies are disseminating the concepts to their clientele.

It is to be hoped that people will use this new information to evaluate the advantages of change and the inherent risks of change. Although some life changes cannot be avoided, others are a matter of choice. People might learn to regulate to some extent the circumstances to which they must adapt. It must be remembered that man has only so much energy. If most of one's energy is used to cope with a hectic environment he has less to spare for preventing disease. Illness can be the unhappy result (Holmes and Masuda 1972).

In summary, the life change concept has an important relationship to the onset and severity of disease. The research documenting these correlations has had significant influence on professionals and laymen alike. For psychosocial nurses the SRE itself can be a valuable assessment tool in clinical practice.

CLINICAL ASSESSMENT OF PSYCHOLOGIC AND PHYSIOLOGIC ADAPTATION TO LIFE CHANGE

Assessment of the linked psychologic and physiologic responses to anxiety-producing situations is essential in clinical practice. In an interview a client will often discuss life changes or conflict-producing situations that he has experienced. It is important to be aware of the physiologic adaptation accompanying these circumstances. One example is the response of the endocrine system. When an individual adapts to environmental change or conflict-producing situations stimuli travel to the hypothalamus via neural pathways and cause the secretion of corticotropin-releasing factor. This substance then reaches the anterior pituitary gland and triggers the release of adrenocorticotropic hormone, or ACTH (Paschkis et al 1967, Selye 1960, p 67). ACTH stimulates the adrenal cortex to produce corticosteroids; these chemicals then prepare the body to adapt to life change or conflict (Masuda et al 1972, Masuda 1966, Nelson et al 1966).

Although the body's physiologic responses can function for long periods of time, they cannot persist indefinitely. The adaptive mechanisms can themselves produce untoward effects on body tissues when functioning to excess. In other words, they can predispose the body to the production of morbid physical changes or illness itself (Selye 1960, Wolff 1960).

Why is it necessary to apply the linked psychologic and physiologic adaptive responses in a client interview? For one thing, it is not uncommon for clients to discuss symptoms or specific diseases they are experiencing. Many illnesses are directly affected by psychosocial factors; examples include ulcerative colitis, cardiac disease, and asthma (Grace et al 1950, Fisher et al 1964, de Araujo et al 1973). As the client's psychosocial-emotional status deteriorates the disease process often worsens; the inverse can also occur. The counseling relationship can be a contributing factor in improving the course of a client's illness.

CLINICAL EXAMPLE

A 52-year-old man sought mental health counseling to help him deal with an impending divorce and the many consequent life changes. He was tense. During the interview he chain-smoked cigarettes, talked rapidly, and frequently got up to have a drink of water. He described himself as being generally an "uptight" individual. At the conclusion of the interview he mentioned that he had a doctor's appointment in the afternoon. The interviewer, who had an understanding of life change and physiologic adaptive responses, questioned him about his health. The client reported having a problem with hypertension that had become worse during periods of marital discord. In conjunction with the physician's treatment approach of weight reduction and limited salt intake the counselor taught the client various relaxation exercises as one type of therapeutic intervention. The client eventually experienced a decrease in his blood pressure.

USE OF SRE AS AN INTERVIEWING TOOL

The SRE itself can be used by the psychosocial nurse as an interviewing guide in the counseling relationship. As an example, the client can be asked about the occurrence of the life change items. This often provides an avenue for the client to ventilate his thoughts and feelings about the changes in his life. Another approach is to ask the client to rank the life change items he has experienced according to how difficult they have been for him. The client might then focus on a specific life change item or on the circumstances causing a series of emotion-producing life changes. An elderly man might discuss retirement and all its associated life changes. Another client might focus on his sexual difficulties and later identify some of the contributing problems in his marriage.

The SRE has also been found to be a helpful interviewing guide when counseling pregnant women. Women often experience major life crises during pregnancy (Williams et al 1975). Many changes are associated with the physical fact of being pregnant; others are not. Women who are unable to cope with these life changes may be referred for mental health counseling. During interviews the therapist can use the SRE to identify the degree and type of life changes experienced. Life changes associated with pregnancy might encompass eating habits, sleeping patterns, recreation, and personal habits. Pregnant women, often on medical recommendation, must adhere to a stricter dietary regime than when in the nonpregnant state. Others feel tired and subsequently curtail their involvement in recreation and social activities. Anticipatory guidance or educational preparation by the nurse that addresses the causes of these and other changes may prove useful, particularly for the primigravida. The nurse can also detect maladaptive coping mechanisms in the assessment process. Further intervention can be initiated to assist each woman individually in resolving the reactions induced by multiple life changes.

SRE: CLIENT ASSESSMENT, TREATMENT, AND PLANNING

The specific interrelationship of health change, LCU magnitude, and life change items can be determined for clients by using the SRE. One's current life situation, as an example, can be assessed by calculating life change scores for the preceding 6 months to 3 years. After the client indicates which items on the SRE were experienced, the mean values of the life change items experienced during specific time periods can be added for the total LCU score. To illustrate, a 35-year-old woman in group therapy, Ms. M, discussed the feelings she experienced when separating from her husband (65) a year previously and when later attempting to reconcile their marriage (45). She and her husband had even tried to settle their differences with the assistance of a marriage counselor. As time passed, however, the number of their arguments increased (35); both thought that divorce (73) was the only realistic resolution for them. With the divorce came financial problems (38) for Ms. M and a move to an apartment (20). It also became necessary for Ms. M to go back to work (38) as an LPN. Another difficult adjustment was her declining social life; the couples she associated with during her marriage rarely asked her to join them in social events (18). Changes in life style accompanying a recent divorce are not unusual. In a year Ms. M accumulated a life change score of 332 LCU; the score is indicative of a major life crisis.

The LCU score is not an absolute indicator that everyone who scores high will become ill. Much change in a short period of time, however, increases the likelihood of developing an illness. Ms. M, with an LCU score of 332, is in the high-risk group; the odds are 8 out of 10 in favor of her becoming sick in the following 2 years. Although the numerous changes Ms. M had experienced in her past could not be reversed, her therapists in the group helped her deal with her current circumstances and future plans. Many of the life events on the SRE are changes one can either choose or reject; getting a new job, moving to another house, or applying for admission to a new college is often purely a matter of choice.

Since change is so much a part of our society it cannot always be avoided, but people can learn to regulate to some extent the circumstances to which they must adapt (Table 4.4). As Ms. M became more involved in group therapy she shared her desire to return to school to become a physical therapist. To accomplish this goal several changes would be necessary immediately: (1) move to an apartment closer to the school, (2) work on the night shift to permit daytime classes, (3) reduce expenses to accommodate lowered financial status brought on by costs of tuition, books, and other school items, and (4) change sleeping habits. The disadvantages of these added life changes were weighed against the long-term benefits, and the possible risks of health change were considered. With this information Ms. M returned to the group a week later and announced that she had decided to postpone returning to school for awhile. She commented, "I think I'll try to save some money first and then go back. It really isn't that big of a deal to wait. Besides, knowing me, I'm likely to go skiing and break my leg!"

Another important aspect of intervention with Ms. M was strengthening her coping techniques following the divorce. In dealing with past crises and conflict-producing situations Ms. M was typically nonassertive. She had relied on her husband to deal with annoying circumstances for her. In their relationship she had had difficulty defending herself, and she often felt victimized. Ms. M's nonassertive attitude was causing much difficulty as she attempted to cope with her changed life style. In relation to illness onset, Holmes and Masuda (1972, p 106) have emphasized that "the

Table 4.4. HELPING CLIENTS TO COPE WITH LIFE CHANGE

The following suggestions using the SRE can help clients maintain their health and prevent illness:

1. Orient clients to the life event items and the amount of change they require.
2. Have clients place the SRE where they can see it easily several times a day.
3. Help clients to recognize when a life change occurs.
4. Encourage clients to think about the meaning of the change and identify some of the feelings experienced.
5. Discuss with clients the different ways they might best adjust to the event.
6. Encourage them to take time in arriving at decisions.
7. If possible, encourage clients to anticipate life changes and plan for them well in advance.
8. Encourage clients to pace themselves. It can be done, even if they are in a hurry.
9. Encourage clients to look at the accomplishment of a task as a part of daily living and to avoid looking at such an achievement as a stopping point or a time for letting down.
10. Remember that the more changes clients experience the more likely they are to get sick. Of those people with over 300 LCU for the previous year almost 80% get sick in the near future; of those with 150 to 299 LCU about 50% get sick in the near future; of those with less than 150 LCU only about 30% get sick in the near future. Thus the higher the LCU score the harder one should work to stay well.

activity of coping can lower resistance to disease, particularly when one's coping techniques are faulty, when they lack relevance to the type of problems to be solved." One intervention approach was to work with Ms. M's nonassertive behavior in the group and teach her some assertive skills. She later attended a workshop on assertiveness training for women.

High LCU scores have also been correlated with an increased probability of accidental injury (Bramwell et al 1975). Individuals experiencing many life changes may focus their attention on these events to the exclusion of what may seem to be less significant aspects of their environment. Many a person has had the experience of driving along in his car thinking about an important problem, then suddenly realizing he has just run a red light. As an individual becomes increasingly preoccupied he may pay less attention to environmental clues indicating danger. The following account is a good example of this phenomenon.

CLINICAL EXAMPLE

A 23-year-old man, Mr. B, was involved in a severe motorcycle accident; eventually he had his right leg amputated below the knee. Several days after the amputation he secluded himself in his room; he wept and refused to eat. A mental health professional received a consultation request from the surgeon to evaluate the patient's depression. In the initial assessment, Mr. B related many life changes before and after his accident. The emotions he was experiencing during this crisis also made him wonder if he was "going crazy" (see Chapter 10). In the second session the SRE was used as an interviewing guide. The report of life events summed to 472 LCU during the 6 months prior to his accident. Examples include the following: (1) death of his brother, (2) quit school, (3) found a new job near home, (4) change in financial state, (5) fired from work, and (6) met a young woman he wanted to date. Mr. B described the occurrence of the accident in the following statement: "You know, I was just riding along the highway. It was a Sunday—good weather, nice day, the whole bit. This guy in a car was on a side road—you know, perpendicular to the highway. I don't know why I didn't see him. Guess my mind was on other things. Anyhow, he pulled right out, and I ran into him."

Following the accident Mr. B experienced another significant cluster of life changes (392 LCU). Many of the life events were related to his long-term hospitalization (eg, changes in his personal habits, sleeping patterns, residence, recreation). However, another group of life events was not related to the accident. Mr. B and his girlfriend had previously decided to get married. Although his hospitalization interfered with their plans for a home wedding, they were married (50) in the hospital cafeteria. Soon afterward he found out that his wife was pregnant (44). Despite their worsening financial status (38) his wife quit work (26) because of constant nausea.

Using the SRE gave Mr. B an opportunity to discuss items on the scale that concerned him. One area he dealt with extensively was what his sexual relationship with his wife would be like without his leg. He expressed much worry about how his wife would respond. Because of their lack of income she was living with his parents in another state and had not seen him since the amputation. The intervention approach was to make arrangements for his wife to live in an inexpensive apartment near the hospital. Mr. B later confided that this aspect of their relationship had worked out well.

Other life change items that Mr. B dealt with concerned his plans for the future. Prior to his accident he had been employed as a laborer in a sawmill. He questioned whether he could return to this type of employment. After consultation with a vocational rehabilitation specialist he applied for college and received financial assistance through the G.I. Bill.

Another intervention approach was to discuss with Mr. B the relationship between life change and emotional reaction. As he began to understand and discuss the magnitude of the life changes he had experienced in the past year his comfort and satisfaction significantly increased. Ten months after his hospital discharge Mr. B, his wife, and their baby visited with the hospital staff. They seemed reasonably satisfied and comfortable. Incidentally, their lives have also been significantly stable, with little life change.

SUMMARY

Research has shown that people can get sick when experiencing significant changes in their lives. Many of these changes are events of everyday life; others are uncontrollable and highly undesirable. Prolonged physiologic adaptation to change, however, can produce untoward effects on body tissue and eventual illness.

To determine the magnitude of life changes experienced in specific time periods the SRE was developed. This scale is an invaluable clinical assessment tool for psychosocial nurses. The interrelationship among health changes, LCU magnitudes, and specific life change items can be determined for clients. The SRE itself also is helpful in the treatment process and in planning for the future. Using the scale, clients can learn "to regulate to some degree the situations in which they have to adapt, they can achieve considerable responsibility and skill in weighing the advantages of change against its risks" (Holmes and Holmes 1975, p 51). The SRE can also be a valuable interviewing guide for psychosocial nurses. It can provide an avenue for ventilating thoughts and feelings about specific life changes and the circumstances causing them.

References

Bramwell S T, Masuda M, Wagner N N, Holmes T H: Psychosocial factors in athletic injuries: Development and application of the social and athletic readjustment rating scale (SARRS). J Human Stress 1:6, 1975

De Araujo G, Van Arsdel P P, Holmes T H, Dudley D L: Life change, coping ability and chronic intrinsic asthma. J Psychosom Res 17:359, 1973

Fischer H K, Dlin B M, Winters W L, et al: Emotional factors in coronary occlusion. II. Time patterns and factors related to onset. Psychosomatics 5:280, 1964

Grace W J, Wolf S, Wolff H G: Life situations, emotions and chronic ulcerative colitis. JAMA 142:1044, 1950

Graham D T: The pathogenesis of hives: Experimental study of life situations, emotions, and cutaneous vascular reactions. In Wolff H G, Wolf S G, Hare C C (eds): Life Stress and Bodily Disease. Baltimore, Williams & Wilkins, 1950, pp 987–1009

The Hazards of Change. Time 97:54, 1971

Hinkle L E et al: An investigation of the relation between life experience, personality characteristics and general susceptibility to illness. Psychosom Med 20:278, 1958

Holmes T H, Goodell H, Wolf S, Wolff H G: The Nose: An Experimental Study of Reactions Within the Nose in Human Subjects During Varying Life Experiences. Springfield, Ill, Thomas, 1950

Holmes T H, Masuda M: Life change and illness susceptibility. In Scott J P, Senay E C (eds): Symposium on Separation and Depression. Washington D C, American Association for the Advancement of Science, 1973, pp 161–86

Holmes T H, Masuda M: Psychosomatic syndrome. Psychology Today 6:72, 1972

Holmes T H, Rahe R H: The social readjustment rating scale. J Psychosom Res 11:213, 1967

Holmes T S: Adaptive behavior and health change. Medical thesis. Seattle, University of Washington, 1970

Holmes T S, Holmes T H: Risk of illness. Continuing Education May 1975, pp 48–51

Holmes T S, Holmes T H: Short-term intrusions into the life style routine. J Psychosom Res 14:121, 1970

Jacobs S C, Prusoff B A, Paykel E S: Recent life events in schizophrenia and depression. Psychol Med 4:444, 1974

Lamott K: What to do when stress signs say you're killing yourself. Today's Health 53:30, 1975

Lief A (ed): The Commonsense Psychiatry of Dr. Adolf Meyer. New York, McGraw-Hill, 1948, p 420

Masuda M: Differing adaptive metabolic behaviors. J Psychosom Res 10:239, 1966

Masuda M, Holmes T H: The social readjustment rating scale: A cross-cultural study of Japanese and Americans. J Psychosom Res 11:227, 1967

Masuda M, Perko K P, Johnston R G: Physiological activity and illness history. J Psychosom Res 16:129, 1972

Nelson G N, Masuda M, Holmes T H: Correlation of behavior and catecholamine metabolite excretion. Psychosom Med 28:216, 1966

Paschkis K E, Rakoff A E, Cantarow A, Rupp J J: Clinical Endocrinology, 3rd ed. New York, Harper & Row, 1967

Pasley S: The social readjustment rating scale: A study of the significance of life events in age groups ranging from college freshman to seventh grade. Tutorial in psychology, Chatman College, Pittsburgh, Pa, 1969

Paykel E S, Myers J K, Dienelt M N, et al: Life events and depression. Arch Gen Psychiatry 21:753, 1969

Rahe R H: Life-change measurement as a predictor of illness. Proc R Soc Med 61:1124, 1968

Rahe R H, Meyer M, Smith M, et al: Social stress and illness onset. J Psychosom Res 8:35, 1964

Ruch L O, Holmes T H: Scaling of life change: Comparison of direct and indirect methods. J Psychosom Res 15:221, 1971

Selye H: The concept of stress in experimental physiology. In Tanner J M (ed): Stress and Psychiatric Disorder. Oxford, Blackwell, 1960

Stevens S S, Galanter E H: Ratio scales and category scales for a dozen perceptual continua. J Exp Psychol 54:377, 1957

Toffler A: Future Shock. New York, Bantam, 1970

Tollefson D J: The relationship between the occurrence of fractures and life crisis events. Master of Nursing thesis. Seattle, University of Washington, 1972

Williams C C, Williams R A, Griswold M J, Holmes T H: Pregnancy and life change. J Psychosom Res 19:123, 1975

Wolfe S W: Avoid sickness—how life changes affect your health. Family Circle May 1972, p 30

Wolff H G: Stressors as a cause of disease in man. In Tanner J M (ed): Stress and Psychiatric Disorder. Oxford, Blackwell, 1960

Wyler A R, Masuda M, Holmes T H: Magnitude of life events and seriousness of illness. Psychosom Med 33:115, 1971

CHAPTER

5

ANXIETY: A MENTAL HEALTH VITAL SIGN

Helen Hope Graves
Elaine Adams Thompson

PEANUTS
IS IT CHRISTMAS YET?

CHRISTMAS?! GOOD GRIEF, NO! THIS IS STILL FEBRUARY...

I LIVE IN CONSTANT FEAR THAT CHRISTMAS WILL COME, AND I WON'T KNOW ABOUT IT...

WE ALL HAVE OUR ANXIETIES

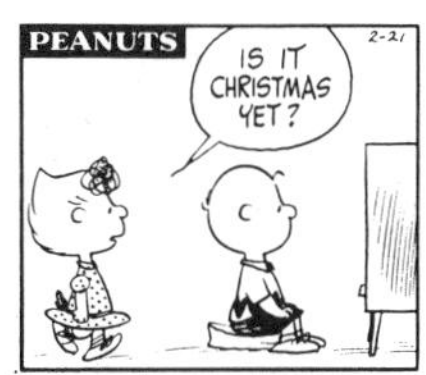

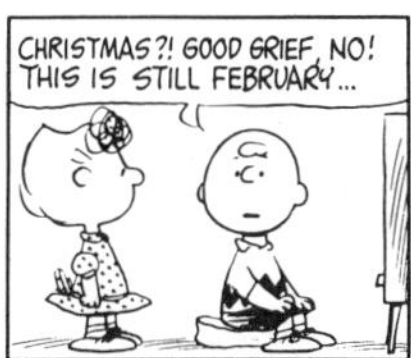

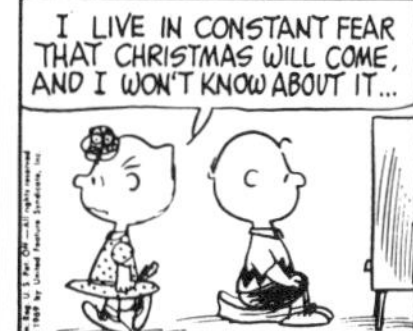

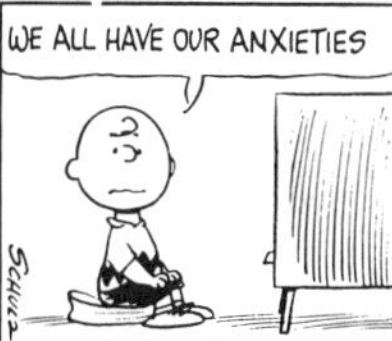

Anxiety has approximately the same relationship to emotional well-being as the common cold has to physical well-being: each is a nearly universal experience; each may be mildly or severely incapacitating; neither is lethal to the organism (although each has the potential for serious consequences if ignored); lay remedies and professional remedies for each are legion. Although some degree of anxiety is present in most individuals a good part of the time (so-called normal anxiety), this emotion can increase to the state of complete, immobilizing panic. The degree of anxiety is an indicator of the degree of distress that an individual is experiencing; estimation of that degree requires that the professional nurse be able to work with the patient to identify the experience known as anxiety and be able to help the patient cope with the difficulty.

This chapter will be an exploration of the concept of anxiety, including its etiology, effects, and ramifications and the appropriate interventions. This presentation will also consider anxiety in the counselor as a variable in the interactive process.

DEFINITION OF ANXIETY

May (1950, p 191) has defined anxiety as "an apprehension cued off by a threat to some value which the individual holds essential to his existence as a personality." Thus anxiety usually occurs when a person is confronted with or anticipates a situation that he perceives as threatening to his physical, social, economic, or emotional security. The perception or anticipation need not be consciously perceived; it may for a time lie outside of the individual's awareness. This helps to explain the phenomenon wherein a client becomes vaguely aware that there is "something wrong" because he experiences physical symptoms seemingly inappropriate to the situation and assumes that he is about to experience a catastrophic, life-threatening event.

CLINICAL EXAMPLE

Mrs. A, a 41-year-old suburban housewife, spent an exhausting day canning peaches. The canning paraphernalia has been cleaned up, dinner for herself and her husband prepared and eaten, and she and her husband are now finishing the meal with coffee and a cigarette. Mr. A takes his paper to the living room, while his wife continues to sit at the table enjoying her coffee and respite from her strenuous day. As Mrs. A sits there she begins to be aware of a vague inner restlessness and a sense of foreboding. She feels her heart rate pick up; the beat becomes stronger. She feels a bit nauseated, her tension increases, perspiration pops out on her upper lip, and her heart beats harder and faster. At this point Mrs. A concludes she is about to die of a heart attack brought on by overwork.

A hurried trip to the hospital emergency room follows with Mr. A now visibly upset, thus further alarming his wife. Curiously, the closer they get to the hospital the less Mrs. A is frightened. By the time the emergency physician checks her over and gives his impression that she has not experienced a heart attack but rather has experienced a sharp attack of anxiety, Mrs. A is about half ready to believe him, but half not ready. She cannot understand the reasons for feeling anxious, if indeed that was the situation; but it seems to her quite reasonable that a day of unusually hard work might lead to heart failure.

In this example we have a rather typical situation that prepares the way for further somatization of anxiety involving peaks of tension and anticipated catastrophe.

Not all first experiences of anxiety are as dramatic. For instance: A young mother on her first trip to the grocery with her new baby sensed an irrational and consuming idea that someone was about to take away her infant; in panic she fled from the store. Later, feeling somewhat embarrassed by her panicky behavior, she puzzled over its possible cause. No real, objective external threat existed; yet she felt threatened.

Normal and Abnormal Anxiety

Even less dramatic than the previous example are the everyday life experiences accompanied by tension and apprehension. Taking a test, going to a job interview, meeting new people, giving a first dinner party, trying out for a part in a play, approaching a new class of students—all of these tend to add to the baseline emotional titer each of us carries. The literature commonly identifies normal anxiety as that degree of arousal appropriate to the situation as validated by others conversant with the situation. A test for a driver's license will usually occasion increased alertness, mild tension, and perhaps increased heart rate, sweating, and internal trembling. The applicant may score better on the test in this keyed-up state than if he were totally relaxed.

Morbid anxiety, on the other hand, moves the person away from his usual, optimal level of performance toward noncoping behavior that is maladaptive and nonfunctional. Although there may be an objective threat present, it tends to be misperceived by the anxious individual. In the example of the driving test the individual could become so severely anxious as to compromise his ability to perform the required behaviors. The reaction would then be inappropriate to the situation, and it is this element of exaggerated response that defines abnormal anxiety.

Pure anxiety is rarely seen, except perhaps in some episodes of psychotic behavior. Rather, anxiety is usually observed as part of a pattern of emotions or as an underlying specific behavioral response, as noted in the previous examples. Behavioral responses are frequently relied on to disguise, defend against, or ward off feelings of anxiety. In psychoanalytic theory the classic defense mechanisms are seen to have as their function the protection of the individual from the pain of anxiety in its pure state. For example, the student who fears he has done poorly in an examination may attack the instructor's presentation. Anger, denial, somatic complaints, and withdrawal are additional behavioral responses utilized to temper anxiety or avoid awareness of anxiety, and although they may effect this result, the cost in psychic energy can be higher than the benefit derived.

Energy used to maintain avoidance patterns can better be utilized by the individual to identify and deal with the underlying anxiety. A phobic individual, for example, spends a great deal of energy avoiding the phobic object or activity and may involve everyone around him in the activity, thereby creating further difficulty for himself. Although he remains free from the experience of anxiety as long as the phobic behavior persists, the cost can be enormous. Energy directed into phobic behavior cannot be used more productively to help the individual cope successfully.

Thus anxiety is painful, emotionally crippling in its more severe manifestations, and maladaptive in terms of benefit to the individual versus the cost in psychic energy for protection from the conscious experience of its discomforts. Inherent in the previous statement is the implication that there are indicators the nurse can utilize as she works with the distressed client to help him identify what he is feeling and to explore with him what might be undertaken to produce behavior that is more adaptive.

Fear and Anxiety Differentiated

Physiologic responses to objective threat and to psychologic threat may be difficult for both patient and nurse to differentiate. Schematically, fear and anxiety can be analyzed as shown in Table 5.1.

Table 5.1. ANALYSIS OF FEAR AND ANXIETY

FEAR	ANXIETY
1. Developmentally occurs later than anxiety.	1. Experienced before language is acquired and hence cannot be named.
2. Usually a specific stimulus can be identified.	2. Its effect is a strong sense of impending disaster or doom without identifiable stimulus.
3. Direct action to relieve the pain and discomfort is theoretically possible.	3. Absence of identifiable stimulus makes it difficult or impossible to take direct action for relief.
4. The subjective feeling is that of being in danger from threat to life or limb. The danger is external to the person.	4. Without recourse to an action for relief the anxious individual feels helpless, isolated, and insecure.

Fear and Anxiety Mixed

Fear and anxiety are likely to occur together, and they may potentiate one another. An important task for the nurse consists in assessing with the patient what he is experiencing and then helping him to sort out one emotion from another.

Although the physiologic responses to anxiety appear to differ little from those to fear, there may be substantial differences in the state of the organism itself when the anxiety episode occurs. Spielberger (1972) has hypothesized two forms: state anxiety and trait anxiety. The former is the state in which a person exists at the time of an anxiety episode relative to sympathetic arousal. Trait anxiety, on the other hand, refers to the situation of habitual anxiousness (degree of arousal) as reflected in the common observation of clinicians that "he carries a high level of anxiety," plus the fact that this individual seems prone to episodes of acute anxiety. State anxiety has been further analyzed into what other investigators have called psychic anxiety and somatic anxiety. Psychic anxiety in this schema includes "muscular tension and worry," while somatic anxiety, as one might surmise, includes "somatic complaints, distractability, and a 'feeling' component, disquietude and mental distress" (Schalling and associates 1975, p 614).

A further interesting speculation in some of the recent studies of anxiety involves the notion that original arousal (from grade +1 to +4, Table 5.3) may not adequately explain the phenomena under investigation and that there are mechanisms operating in addition to the sympathetic system. Cortical monitoring of sympathetic function is well documented (Miller 1969), and this may play a role in the different affective perceptions of fear and anxiety. Schalling and associates (1975) suggested that the reticular activating system may help to organize responses and "maintain vigilance," while the limbic system may have a function in "providing control of responses through incentive-related stimuli'' (p 604). Each of these ideas represents an approach that may be pursued in developing interventions to ameliorate morbid anxiety.

GENESIS OF ANXIETY

Interpersonal Approach

From the perspective of interpersonal theory the genesis of anxiety can be understood as a response to the absence of tenderness in the caring adult that the infant has learned to expect and that has the force of physiologic need. The infant's needs for oxygen, fluids, food, warmth, and rest are met by the caring adult, not only directly in a physical way but also with what Sullivan (1953) has called tenderness—the affective response of the mothering adult. In this process the baby develops tensions that express a need for tenderness and that are relieved by the mother's behavior. Thus there are physiologic needs that must be satisfied for the infant's emotional security. If those security needs are unmet the infant manifests symptoms of classic anxiety.

Further, if the mothering adult is herself anxious when ministering to the child her anxiousness is communicated to the child, and he in turn becomes anxious. ''The tension of anxiety, when present in the mothering one, induces anxiety in the infant. . . . How the anxiety in the mother induces anxiety in the infant is thoroughly obscure'' (Sullivan 1953, p 41).

If one accepts this explanation for the beginnings of anxiety the affective components of severe apprehension and the feelings of helplessness and isolation are more easily understood.

Behaviorist Approach

Learning theory conceptualizes the experience of anxiety somewhat differently. For the behaviorist the capacity for an anxiety response is innate (Fisher 1970) and accompanies situations in which an individual experiences punishment. Early behavior is motivated by internal stimuli that disrupt the body's physiologic equilibrium. Hunger, thirst, and lack of body warmth are conditions in which disequilibrium is present, and the infant instinctively seeks to satisfy these needs. The reinforced response (food, milk, being bundled) is coupled with social behaviors from the caring person that in themselves can be either rewarding or punishing. Some of these social behaviors become reinforcers: a smile from the mother, a warm soft voice, and smooth gentle handling. Others become punishers: withdrawal of attention, spanking, social disapproval. The latter are associated with signs of physiologic arousal (increased pulse, glandular reflexes, increased blood pressure, respiration, and muscle tension), which are referred to by the behaviorists as respondent behaviors (Burgess and Bushell 1969).

A stimulus (behavior of a child) followed by a punishment response acquires aversive properties and in turn acts to suppress the original behavior in the child.

CLINICAL EXAMPLE

Michael, a 16-year-old boy, decided to use the family car without conferring with his parents. He ran a few errands, and in the process he met some friends who talked him into joining them at the local hamburger joint. When he returned home his father was irate. His driving privileges were revoked for 3 days, which included the subsequent Friday evening on which he had planned an important date. Michael was visibly upset; he felt angry and at the same time helpless.

Stimulus behavior (taking car without permission)

↓

Response (punishment and anxiety; driving privileges revoked)

The stimulus behavior becomes a conditioned aversive stimulus that in the future serves to suppress the original behavior (taking the car without permission) (Reese 1966). Aversive stimuli evoke anxiety, and this anxiety in itself becomes a stimulus for escape and avoidance behaviors. A child readily learns to recognize cues in a situation that in the past has led to punishment from the parent. Situational cues create anxiety in the child, who in turn develops patterns for avoiding the punishment. Thus the power of the threat of punishment is learned.

Normally the anxiety generated by aversive stimuli has limited effects and is of short duration. However, stimulus generalization (behavior that is strengthened in one situation is likely to occur in another) is a behavioristic explanation of prolonged and/or recurrent anxiety responses (Burgess and Bushell 1969). Patterns of behavior developed to avoid anxiety-provoking situations can in extreme cases lead to phobic behavior. Table 5.2 provides a schema of the conceptual approaches in interpersonal and learning theories.

PHYSIOLOGIC AROUSAL

The result of the bodily effects of sympathetic nervous system activation may be fear or anxiety. Each is characterized by predominantly sympathetic discharge, which produces measurable behavioral responses such as rapid pulse, increased blood pressure, pupil dilation, and increased perspiration. For any species physiologic arousal is an adaptive response, as it prepares the animal to either flee or fight a threatening

Table 5.2. SCHEMA OF CONCEPTUAL APPROACHES

INTERPERSONAL THEORY	LEARNING THEORY
Anxiety is communicated interpersonally.	Capacity for anxiety is innate.
Infants have two basic needs: 1. Need for satisfaction of physiologic requirements for survival 2. Need for security (lack of security produces anxiety).	Infant recognizes cues of anxiety in the parenting figure associated with stressful situations.
In seeking need satisfaction the infant meets with social disapproval and lack of tenderness.	Internal stimuli disrupt physiologic equilibrium of the infant's body. Disequilibrium motivates behaviors by which the infant seeks to satisfy basic needs (hunger, thirst).
As the child's cognitive abilities develop, anxiety is experienced insofar as it is anticipated that a significant other will disapprove the way in which satisfaction is achieved. Ability to feel anxiety depends on the child's ability to perceive and anticipate another's feelings. A child will not feel anxious if he is not capable of anticipating disapproval.	Need-satisfying behaviors are both rewarded and punished. Punishment is coupled with the emotional response of anxiety. Behavior followed by punishment 1. Acquires aversive properties 2. In future situations acts to suppress the behavior.
In response to anxious feelings in social interactions a child develops avoidance patterns. He learns to 1. Alter the meaning of social interaction 2. Deny the existence of disapproval or deny the existence of anxiety 3. Selectively inattend.	Anxiety itself becomes a stimulus for escape and avoidance behaviors.
Anxiety is perceived as a sense of failure as a human being (Sullivan 1953).	

stimulus. However, for the human being in a social context the response is often inappropriate and disorganizing. Preliminary evidence from the field of neuroendocrinology indicates that man has the capacity to override emotional and physiologic responses via cortical functions.

The autonomic nervous system, which is comprised of the sympathetic and parasympathetic nervous systems, is activated by the hypothalamus, brainstem, and spinal cord. Sympathetic discharge is a mass response in which many portions of the body are stimulated simultaneously. The adrenal medulla, which is under the control of the sympathetic nervous system and which on stimulation secretes two hormones (epinephrine and norepinephrine), also contributes to the physiologic effects observed in the fight–flight response (dilation of arterioles of the heart and skeletal muscle, increased heart rate, etc) (Guyton 1976, Cannon 1939). In contrast, the parasympathetic nervous system is relatively selective; it acts on specific organs and elicits such responses as digestion, salivation, and muscular relaxation.

The hypothalamus, which is located in the central portion of the brain, mediates adrenal cortical and autonomic responses in the body. Although the interrelationship of the hypothalamus and other organs of the brain is only partially understood, it is known that the hypothalamus has connections with the limbic system (Pribram 1967, Oken 1967). The cerebral cortex, including the limbic cortex, is known to activate the hypothalamus (Pribram 1967). Extrapolating primarily from animal research, scientists have suggested that the limbic system is related to emotional behaviors and that there appears to be a feedback system between the cortex and the hypothalamus.

ASSESSING DEGREE OF ANXIETY

The degree of anxiety evoked by a stressful situation can partially be inferred from direct observation of an individual's behavior. Such observations reflect ongoing mental, emotional, and physiologic processes that can be used as guides in assessing an individual's ability to deal with anxiety. In Table 5.3 anxiety has been categorized as to its relative effects on human behavior, that is, in relation to the degree of increasing arousal, with anxiety as the concomitant affective state. The manifestations of anxiety are organized under (1) physiologic, (2) cognitive, and (3) behavioral and emotional responses.

The phases of anxiety (designated as + to ++++) tend to be sequential, and the characteristics of one phase may overlap with those of adjacent phases. Although the nurse may observe increases ranging from mild anxiety to panic in an individual, it should be noted that anxiety need not always progress in that order. That is, a patient may very well reach a state of panic without ever having exhibited the progression implied in this schema (Table 5.3).

Another important point about the observation of the anxious patient is that there may be nonuniformity in types of responses. A patient may verbally express a moderate degree of anxiety and at the same time show signs of severe anxiety in his physiologic responses: pacing, perspiring, flushing, breathing rapidly. In any situation the degree of anxiety should be determined as the highest degree observed in the patient's response (Lesse 1970).

Table 5.3. RESPONSE CATEGORIZATION TO ANXIETY LEVELS

LEVEL OF ANXIETY	PHYSIOLOGIC	COGNITIVE	BEHAVIORAL AND EMOTIONAL
Minimal	Relaxation response: ↓ Pulse ↓ Respirations ↓ O_2 consumption Pupillary constriction ↓ Muscle tension ↓ Blood pressure	States of altered awareness: Daydreaming Yoga Relaxation Biofeedback Transcendental meditation Some stages of sleep Emotional and cognitive activity minimal Focus typically on single mental image	Disregard for environmental stimuli; no attempt to deal with external stimuli No verbal interaction Muscles relaxed; passive movement easy
Mild (+)	Muscle tension at minimum; passive control of interaction between psychologic processes and muscular activity	Perceptual field broad Ability to take in multiple stimuli Passive awareness of environment	Feelings of safety and comfort Behavior primarily automatic: carrying out well-known habits and skills, noncompetitive games and pastimes Solitary activities Facial muscles appear relaxed Voice calm

(continued)

Table 5.3. RESPONSE CATEGORIZATION TO ANXIETY LEVELS (Continued)

LEVEL OF ANXIETY	PHYSIOLOGIC	COGNITIVE	BEHAVIORAL AND EMOTIONAL
Moderate (++)	Increased tension that is tolerable, even pleasurable	Perceptual field narrowed	Feelings of challenge and the need to handle the situation at hand
	Maximum conscious interaction between mind, body, and emotions	Ability to solve problems at all levels, optimal level for learning	Competitive games; carrying out less familiar skills and habits, learning new skills
	Attention focus: sees, hears, and grasps fewer stimuli than +1 anxiety	Can attend to specifics if directed to do so	Voice denotes concern and interest with environment
	↑ alertness		
Severe (+++)	Survival response (fight or flight)	Perceptual field greatly reduced	Feelings of increasing threat; need to respond to situation is heightened
	Sympathetic nervous system activation: ↑ Epinephrine ↑ BP, P, R Skin vasoconstriction ↑ Body temperature	Time sense distorted	Personal space is extended.
	Diaphoresis	Selective inattention operates: stimuli threatening to self-system and biologic integrity or expectations may be filtered out	Physical activity may increase with decreasing organization and purposefulness (pacing, wringing of hands, running away, freezing on the spot, trembling, stammering, fidgeting)
	Dry mouth		
	Urinary urgency		May feel nauseated

	Loss of appetite: ↓ Blood to digestive system ↑ Glucose production by liver Sensory changes: ↓ Hearing perception Pain perception lessened Pupils dilate; vision fixed Muscles tense, rigid (may be fixed)	Dissociating tendency: events and/or feelings are denied existence in awareness Selective enhancement operates: focus on one particular or many scattered details Problem-solving difficult	May experience "cold sweat" Anxiety easily increased with new stimuli such as noise or people approaching patient Verbalization typically rapid and/or characterized by blocking Flight behavior may be manifested psychologically with withdrawal, denial, depression, somatization
Panic (++++)	Continued physiologic arousal Eventual release of sympathetic discharge: Blood returns to major organs (individual may appear pale) May be hypotensive Ability to respond to pain, noise, external stimuli at minimum Motor coordination poor ↓ Blood flow to skeletal muscles	Perceptual field closed, may be distorted Thoughts are random; logical thinking impaired Details may be "blown up" or the speed of scattering increased Unable to solve problems; new stimuli tend to overload mental functioning	Feelings of anger, helplessness emerge; may be experienced as rage, dread, awe, terror Individual may strike out physically or verbally or may withdraw Behavior may be primitive: crying, biting, flailing, curling up Physical activity increasingly disorganized Voice pitch higher, louder; flow of words rapid; sometimes may experience blocking of speech Facial expression of terror, grimacing

This table is a compilation of the authors' ideas as well as those drawn from Benson (1974), Carson (1969), Lesse (1970), Nelson (1971), Peplau (1963), and Sullivan (1953) and from Concept of Anxiety (1968).

PROBLEM-SOLVING PROCESS

The paradigm that follows is frequently cited in delineating the problem-solving process. It can serve as a guide in dealing with clients experiencing various degrees of anxiety.

I	II	III
BEHAVIOR	**COGNITION**	**PROCESS**
Actions	Concrete	Assess
Thoughts	↓	• Describe
Feelings	Abstract	• Define
		• Analyze
		Plan
		Implement
		Evaluate

This diagram represents the direction in which communication with the anxious person is most readily achieved. That is, it is generally easier for a person to talk about his actions in a situation than it is for him to elaborate on his feelings (column I). As language develops in the toddler his first words are action-oriented. The child is somewhat older before he is capable of verbalizing his thoughts about any given situation, and it is even later before the child learns to associate and express the emotions that he experiences. Thus with anyone experiencing moderate to severe anxiety, the cognitive and perceptual demands are less when one is asked to describe one's behavior than when one is asked to describe one's emotions.

Similarly, in cognitive development (column II) a child learns first to identify concrete entities in the world. As is described in Piaget's theory, the ability to think in abstract terms emerges in the second decade of life and is maximal by the end of that decade (Phillips 1969). Under stress we tend to fall back on earlier patterns of functioning, including cognitive and verbal skills.

INTERVENTIONS

When clients are experiencing moderate to severe anxiety, communication can be facilitated and anxiety lessened if the nurse focuses first on a description of client behaviors, then on related thoughts, and finally on feelings. This systematic process also minimizes any anxiety that might be experienced by the counselor in dealing with an anxious individual.

Column III delineates the steps in the problem-solving process. The hierarchical order of the words from "assess" to "evaluate" implies that the steps are successive and that moving prematurely from one step in the process to the next can lead to inaccurate, inefficient, or inappropriate problem-solving. It is essential that the nurse develop skills with which she can evaluate the client's readiness to progress in the problem-solving process.

In talking with a moderately anxious person in an attempt to elicit descriptions of stressful events that precipitated his anxiety, the nurse should ask such questions as these: Where were you? Who was there? What did he say? What did you tell him? As the nurse elicits more and more description of the behaviors that occurred, she moves toward eliciting information about the client's thoughts both at the time of an incident and at the time of questioning. Communication at this early phase should still be on the descriptive level (eg, What did you think when he said that?).

As the client relates descriptively the nurse must employ observational skills, for as the client talks he will deliver cues that reflect his anxieties, fears, and hopes about the event and its consequences. As the client describes a stressful situation, the nurse may well observe bodily cues (flushing, blanching, tenseness, rapidity of speech) that suggest that the client's anxiety is increasing. Even as the client relates a stressful situation his anxiety may mount to the point where it becomes incapacitating. Recognition of increasing anxiety alerts the nurse to analyze the interaction in progress. Has she moved prematurely toward asking the client to define a situation that for him is still vague? Is the dialogue approaching a particularly emotion-laden topic? Has the nurse asked the client to analyze before his conscious awareness of the situation has been clearly mapped? Has the dialogue moved too rapidly to include thoughts and feelings? At such a time the nurse can utilize any number of alternative approaches:

1. She can slow down and obtain more descriptive, behavioral information.
2. She can utilize her observation of heightened anxiety as the cue to attempt to draw out content of a particularly stressful nature.
3. She can use the opportunity at hand (the client's increased anxiety) to bring related sensations and behaviors into the client's awareness in order to teach him to perceive early signs of heightened anxiety.
4. She can offer a temporary escape either verbally (by offering to talk about it later) or physically (by suggesting a change of scene); this option is particularly useful if the client's anxiety mounts rapidly.
5. She can simply pause (interject silence) in her pursuit of descriptive content to allow the client to regain equilibrium; she may set a new pace for the interaction.

Whatever the nurse decides she must stay within the problem-solving process. Often her zeal to help a client discover his inner tensions becomes anxiety-producing in itself. Frequently the nurse may jump enthusiastically to the analytic phase and ask "why" questions that annoy, frustrate, or confuse the client. To her dismay she may be confronted with silence, an angry retort, or a bewildered "I don't know" accompanied by cues to increasing anxiety.

CLINICAL EXAMPLE

A young mother brought her 3-year-old to the emergency room for lacerations of the hands, forearms, and face. She was obviously distraught, and when the resident physician asked her why this had happened she proceeded to exhibit signs of severe anxiety. She became too confused to speak. Later, in recounting the situation, she stated, "He really got me, I was so anxious . . . then when he asked me why it had happened it was as though I couldn't think. . . . If he had only asked me what had happened I could have told him."

Although this example is not an illustration of delving into deep-seated conflicts it does illustrate that the "why" approach can heighten one's anxiety in a stressful situation. Also implied is the attack element that is inherent in "why" questions. A factor in the mother's increased tension was her perception of the physician's question.

Nursing Action in 4+ Anxiety

Flight. Sometimes an individual's anxiety is so severe (3+, 4+) and his feeling of helplessness so great that flight seems the only way to survive ("I've got to get out of here"). Actual flight, as opposed to freezing or withdrawing psychologically, poses a problem for the counseling person. Is it best for the patient to permit him to flee the situation? His cognitive functions are sluggish, impaired and so blurred by anxiety that decisions are unlikely to be rational. Nevertheless, the client is physiologically mobilized for action, and some helpful intervention is required. The possibilities include the following:

1. Provide means for expenditure of physical energy: walking, running around the grounds or around a gymnasium, pounding a punching bag, yelling loudly (warn others about what's happening).
2. Keep communication simple and direct. Complex, analytic cognitive function is impossible at this time.
3. Allow ample personal space for the client. There is a direct correlation between the amount of personal space needed and the level of anxiety. It is usually not a time for closeness and touching. However, occasionally a highly panicky person may be helped to control his extreme restlessness by being held gently but firmly by a nurse quietly expressing reassurance.
4. In some situations anxiety mounts so rapidly and circumstances are so unfavorable that interpersonal interventions are not effective. Medication of the client for the acute episode may help to reduce the anxiety to a level at which he can deal with it and its concomitant manifestations rationally.

5. When the client is under control the nurse should work with him to describe the situation: what he was doing, who was there, what was said, what happened, etc.

Fight. Physiologic arousal prepares the body to either fight or flee in a stressful situation. When an individual demonstrates anger, hostility, or agressive behavior in a relatively neutral situation, the nurse should be aware that anxiety expressed as anger is a common response. Anger is less painful than are feelings of powerlessness and helplessness. Anger actually generates feelings of powerfulness, which is one step closer to self-preservation. If the client appears angry or ready to fight the nurse can consider the following approaches:

1. Assess the probable level of anxiety:
   a. What is the client doing physically? (Yelling, throwing furniture, pounding his fists on the wall.)
   b. To what extent is the neuromuscular system activated? Does the client need an outlet for his physical energy? (Taking a walk, slamming a door, yelling at a neutral person.)
   c. What are the client's cognitive abilities? Can he focus on his actions? Does this increase his anxiety level?
2. In attempting to reduce the client's level of anxiety the nurse might:
   a. Create a diversion for the client. If asking the client to focus on his behavior increases his anxiety, it may be necessary to offer him an alternate focus of awareness until the anxiety decreases to a level at which he can learn (eg ++ anxiety).
   b. Offer an external source of energy release.
   c. Decrease situational stimuli by speaking in short, direct phrases, avoiding detailed explanations of what she is doing.

Then, in helping the client to learn to deal with anxiety it is imperative to return to focus on the anger:

3. The nurse should work at describing the situation to help the client understand his anger:
   a. What was he doing? Who was there? What did he say? What had just happened? Where was he? What did he think? What feelings was he experiencing?
   b. Define the situation. What was its meaning to him?

DEALING WITH ANXIETY IN ONESELF

Nurses and other counseling people can also be anxious. It has been well documented by many studies and much experience that anxiety is communicable. It has been said that the only disease more easily spread among exposed persons is measles. Following are some steps the nurse can take to deal with her tension in order not to complicate the situation for the client and in order to allow optimum helpful interaction in a situation that requires professional expertise:

1. She should learn to recognize when anxiety is present and accept the fact that everyone is anxious at some time.
2. She should bring to bear maximum cognitive effort in enlarging perception of the situation. It is best to look beyond what is obvious for additional information about one's behavior.
3. She should consciously and purposefully change her behavior and observe for a diminution in anxiety. Forcing oneself to breath slowly and deeply, to speak deliberately, and to move quietly will often promote an astonishing change toward lowered anxiety. Also, when it is appropriate to do so, a few minutes alone to get one's head together may be helpful.
4. If her anxiety persists despite efforts to get it under control she should seek help. Feelings of helplessness, insecurity, and isolation should not be passively endured; they are inimical to optimum nursing function. Colleagues are good resources for assisting with anxiety-provoking episodes.

SUMMARY

In order to work effectively with an anxious client the nurse should take the following steps:

1. Assess the situation
   a. Obtain a detailed description of events and behaviors.
   b. Analyze her observations and what the client is telling her: What hurt? Why? (Decreased self-esteem, fear of failure, lack of coping skills.)
2. Plan interventions
   a. What can the client do for himself, by himself? Determine with the client what new or modified behaviors would be more effective in dealing with his anxiety.
   b. Determine to what extent and in what ways the nurse should be involved in testing these new behaviors. Who else might be involved?
3. Implement intervention
   Note that the process is primarily in the client's hands at this point. The nurse must try out new behaviors and evaluate them. She must recognize that in this process it is often necessary to solicit help from significant others.
4. Evaluate results
   a. Review the implementation phase with the client, beginning with the description of the behaviors the client was trying out. What did he think and feel in regard to his actions?
   b. One cannot evaluate new perspectives without new and old patterns of responses being clearly delineated.

CLINICAL EXAMPLE

Mrs. J was a 45-year-old woman who had been scheduled for an elective abortion, but she was informed only an hour before the scheduled surgery that it would have to be postponed a week until the physicians could perform more laboratory tests concerning her thyroid condition.

ASSESS She broke into tears, saying that she didn't know whether she could stand to wait another week to go through the surgery. She began pacing up and down the hallway wringing her hands. She appeared flushed; her pace continued to increase. The staff nurse suggested that they both take a walk downstairs and get a cup of coffee. Mrs. J's motor activity level was reduced by the long walk, and she was able to sit down and drink her coffee.

Describe She still exhibited signs of + + and + + + anxiety, in that she spoke very rapidly, smoked several cigarettes in a row, fidgeted constantly in her chair, frequently darted glances about the room, had difficulty in completing her sentences, and repeatedly said, "Oh, what will I do, what will I do?" Mrs. J was able to acknowledge that she was severely anxious, but she was unable to associate the anxiety with anything other than the fact that her surgery had been postponed.

Define Further discussion elicited the information that Mrs. J was ambivalent about having the surgery and had great difficulty in deciding to enter the hospital. She feared that she would have to reexperience the **Analyze** discomfort of the anxieties she initially had in deciding to have the surgery. She was concerned that the intervening week would be anxiety-laden. Ironically, the anticipation of anxiety is anxiety-provoking in itself.

Describe During her description of her behaviors related to the recognition of the pregnancy and the events leading to her decision to have the abortion, Mrs. J was able to verbalize feelings of guilt about her decision. **Analyze** Although guilt feelings prevalied, Mrs. J contended that both she and her husband knew that the decision was the correct one for them. She began sobbing again, wondering how she would survive the week intact.

PLAN The nurse and patient explored the ways in which Mrs. J usually deals with her anxieties. She finds relief and comfort in having someone to talk with, usually her husband's sister who lives nearby. When she is severely anxious she finds relief in engaging in physical acti- **IMPLEMENT** vities. She decided, with the assistance of the nurse, to repaint her living room, which she had been intending to do for some time, and to enlist the support of her sister-in-law during the ensuing week.

Mrs. J returned to the hospital the following week for the abortion. **EVALUATE** She was neatly dressed, smiling, and relatively relaxed as she entered the ward. She related that she had managed to paint not only her living room but also the guest bedroom. Her week had gone much smoother than she had anticipated, and she was feeling confident about her decision to have the abortion. She had had a few anxious periods, but both her husband and her sister-in-law had been supportive and had been good listeners. She thought that she was in much better condition for the surgery than she had been the week before.

Finally, talking with someone who listens empathetically tends to lessen painful anxiety. Accepting anxiety, a client's, a colleague's, or your own (the right to have feelings without making value judgments about them), makes it possible to analyze the anxiety through a process of communication. The psychic energy of anxiety can be channeled and directed into adaptive behaviors.

Everyone experiences anxiety. It is anxiety disproportionate to the situation that gives rise to interpersonal and intrapsychic problems. Definition of the disproportion requires effective communication between the counseling person and the anxious client so that the problem resolution can follow.

References

Benson H, Beary J, Carol M P: The relaxation response. Psychiatry 37:37–46, 1974
Burgess R L, Bushell D Jr: Behavioral Sociology. New York, Columbia Univ Press, 1969
Cannon W B: The Wisdom of the Body. New York, WW Norton, 1939
Carson C: Interaction Concepts of Personality. Chicago, Aldine, 1969
Concept of Anxiety (film). Video Nursing 1968
Fisher W: Theories of Anxiety. New York, Harper & Row, 1970
Guyton A C: Textbook of Medical Physiology, 5th ed. Philadelphia, WB Saunders, 1976
Lesse S: Anxiety: Its Components, Development, and Treatment. New York, Grune & Stratton, 1970
Longo D, Williams R A: Psychosocial Assessment and Intervention in Clinical Practice. Seattle, Univ Washington, 1974, pp 58ff, 64ff
May R: The Meaning of Anxiety. New York, Ronald Press, 1950, p 191
Miller N E: Learning of visceral and glandular responses. Science 163:434, 1969
Nelson P: The effects of stress on human behavior (unpublished paper). Seattle, Harborview Medical Center, University of Washington, 1971
Oken D: The psychophysiology and psychoendocrinology of stress and emotion. In Appley M H, Trumbull R (eds): Psychological Stress. New York, Appleton-Century-Crofts, 1967
Peplau H: A working definition of anxiety. In Burd S F, Marshall M A (eds): Some Clinical Approaches to Psychiatric Nursing. London, Macmillan, 1963
——— Interpersonal Relations in Nursing. New York, Putnam, 1950
Phillips J L Jr: The Origins of Intellect: Piaget's Theory. San Francisco, Freeman, 1969
Pribram K: Emotions: Steps toward a neuropsychological theory. In Glass D C (ed): Neurophysiology and Emotions. New York, Russell Sage, 1967
Reese E P: The Analysis of Human Operant Behavior. Dubuque, Iowa, Brown, 1966
Schalling D, Cronholm B, Asberg M: Components of state and trait anxiety as related to personality and arousal. In Levi L (ed): Emotions—Their Parameters and Measurement. New York, Raven, 1975, p 603ff
Spielberger C D: Anxiety as an emotional state. In Spielberger C D (ed): Anxiety and Behavior. New York, Academic, 1972
Sullivan H S: The interpersonal theory of psychiatry. In Perry H S, Gawel M L (eds): The Interpersonal Theory of Psychiatry. New York, WW Norton, 1953

CHAPTER

6

HUMAN SEXUALITY

Marie Annette Brown

Human sexuality is an integral and powerful factor in the individuality of each person, and it has had considerable impact on our society. The noted sex researchers Masters and Johnson (1975) stated that "sex is a natural function," emphasizing that sexual functioning, like respiration, is an essential part of human nature from birth to death (p. 28). While study of the biologic aspects of sex is extremely important, it provides only a foundation from which to explore the more complex aspects of human sexuality. The rich human meanings of sexuality are developed and influenced by personal life experiences, especially interactions with others in what society deems to be socially scripted behavior (University of Minnesota Medical School report 1975).

A tremendous amount of information has been gathered in the past two decades to expand existing knowledge about sexuality. People are becoming more sophisticated and are demanding information about the more personal and formerly taboo aspects of sexual response, often from health care professionals. This turning to health care professionals for assistance in sexual matters has caused concern about the quality of their responses, since in the past our social attitudes limited these professionals to more traditional (and less controversial) areas of sexual concerns, such as reproduction, family planning, and child development. However, with sexual awareness growing and attitudes changing health care professionals must be prepared to treat sexuality as a distinct entity that is worthy of their professional attention.

In primary and secondary health settings the nurse is often the most accessible member of the health team. Consequently the nurse is the professional most frequently asked to formulate a comprehensive plan of care and biopsychosocial assessment for sexual concerns. Providing an adequate response to this need is particularly important in psychosocial nursing. The nurse in the psychosocial area is dealing with individuals in one-to-one or group settings where nursing intervention is focused on persons exploring themselves and their relationships with other people. Being confronted with sexuality and sexual behavior is inevitable in such an environment, and in order to respond to these issues the nurse must have accurate information about the human sexual system as well as sensitivity derived from a good understanding of her own feelings as a sexual being.

In this chapter we will outline the elements of the sexual system (physiologic, partner interaction, autoerotic) and consider some of the sociocultural and psychosocial influences and their interrelationships. In the section devoted to assessment and intervention we will utilize this basic information to formulate ways in which nurses can respond to sexual concerns. Given the complexities of human sexuality, this chapter can only provide an introduction; a basic course in human sexuality supplemented by self-awareness/values-clarifying seminars is necessary for a fuller understanding. Nurses with adequate information and self-awareness will be better able to contribute to the sexual health of the people with whom they have contact.

NURSING CARE AND THE SEXUAL SYSTEM

Everything that is sexual about a person, including sexuality, sex, and sexual functioning, will be designated the sexual system. Like other biologic systems its basis is anatomic structure with physiologic responses, both of which are affected by psychosocial and environmental factors. The sexual system is a recently legitimized term; previously its elements were subsumed under the reproductive system because reproduction was considered to be the desired result of sex. These systems clearly overlap. Having control over one's reproductive functioning and being comfortable with it can contribute to a sense of sexual well-being. Reproductive health must be viewed as only one component of sexual health, although other components of sexual health have not yet been agreed on. General health was at one time narrowly defined as the absence of disease. Today our conception of health is expanding in a positive sense to include emotional and social well-being. Similarly, sexual health might be narrowly defined as the absence of sexual problems. Any expansion of this basic definition must be influenced by predetermined individual value judgments. For example, the various points of view regarding sex education, comfort with nudity and one's own body, minimal guilt, and freedom to experiment all stem from the various opinions of what constitutes optimal sexual well-being. Consequently the stated and implied aspects of sexual health in this chapter are representative of the writer's own value system. Thus it is each nurse's responsibility to examine her value system and determine her personal definition of optimal sexual health. Also, nurses must be prepared to facilitate intelligent self-awareness in their patients, and be accepting and supportive despite any differences that may exist between their own values and those of their patients.

In order to communicate clearly with her patients the nurse must understand the subtle differences in meaning among the basic terms commonly used to define the sexual system:

Sexuality: a dimension of personality; physiologic and psychologic processes inherent in the sexual development and sexual response of the individual, male or female.

Sex: Physical activity or behavior such as intercourse, oral or manual stimulation of the genitals, or masturbation (self-stimulation).

Sexual functioning: A natural bodily function (like that of the bowels or bladder) that begins at birth and can be consciously controlled for a lifetime (unlike those of some other organ systems). Despite conscious control of sexual behavior some aspects of sexual functioning remain involuntary. For instance during sleep every male has an erection, and every woman produces vaginal lubrication every 80–90 minutes, in or out of a dream sequence (Masters and Johnson 1974).

Physiologic Aspects

Intricate physiologic processes take place during human sexual response. Masters and Johnson (1966) have categorized sexual response in four distinct phases: (1) excitement; (2) plateau; (3) climax or orgasm; (4) resolution. The two main variables in these stages are gender (male/female) and aging (past the approximate age of 50 years). Table 6.1 provides a summary of the basic physiologic changes in human beings that occur during sexual activity. This process of physiologic change in the four-phase cycle provides an expanded psychophysiologic perspective from which to consider sexual functioning. The following discussion is by no means complete. Its purpose is to emphasize that the nurse needs specific and relatively simple information about sexual functioning, which at present is rarely found in formal nursing education. However, the development of sexual self-awareness and basic communication skills will prepare the nurse to become at least minimally involved in promoting sexual health when responding to common questions and concerns.

Sexual functioning can be inhibited by unrealistic expectations (both of oneself and of others), inadequate information, or inaccurate assumptions about sex. The following three sections address some common misconceptions about sexual functioning by focusing on concerns that people commonly express regarding their bodies, sexual interaction, and self-stimulation.

Table 6.1. PHYSIOLOGY OF HUMAN SEXUAL RESPONSE*

	FEMALE RESPONSE	MALE RESPONSE	BOTH MALE AND FEMALE RESPONSE	AGING FEMALE RESPONSE	AGING MALE RESPONSE
Phase I (Excitement Phase)	Vasocongestion: clitoris increases in length and diameter; labia minora thicken, flatten, separate, and move away from vaginal opening Vaginal lubrication Vaginal barrel elongates and widens Breast size increases; nipples become erect; areolae engorge Maculopapular rash (sex flush) may appear over breasts and epigastrium Uterus begins elevation into false pelvis	Penis becomes erect through vascular engorgement Scrotal sac tenses and thickens Elevation of testes closer to body Nipples of breast may become erect	Increased blood pressure, heart rate, respirations; peak rates at orgasm (systolic plus 30–80, diastolic plus 20–40) Muscles become tense (myotonia)	Vaginal lubrication occurs more slowly and in lesser amounts Reduction of clitoral size and expansion potential of the vagina Loss of tissue elasticity, ie, disappearance of elevation and flattening reactions of labia majora	May be slower to erect because of minimal deep vascular engorgement Negligible amount of scrotal sac congestion; little if any testicular elevation
Phase II (Plateau Phase)	Clitoris retracts underneath clitoral head Bartholin's glands secrete 2–3 drops of two mucoid-like substances to lubricate vaginal outlet and perineum Labia majora more congested	Increase in size and circumference of penis Size increase and marked elevation of testes Penile emission of few drops of fluid from Cowper's glands Sex flush may appear		Uterine elevation reduced Sex flush less common Minimal color change of labia	Reduction in or absence of preejaculatory fluid Increased ejaculatory control Duration of phase may be longer, especially if there is no ejaculatory demand (ie, a physiologic urge to ejaculate available seminal fluid)

	Labia minora change color from bright red to burgundy Outer one-third of vagina more congested and therefore shrinking (referred to as orgasmic platform) Inner two-thirds of vagina increases its width (balloons) while uterus con tinues to elevate, thus creating chamber and tenting effect			
Phase III (Orgasm)	Peak of pelvic congestion and myotonia Uterine contractions Rapid contraction of orgasmic platform 4–10 times at 0.8-sec intervals	Feeling of ejaculatory inevitability, then within 2–4 sec regular expulsive contractions (2–4 times at 0.8-sec intervals) of the entire length of the penile urethra	Duration and intensity of phase reduced Reduction of number of contractions of orgasmic platform Possible spastic uterine contractions rather than usual rhythmic contractions	Ejaculatory inevitability phase shorter or unrecognizable Decrease in number of ejaculatory contractions Expulsion force of ejaculation diminished Amount of seminal fluid greatly reduced
Phase IV (Resolution Phase)	Uterus expands Rapid loss of congestion from orgasmic platform; gradual loss of congestion from clitoris and breasts Clitoris returns to usual position No refractory period; can be restimulated immediately unless clitoris is very sensitive	Loss of erection in two-stage response: first stage is rapid but incomplete (only to about 1.5 times unstimulated size); second stage of complete return to unstimulated size is slower Loss of congestion and descent of testes and scrotum	More rapid return to nonstimulated state in all respects	Extremely rapid return to nonstimulated state Loss of erection immediately after ejaculation (usually no two-stage response) Refractory period usually lengthens

*Adapted from Masters W, Johnson V: Human Sexual Response, 1966. Courtesy of Little, Brown & Co.

Human Bodies. The human body is not a machine; therefore human sexual response cannot be elicited on demand. Sex is a natural physiologic function, and it varies in much the same way as do other natural functions when they are influenced by the psychosocial aspects of daily living. Feelings of fatigue, anxiety, sadness, or irritation can affect the intensity of sexual response as well as the libido (interest in sex). Illness and injury may also affect sexual functioning, since human sexual response is physiologically dependent on an intact circulatory system to provide for vasoconstriction responses, an intact central and peripheral nervous system to provide for sensory appreciation, and muscular innervation to support vasoconstrictive changes (Woods and Mandetta 1975). Depending on the nature and extent of the injury or illness, sexual functioning may decrease or increase, or it may vary from its usual manner of expression. For instance, many physically disabled persons continue their sexual functioning by developing variations in movements and positioning and by creating new erogenous zones.

Aging obviously brings certain changes in sexual functioning (Table 6.1). However, sexual activity and desire do not automatically cease at middle age; people can and do continue to function sexually as long as they live. Like the disabled, the aging are challenged to create their own individual modifications and styles of experiencing and expressing their sexuality.

The subjective experience of sexual response varies from one individual to another, and at different times it varies within any one individual. Physical stimulation of any sensitive area produces varying amounts of response and pleasure at different times, and the level of response is influenced by the person's psychologic response, energy, thoughts, and experience at the time of the physical stimulus.

Contrary to popular belief, a person's sexual capacity, ability, and performance are not directly related to vaginal or penile size. Anatomically, the vaginal barrel is a collapsible canal of elastic tissue that expands only as needed to accommodate whatever is being inserted, whether it be tampon, finger, or penis. The highest concentrations of nerve endings in this area are in the labia (especially the inner labia), the introitus vaginae (vaginal opening), and the clitoris. Some changes in the tightness and elasticity of the vagina do occur with childbirth and aging; however, the pubococcygeal muscle surrounding the introitus vaginae can be strengthened and tightened like any other muscle through specific exercises. During sexual excitement the inner two-thirds of the vagina expands and the outer one-third and the introitus vaginae swell and press together to grasp the penis more firmly. Thus a longer penis (which would penetrate deeper) actually has little effect on the degree of physiologic stimulation during intercourse. In the male the size of the flaccid (nonstimulated) penis varies considerably, but there is much less variation when the penis is erect. The average size of an erect penis is 5 to 7 inches. In general, the smaller the penis when flaccid the greater its percentage increase with erection; conversely, the larger its flaccid state the smaller its percentage change with erection.

Just as penis size is of concern to many men, breast size is a concern for some women. There is considerable variation among women in the amount of pleasure and erotic sensation produced by breast stimulation. Whatever the response it is an individual and subjective experience that has no direct relationship with actual breast size.

Sexual Interaction. The physiologic responses that occur during the four-phase cycle (Table 6.1) usually require some kind of stimulus. Frequently this stimulus is provided by physical and/or mental interaction between two persons, whether heterosexual or homosexual. Thus sexual interaction is something that transpires between two people. To be effective sexual stimulation must occur in both people; it occurs *with* another person, not *to* another person. Doing it to a partner rather than with a partner negates any kind of sharing and tends to turn the human being into an object or an impersonal receptacle. Careful choice of a partner can facilitate effective sexual functioning, for having an interested and interesting partner is an important positive aspect of sex. Sharing with another person, however, does not mean that one is responsible for the other person's sexual functioning. Furthermore, it should not be assumed that both partners will experience the same kind and the same intensity of arousal or pleasure at exactly the same moment. For example, simultaneous orgasm occurs infrequently. Striving for it can make sex a task and can create performance anxiety. When people are not overinvolved in their own orgasms they are better able to enjoy the orgasmic responses of their partners.

The psychophysiologic experience in sex is enhanced when individuals assume responsibility for their own sexuality and honestly communicate their individual sexual desires or needs to their partners. Responsible behavior also includes a sensitivity toward one's partner and a commitment to cooperate in whatever ways necessary to facilitate the other person's sexual satisfaction. Taking individual responsibility can promote acceptance and freedom in a sexual relationship. For example, most males at some time experience periods of transitory loss of interest, impotence, premature ejaculation, or reduction of ejaculatory demand. Most females at some time experience periods of transitory loss of interest, lack of responsiveness, discomfort with intercourse, or orgasmic impairment. When these periods occur people who have adequate information and who accept responsibility for their own occasional variations can avoid the destructive consequences that blaming or finding fault with their partners can create.

Self-Stimulation. The physiologic responses produced by partner interaction can also be brought about by self-stimulation (masturbation) or various autoerotic behaviors. Self-arousal and self-satisfaction of sexual desire have in the past had considerable negative judgment passed on them. Fraught with misconceptions, this is one of the most troubling areas of sexual behavior and probably the most difficult one to discuss. In fact, the opportunity for sexual partners to have a frank discussion and a sharing of experiences and concerns about masturbation may never arise, even between partners involved in an intimate relationship for years. The secrecy surrounding this particular area of sexuality creates overtones of anxiety, embarrassment, and fear. The nurse must be aware of the patient's reluctance to initiate discussion in this area; she can facilitate sharing, if appropriate, and allay apprehension with factual information.

Much of our literature in the past was filled with warnings about the harmful effects of masturbation; such warnings have not been supported by the more recent findings of scientific investigations. We now know that masturbation does not cause acne, warts, mental illness, or inability to respond to a sexual partner. Today it is difficult for us to realize how deep-seated the fear of masturbation was in our society; cases of female children undergoing surgical removal of the clitoris to prevent any kind of self-stimulation have been documented. Unfortunately this intense fear did not dissipate but rather evolved into a diffuse anxiety and today we have feelings of embarrassment when the subject is raised. In some quarters there is still anxiety and fear that masturbation may be addictive, although people may masturbate once or 1000 times during their lifetimes, depending on their personal situations, levels of sexual interest, and comfort with touching their own bodies.

The motivation to masturbate is enormously varied, and any requirement for a "legitimate" reason is irrelevant and restrictive. One common myth is that self-stimulation is acceptable and necessary only when one does not have a sexual partner available. Actually, partners in a relationship often masturbate as a variation of sexual behavior. People masturbate as a means of sexual expression and affirmation of their own sexuality. The desire or need to masturbate may or may not relate to any stimulus from another person; in fact, people may masturbate because of conflicts in their lives that are not sexual, eg, boredom, frustration, loneliness, or anxiety. Masturbation can provide a comforting and pleasurable release from the tensions these feelings create. In fact, for those who are adept, masturbation seems to produce the most intense physiologic sexual response, although most people report the experience of partner sex to be the most subjectively satisfying (Masters and Johnson 1966).

Despite anxiety and prohibition the fact remains that masturbation is an extremely common behavior in our society. Approximately 99 percent of all males and 75 percent of all females masturbate at some time during their lives (University of Minnesota Medical School report 1975), and if masturbation were loosely defined as caressing or stimulating one's genitals we would need no statistics. Self-stimulation is a universal experience of infancy, and young children often masturbate openly until socialization in regard to sexuality begins to control their behavior. During adolescence most males experience their first orgasm through masturbation or nocturnal emission (wet dreams). Many females stimulate their own genitals for a long time before they attach a label to what they are doing. With increasing age females more often report orgasms during sleep.

Despite the obvious frequency of this behavior a lack of explicit printed material and an inability to share experiences and concerns about masturbation leave many people relatively uninformed about the countless activities that actually occur. For example, males commonly believe that female masturbation simulates intercourse; however, when females masturbate only a small percentage of them actually insert something into their vaginas. Generally, masturbation is a direct or indirect clitoral stimulation. The psychologic experience of masturbation also varies considerably. Some people create sexual fantasies during masturbation, while others appear to concentrate on the sexual sensations alone.

The considerations that have been discussed should prepare nurses to respond thoughtfully and enable them to provide some reassurance to patients who articulate concern about masturbatory behavior. For a patient to initiate a discussion of masturbation at all often reflects a high level of trust. It is hoped that the nurse will be adequately prepared to make optimal use of this opportunity to help alleviate pain or discomfort in another human being.

Sociocultural Aspects

To a significant degree culture and subculture dictate the way we are as sexual beings. Our culture has separated sexual functioning from other natural processes, assigned sexual roles, defined sexual practices, and created sexual restrictions. Because nurses cannot help but reflect their cultural background it is necessary to look at the ways in which attitudes and values influence patient–professional interaction.

Most people experience varying degrees of anxiety when confronted with values, behaviors, or points of view different from their own. Whatever the source of anxiety it may limit an open and honest discussion of sex. Certainly the inability to confront and discuss sex and sexuality works a disservice on both the professional and the patient. Anxiety about sexual discussion serves to block communication, thus preventing the nurse from expanding her own professional role; it also serves to perpetuate misinformation, especially (but not exclusively) for the patient. Because of these communication barriers patients may also be denied essential services, since they may not know what to ask for or may not be assertive enough to demand care. Furthermore, patients may in the past have been in situations where they experienced discomfort and embarrassment and had their concerns discounted by health professionals, and they may be reluctant to risk further questions. It must be noted that having a sound information base and self-awareness does not guarantee a completely comfortable, nonproblematic interaction about sexuality with a patient or peer. However, it is imperative to have this foundation from which to begin, since without it any commitment to the preventive aspects of nursing care is thwarted.

In order to appreciate and deal with sexual concerns it is important to be aware of cultural prescriptions and proscriptions about sexuality, ranging from sex roles to specific sexual practices. Because of the complexity of our culture an examination of one's sexuality in relation to the culture is a more extensive process than this section can provide. Instead, some examples of the kinds of sociologic information that nurses need to consider are presented.

Because of ongoing cultural change the sexual practices that are considered acceptable vary among subcultures and different age groups. For example, Kinsey's study in 1953 indicated that half of the women interviewed had experienced fellatio and cunnilingus (oral sex). A 1975 study reported that 91 percent of women between the ages of 20 and 39 years had experienced oral-genital sex—clearly a dramatic change. The survey also reported that strongly religious women in all age groups were usually less likely than nonreligious women to experience cunnilingus or fellatio. However, in strongly religious women over 40 years of age (the group least involved with oral sex), 8 of every 10 women had experienced cunnilingus, with similar proportions applying to fellatio. Also, it has been found that the frequency of nonmarital sexual activity has increased progressively over the past two decades (Levin 1975). Hunt's study (1973) indicated that of the single women interviewed 75 percent had experienced intercourse before the age of 25 years.

To understand the impact of this cultural change on awareness of our traditional norms is important. The changing status of women and their new roles in our society have had a dramatic effect on sexuality. The female sexual role was formerly considered to be that of a passive receptacle for semen, and the cultural assumption was that "nice" women had no sexual feelings (Masters and Johnson 1975). In many cases male sexuality has suffered because of our changing cultural expectations. As cultural permission for mutual sexual enjoyment within marriage developed the male came to be designated the one responsible for the pleasure experienced by both partners, and the fault or blame for any sexual dysfunction that developed usually was considered his. While the feminist movement has brought some significant changes, many aspects of female sexuality remain restricted, and expression of female sexuality is still unequal to that in males. Levin's 1975 survey of 100,000 women revealed the part that women themselves play in perpetuating inequality of sexual expression. A marked hesitancy to accept and allow for freedom of sexual experience was reflected in the fact that 24 percent of the women objected to their daughters engaging in premarital sex while only 12 percent objected to their sons having that freedom of expression (Levin 1975).

Sometimes labeled the sexual revolution, this sweeping alteration in cultural attitudes and mores regarding sexuality has brought with it a whole new range of life-style options for women and young people. Essentially, our society is witnessing a struggle among the advocates of basically three possible value positions on the meaning and function of human sexuality. Each of us may support concepts taken from more than one of these value positions. Although the divisions between positions constitute an oversimplification, they set up a framework for discussion and a tool for later assessment and intervention.

Position I. This traditional value position attempts to deny and repress all sexual expression except that between heterosexual married adults, and even there it attempts to impose certain restrictions. Some typical attitudes of this position are as follows:

1. Sexual instincts need controlling.
2. The purpose of sexual behavior is reproduction.
3. Explicit sexual references, whether visual or verbal, should be prohibited.
4. Sex education of children should be provided only by parents and religious institutions in order to instill "responsibility."
5. Prostitution and pornography should be unconditionally prohibited.
6. Homosexuality is repulsive and abnormal.
7. Attitudes regarding birth control may vary from avoidance of discussion to acceptance within certain limits.
8. Communicating about sex should be discouraged because it takes away the mystery and holiness of the act.
9. Two codes of ethics should be maintained: one for males and another for females.
10. Traditional sex roles for men and women should be supported with regard to dress, education, and employment.
11. Masturbation, premarital sex, and extramarital sex are to be condemned.
12. Sex is linked with sin and immorality.

Position II. Growing in popularity is the value position that basically represents accommodation to a wider range of sexual activities with a greater tolerance of deviation from traditional sexual norms. Its characteristic attitudes are as follows:

1. Sex is a reality to be considered rationally rather than spiritually or supernaturally.

2. Sexual urges and needs are normnal.
3. Some sexual activities may be seen as symptomatic, as caused by underlying problems (eg, homosexuality is an indication of emotional immaturity).
4. The research of Masters and Johnson is accepted, as is their belief that sexual problems in a relationship must be dealt with rather than ignored or denied. Sex is seen as a form of communication, and open communication about sex between partners is highly valued.
5. Masturbation is understandable and probably not destructive.
6. Sex education is accepted and may even be supported in the schools.
7. The use of birth control is sanctioned; thus there is a departure from traditional religious attitudes.
8. Prostitution, pornography, divorce, and abortion are viewed in a more relaxed manner. Nonintervention in the private sexual activities of consenting adults is valued.
9. Cohabitation or living together is accepted; further sanction is extended if it results in marriage.
10. Sex is rarely linked with sin or immorality. Situational ethics are used to evaluate morality rather than absolute standards.

Position III. This position is sometimes called the libertarian or hedonistic value position. Some typically held views are the following:

1. Sexual intercourse is a positive good in itself.
2. Sex is basic to a happy life, as is good food, exercise, rest, and other essential ingredients.
3. One's sexuality should be cultivated.
4. Sexual pleasure is desirable in its own right.
5. The goal of sex education is the development of sexual skills and techniques. Books like *The Joy of Sex* and *More Joy* are readily accepted.

Lost in the midst of this struggle among value positions are many people who have never considered the differences between sex and sexuality or who are confused about the differences. The various communications media tend to emphasize sex and all the behaviors that have to do with intercourse, reproduction, and physical gratification; but human sexuality is a much more encompassing phenomenon than they display, for it includes all the things about one's personality and one's body that distinguish the masculine and feminine expressions. Examples of the confusion that can result abound: equating the quantity of sexual intercourse with the quality of one's sexual experiences; confusing the frequency of sexual activity with one's feelings about one's sexual partners; thinking that the number of sexual partners is of more importance than the extent of enjoyment derived from sexual occasions.

In our culture both men and women are continually encouraged to value external sexual appearances above the internal quality of their feelings about themselves as men and women. This internal quality is what distinguishes the human being, and it is this dimension of the person that craves warmth and affection, comfort and support, and stimulation and release.

Despite cultural expectations and uncertainties, the universal human reality is that loneliness, pain, and rejection lead people to seek out other people as sources and receivers of tenderness, assurance, and renewal. For many people no human interaction can express these as powerfully as lovemaking. No other kind of being together makes people feel quite as reconfirmed in the joy of their maleness or femaleness or quite as desired, cherished, and approved.

It must also be remembered that there are hundreds of thousands of men and women whose sexuality is intact but who, because of health, situation, or preference, are celibate and do not participate in any form of sexual expression with another person. These individuals are usually as mature, well adjusted, and fully functional as anyone else. They have sexual feelings, they may or may not masturbate, and they are outwardly very much sexual in the sense of being a man or a woman, with all the accompanying concerns, pleasures, and feelings.

Psychosocial Aspects

As in other areas of socialization, our attitudes about sexuality begin in infancy and continue to develop throughout life. Nurses are well aware of the process of human growth and development, and they should utilize that basic information to respond more comprehensively to sexuality issues. This section deals with the especially vulnerable times when sexual concerns are more likely to be experienced or expressed.

Sexuality experienced as a child is obviously different from sexuality experienced as an adult. The adult meanings of sexuality as influenced by cultural values, role modeling, and personal experiences develop gradually during the maturation process. Children usually touch themselves and their genitals, and they often engage in same-sex or opposite-sex body exploration, sometimes even to the point of actual penetration. Parents who become aware of these behaviors are often appalled, or at least seriously concerned. They view the child's sexuality in terms of a collection of adult sexual meanings that took them a number of years to develop. But their motives, feelings, and needs are more complex than those of a child. The traditional assumption is that children are or should be almost asexual. Also, because adults in our society feel discomfort in confronting the normal interest and curiosity that children exhibit toward sex, we have only minimal research data to assist us in assessing the sexual concerns of children and intervening appropriately when necessary.

Adolescent sexuality has been the object of close scrutiny by the communications media, churches, and social agencies. The topic usually arouses intense feelings, and there are no clear-cut norms in this area. In addition to the external cultural struggle and the lack of norms for adolescent sexuality, adolescents are involved in their own internal struggles for self-identity. They expend considerable amounts of energy to separate themselves from parents and to clarify values and behaviors that are compatible with their own individuality. Their ambivalent feelings about the desire for control over their own lives are reflected in their uncertainty about sexuality.

Many parents oppose involvement with alcohol, drugs, and sex for their adolescents. With alcohol and drugs it is possible for adolescents to rebel against parents, respond to peer pressure, test personal limits and values, and still have to deal with only the personal consequences of their behavior. Sex, however, can have more complex consequences: It is a more personal and more emotional experience than those derived from alcohol or drugs. The aspect of social interaction with the sexual partner can further complicate the experience because the other person's feelings and behaviors must be taken into consideration. Also, the adolescent peer group is not experienced in providing a comfortable situation in which to deal as thoughtfully with concerns about sex as with concerns about drugs or alcohol. Because of adult ambivalence and confusion adolescents are rarely provided with growth-producing environments in which to deal with their sexuality. For example, a male adolescent may be concerned about his masturbatory activity. He may have some opportunity to manifest his heterosexual orientation to his peers, but without a chance for significant discussion or support from peers, parents, or others he may experience isolation or intrapsychic turmoil about the appropriateness of his behavior.

Adults tend to view adolescent sexuality in much the same way they view childhood sexuality (using adult cognitive processes, emotional attitudes, and value systems), even though many aspects of sex serve different purposes and meet different needs for the adolescent. Adults also tend to assign adolescent sexuality a lesser status than that of their own sexuality; they refuse to recognize the experiences, feelings, and struggles of the adolescent as serious and important. They may take the attitude that "It's just puppy love." Adolescents face not only the task of confronting and understanding their uncertainty and confusion about their developing sexual thoughts, experiences, and behaviors but also the task of choosing a method of expression that is appropriate for them. Kaufman and Krupka (1973) pointed out that "the anxiety generated by the confrontation is fairly easily coped with by some, while others struggle for years only to emerge exhausted and terrified by the very prospect of sexuality which then has to be dissociated from their experience."

The middle years constitute another potentially vulnerable time. The physiologic changes in sexual response that begin to occur between the ages of 40 and 50 years gradually increase with aging. Menopause can be difficult or even a time of psychosocial crisis for a woman; it increases her awareness of aging, even though she may be relieved about the end of menstruation and the possibility of unwanted pregnancy. We live in a culture that values beauty, youth, and vigor, and we link those attributes with sexuality, often to the exclusion of all other characteristics. People who have tenuous sexual relationships or low self-esteem may experience these sexual changes in a negative and disruptive way. For instance, the increased time spent and the amount of stimulation necessary to bring about erection or vaginal lubrication need not become a problem. If people are prepared for these changes, and if they maintain open communication and a willingness to develop new ways of being together sexually, there exists the potential for growth and increased appreciation of the relationship. Unfortunately, sex education in this country is minimal, undersupported, and ambivalent. People often make incorrect assumptions about the meaning of the physiologic changes in sexual response that occur with aging. Consequently sexual relationships that could have continued until death become minimal or terminate prematurely. The nurse has many opportunities during the delivery of adult health care to intervene and initiate more humane, prevention-oriented sexual health care.

ASSESSMENT AND INTERVENTION

Nursing assessment and intervention can take a variety of forms, depending on the depth and complexity of the sexual concern and the comfort level and preparation of the nurse. Several levels of nursing action will be presented in this section. Nurses dealing in the area of sexual health must rely on their skills learned from education in the nursing process, and they must respond to patients as they would for any other aspect of the delivery of health care.

The basic tool is nursing biopsychosocial assessment. The nurse and the patient collaborate in the assessment process and then together arrive at an acceptable intervention plan. The patient is certainly the expert on his own needs, and has the right to self-determination. At the same time, nurses have a responsibility to provide care that is comfortable for them as well as ethically and professionally consistent with their role.

This approach is certainly applicable to the nurse providing sexual health care. This point is stressed because of the orientation of our culture to sexuality. Other psychosocial issues are treated more seriously and with more respect (eg, depression and suicide); in contrast, our culture's way of dealing with discomfort about sexuality employs humor, informality, exploitation in the communications media, dirty jokes, and avoidance. It is important that nurses be aware of professional ways of dealing with discomfort in themselves and in the persons they care for; otherwise the critical foundation of the assessment process in sexuality will be negatively affected.

The initial step in the assessment process is for the nurse to identify the depth and complexity of sexual issues she feels comfortable and competent to become involved with and respond to. The following framework points out possibilities for assessment and intervention on three levels: providing information, identifying problems, and actual sexual therapy. Each level can be helpful to the patient and can be provided by the same nurse or several different nurses, depending on the sexual problem and the situation within which the nurse is working.

Providing Information (Level I)

Frequently a person's concerns about sexuality and sexual relationships derive from misinformation or lack of knowledge and technique: the world of sexuality, as that person knows it, is limited and confined. It is important to assess the person's openness to new ideas and information; the person's style of sexual expression is also important. Fear of the unknown and some anxiety with new experiences are common in human behavior. These concerns do not usually create problems that cannot be dealt with.

Often a patient is unaware of what help he needs from the nurse to express a sexual concern or issue. The assessment process is therefore initiated by spending time with the patient. The nurse listens to a description of the situation and determines what the issue is, which aspects of the patient's life the issue affects, and what meaning the issue has in the patient's life. This assessment process can take a few minutes or several hours. Even if the interaction lasts only a few minutes the experience of ventilating one's feelings and receiving support from the nurse during that process can be a very helpful intervention. For example, a young man 16 years old walked into a Planned Parenthood Center very anxious and embarrassed and asked to talk with someone. The interaction with the nurse/counselor took 20 minutes. The young man was concerned because in his first experience of attempting intercourse with his partner he had ejaculated at the moment of intromission. Subsequently he became very uncomfortable about his ability as a sexual partner and his masculinity; he was afraid he had a severe sexual problem. His embarrassment had caused him to avoid his partner, and their relationship had become strained. The intervention provided him with adequate information to understand what had occurred and with reassurance that his problem was common in first-time sexual experiences.

For this information to be properly communicated the patient and the nurse must agree on the meaning of the terms used. Technical words can sound cold and clinical, and some people might find slang words dirty and objectionable. It is best for the nurse to use the words she is most comfortable with; being sure to clarify the exact meaning of each word, even those that might be assumed to have standard definitions, such as impotence and orgasm.

During the conversation the nurse needs to ask only relevant questions. It is important that the questions be direct and asked in a form that assumes the patient has experienced everything sexually. For example, the nurse can ask "When did you begin to masturbate?" not "Have you ever masturbated?" This style of questioning enables the nurse to convey personal comfort and acceptance. It also may reduce anxiety in patients who are embarrassed or hesitant to acknowledge their participation in certain sexual behaviors for fear of judgment by the nurse.

Initially ask safer, more general questions, gradually moving toward questions involving specific areas of the problem. Once the nurse thinks that the concern has been adequately expressed and the patient has been heard out she can provide the relevant information the patient needs to understand the problem. The nurse should avoid giving advice even if it is asked for, as in the requests "What should I do?" and "What would you do?" The nurses's response to such questions should be clear and creative: "I have the feeling you don't trust your own judgment and would rather have someone decide for you." "My experience has been that decisions people make for other people turn out to be uncomfortable in the end." "One helpful thing for you right now might be to clarify for yourself what you want so that you will feel comfortable with whatever you choose." "I would feel more comfortable about this if we spent time exploring what you see as the most comfortable option for you." "Each person is unique. What I would do would not necessarily be the most comfortable thing for you or your partner." In these kinds of situations the nurse must be aware of the difference between providing information and giving advice. Information gives people more tools to work with and a greater sense of personal power. Advice can undermine important factors in self-esteem—the sense of control over one's life and the sense of power that comes from deciding what one wants to do and doing it.

Role Modeling. The relationship the nurse establishes with the patient can itself be a form of support and reassurance. If the nurse is comfortable in discussing sexuality and can accept herself as a sexual person, the communication will be enhanced by a positive role for the patient to model. Discussions of sexuality involve body language and nonverbal communication. It is important to remember that even if nothing is said, the nurse's feelings will probably be communicated to the patient.

In discussions such as these a patient often expresses anxiety about being considered normal in his sexual activities. Normal sexuality is an ambiguous concept. Sexuality is an individual experience that is individually interpreted, and the patient should understand this. Less emotionally charged phrases (eg, "That is common" "That is not unusual") are appropriate, and they can lessen the anxiety felt by a patient relating sexual activities.

The nurse must be tolerant of sexual values, behaviors, and life styles that are different from her own. Whether or not she identifies with the patient's thoughts and feelings it is necessary to give periodic reassurance that thinking and talking about sex is acceptable. If the patient initiates the topic the nurse can positively reinforce the fact that he took the risk. However, if the nurse chooses to initiate the topic it is important to convey the message that sexuality is an acceptable area of discussion at that time or in the future, whenever the patient chooses to pursue the topic.

Discussion of sexuality may involve feelings or fantasies the patient has about the nurse. Determining a comfortable way of responding to these feelings before the situation arises can reduce the nurse's anxiety. When she responds the nurse must consider her professional role, ethics, values, and personal feelings and express them honestly and directly. It is best to avoid initial responses such as "I'm married." Such responses don't adequately deal with the situation, and they may serve to block further communication. The nurse should be willing to stay with the issue until the patient feels that it is resolved. The nurse is not responsible for the patient's sexual feelings; she cannot evaluate herself, her therapeutic skills, and her professionalism negatively simply because a patient has sexual feelings or fantasies about her.

When discussing sexual concerns, as when discussing any other problem, the nurse must take the patient and his concerns seriously. She must operate from the premise that if the patient musters up the courage to report a sexual concern then that concern is genuine, even though it may vanish in a moment as a result of information or reassurance.

Identifying Sexual Problems (Level II)

The nurse engaged in clarifying sexual problems may need to consider several major areas of concern: psychophysiologic aspects, partner interaction, attitudes and values, and fantasies. Assessments and interventions can be formulated around a specific sexual issue, or they may be developed in the process of taking a sexual history. A sexual history is used primarily as an assessment tool, but it can also provide a number of opportunities for intervention. A chronologic account of the patient's sexual life allows the patient to become aware of the patterns of growth and change in his sexuality. The act of relating this natural progression of sexual experiences may help the patient to recognize the sources of his current concern and clarify the contributing factors. The channeling and structure of any standard sexual history assist the nurse in obtaining maximum information in minimum time. This specific questioning also may provide an opening for discussion of experiences and feelings that have been outside the patient's immediate awareness. There are many varieties of format for taking a sexual history. The nurse is encouraged to develop content and structure that are most comfortable for her individual style. Masters and Johnson (1970), who are responsible for popularizing the history-taking process, have developed an extensive outline that can serve as an introduction for nurses developing their own formats.

Psychophysiologic Aspects. Often the physiologic aspects of the patient's sexual concerns are readily apparent to the patient but are expressed so vaguely that they are not understood by the nurse. The patient may have a sense of discomfort or may be receiving dissatisfactory feedback from his partner, while he has only a vague idea of what the problem is. The nurse should begin her assessment by gaining specific understanding of the psychophysiologic areas of potency or responsiveness that are outlined in Table 6.2. It must be emphasized that a complete medical examination is a crucial part of a general sexual assessment and that it can influence intervention and treatment.

Female Concerns. The sexual concerns of women that will be discussed have been delineated to cover the topics formerly lumped together under the ambiguous catch-all term frigid. There is no definition of frigidity in the modern human sexuality literature. It is an antiquated pejorative misnomer that tends to promote destructive results.

One frequent concern of women is failure to experience orgasm during intercourse or other sexual activities. Generally orgasm is experienced as

Table 6.2. PSYCHOPHYSIOLOGIC AREAS OF POTENCY OR RESPONSIVENESS

FEMALE	MALE
Lack of orgasm	Erectile failure
Nonarousal or lack of responsiveness	Premature ejaculation
Physical discomfort with intercourse	Ejaculatory incompetence
Conflict about masturbation	Conflict about masturbation
Difference in interest	Difference in interest

a peak of arousal with subsequent total body relaxation. However, there is no specific universal experience of orgasm. It is subjectively experienced, and it varies from woman to woman. The intensity and feelings during orgasms also vary within each woman's experience. The woman may feel any of the following:

1. A desire to continue genital contact
2. Pelvic congestion (a sensation of being aware of her genitals when normally she is not)
3. Disappointment that arousal builds up to a plateau that levels off and never increases—she was expecting a definite peak and ending of arousal
4. A series in which her response excitement builds up and subsides, repetitively, without and definite orgasmic release
5. Contentment and happiness with the pleasure she experienced and feelings of warmth and closeness from intercourse or sexual pleasuring/stimulation.

Nonarousal or lack of responsiveness either with a partner or during self-stimulation is a second concern of women. There is usually no vaginal lubrication, such as would occur in Masters and Johnson's excitement phase as an indicator of the body's response and processing of sexual stimuli. The woman may not feel pleasure or sexual arousal when she touches herself, when her partner touches her body, breasts, or genitals, or during penetration (insertion of the penis into the vagina) and intercourse. She may express this concern directly ("I don't feel anything"), or she may describe discomfort such as anxiety, disgust, boredom, tension, or disappointment during sexual contact.

The third concern, actual discomfort with intercourse, can be a serious problem for women. The importance of the pelvic examination should be emphasized in this situation. Pain associated with intercourse may be a symptom of physical pathology (possibly due to vaginal infections or herpes infection). This concern may be expressed vaguely as discomfort following the completion of intercourse, or it may be expressed otherwise: "He's too big." "I'm too small." "When he thrusts too deep or in certain positions it hurts." A more specific type of pain is dyspareunia, in which the woman experiences pain either part of the time or all of the time that the penis is thrusting inside the vagina. Vaginismus occurs when the muscles around the vaginal opening contract involuntarily and close so tightly that penetration is extremely painful or impossible. This problem usually occurs with initial penetration, and thrusting during intercourse may cause no problem.

Another sexual concern of women centers around self-stimulation or masturbation. The woman may have conflicting attitudes about touching her own body. She may experience guilt or may denigrate self-stimulation as being a second-class experience; she may feel that she would like to incorporate masturbation as part of her sexual behavior were it not for the fact that she is nonresponsive or nonorgasmic while masturbating. In addition, a woman may be struggling with the decision to incorporate variety in her masturbatory activities. She may be inexperienced or unaware of the potential value of incorporating fantasies, or she may be troubled by those fantasies that seem abnormal or nontraditional. Also, the idea of using a vibrator may seem frightening or unnatural to her. She may express disappointment or even fear of being able to experience orgasm only when using the vibrator. Vibrators are becoming increasingly popular and are frequently used in preorgasmic women's groups, but for some women there remains an aura of fear or embarrassment about them or a feeling of distaste for their mechanical nature. Unfortunately there has been little research to provide reassurance.

Male Concerns. Despite our society's efforts to maintain an image of male virility, males also frequently experience concerns about their sexual functioning. In fact, because male sexual functioning is anatomically obvious, men often are more directly confronted with their problems than are women. Thus they can easily develop performance anxiety, which has a further negative effect on their sexual functioning. For example, if a man is unable to have sexual intercourse because of situational factors (eg, alcohol or fatigue) he may feel embarrassed and humiliated, especially if his partner withdraws or responds negatively. He may then enter his next sexual encounter with vivid recollection of having failed. His anxiety about his performance may inhibit his sexual functioning, because anxiety and fear usually preclude sexual arousal. Consequently his worst fears are realized: he does not achieve erection. His concern escalates further. This cycle then repeats itself: from failure to performance anxiety and stress that inhibits sexual function to failure again. This situation, which is common in both men and women, can be dealt with and in many cases prevented by education and communication, by adopting more realistic expectations in sexual functioning, and by removing sex from a competitive arena where perfect performance is valued and any variation is considered failure.

The three most common male concerns about sexual functioning are failure to achieve erection or impotence, premature ejaculation, and ejaculatory incompetence. Impotence is the inability to achieve or maintain an erection. Premature ejaculation is the most common male concern, and it can be described in a variety of ways. Kaplan (1974, p 290) described it as a situation where a man is "unable to exert voluntary control over his ejaculatory reflex, with the result that once he is aroused he reaches orgasm very quickly." The various clinical definitions of the term very quickly cover a wide range: 30 seconds after penetration; 1.5 to 2 mintues; 10 thrusts; any time span, but with him reaching orgasm before his partner 50 percent of the time. Ejaculatory incompetence (retarded ejaculation or inability to ejaculate) may be situational or complete: the man receives sufficient stimulation, he strongly desires orgasm, and yet the orgasmic reflex is not triggered (Kaplan 1974). If this problem is situational the man may be able to ejaculate normally during masturbation but unable to experience orgasm intravaginally or with oral or manual stimulation from his partner. Another situational example involves the man who is unable to ejaculate because of the physiologically depressive effects of alcohol or other drugs. Complete ejaculatory incompetence is unusual; it should be thoroughly investigated medically to rule out any organic basis.

Common Concerns. Some concerns about sexual response or the sexual relationship are shared by men and women. A common problem is that one partner has less interest in sex and less desire for sexual activity (of all kinds) than the other. One partner may wish more foreplay, a greater variety of sexual activities (eg, oral sex) and positions, and longer duration of intercourse than the other.

Whether the patient presents a specific complaint or vague general concerns the nurse must use her knowledge of sexual physiology and the outline of sexual response cycles (Table 6.1) to gather more information for biopsychosocial assessment. The following brief examples illustrate the kinds of questions that can be used to begin an assessment of the physiologic status of the sexual problem:

1. Specific concern ("I can't have orgasm."):
   What do you experience in your body that feels sexual to you?
   Describe the physical sensations you associate with sex.
   Do you notice nipple erections, vaginal lubrication, sex flush, etc?
   How do you feel physically and emotionally after intercourse or other sexual activity?
   Do you experience any sense of pelvic fullness or congestion? (This may indicate that she is aroused to the plateau level but skips orgasm.)
2. Generalized concern ("I don't like sex."):
   What do you experience generally that you could possibly label as sexual feelings or responses?
   What do you experience physically before, during, and after a sexual situation?
   What do you experience emotionally before, during, and after a sexual situation?
   What specific kinds of discomfort are you aware of during a sexual situation?
   At what point in the sexual interaction does this discomfort usually begin?
   When are you first aware of this discomfort?

The woman in example 2 may be overwhelmed by her sexual concern, and she may be unaware of what it is that troubles her. Consequently the nurse must be adequately prepared to ask detailed, specific questions about sexual response to facilitate the woman's clarity about the situation. It is also critical that the nurse feel comfortable in asking these kinds of specific questions; this can ease the patient's discomfort or embarrassment in responding, because most people have had little experience in communicating so directly about sex. The nurse's skill then becomes not only an assessment tool but also an intervention through role modeling; in some cases the initial concern can be resolved during the clarification process.

Nurses sometimes avoid directness and specificity in dealing with sexuality because they are afraid of invading the patient's privacy. There is little potential harm in asking specific questions, if it is done in a thoughtful, concerned manner. The patient always has the option to refuse to answer. Patients rarely get angry or feel violated if the nurse communicates verbally and nonverbally her intention to use specific questioning to assist in resolving the problem. Sharing intimate information about sexuality with a concerned person is a rare experience for many people. Once the patient gets through the initial discomfort, this can turn out to be a positive and powerful experience for both persons involved.

Partner Interactions. Sexual problems are often complex, and they usually have several contributing factors. The sexual dysfunction of one partner may be caused by problems in the interaction with the other. To assess and resolve this kind of problem a careful sexual history of each partner is necessary. The nurse can then assess these factors, which may be basic to the resolution of the initial concern.

The value of taking a history and assessing partner interaction is illustrated in this example: A woman was initially concerned with not being able to attain orgasm. After assessment through sexual histories of both partners the male was found to be experiencing premature ejaculation. The woman was unaware of the significance of his premature ejaculation because he was her first sexual partner. He was unaware of the significance of his premature ejaculation because he "had always been this way and no one else ever complained." He also felt threatened by any questions about his virility, and he found it easier to deal with what he considered to be her problem. Both partners lacked information about the physiology of sexual response. They had not developed good self-esteem about their own sexuality that would facilitate open, honest communication between them concerning sexual issues.

Frequently an overtly expressed physiologic or sexual dysfunction is a symptom of communication problems within a relationship. Kaplan (1974, p 155) pointed out that in the past psychiatry has tried to help patients directly by changing them (ie, by modifying their brain chemistry, their fears and guilt) and has largely ignored the ecologic variable (the sexual system and the relationship to which they are responding). Sexual difficulties must be considered in the context to the partners' relationship, which can be considered their environment.

Many sex therapists now think that the sexual system in which many such couples are involved is not only negative and dehumanizing but also highly destructive. As Kaplan (1974, p 155) emphasized, "for a person to function sexually in such a system where there is fear, rejection, misunderstanding, humiliation, demand, and alienation between spouses would be dysfunctional!" Given such an environment it can be considerably more healthy and more appropriate to withdraw than to continue in such vulnerability.

Probably the most critical aspect of the nurse's biopsychosocial assessment is gaining an understanding of the relationship between the people expressing the concern. For this reason many professionals think that dealing with a symptomatic patient alone is not as productive as working with the couple together.

Another observation about partner relationships illustrates our cultural ignorance and sexual misinformation. A person expressing a sexual concern may be aware of instability or tension in the other partner but may not be able to relate it to the problem. The old platitudes about marriage not being a bed of roses, etc, derive from the unfortunate reality that marital problems are normal in our society. Most relationships have periods of stress and instability that can be worked through. Many couples engage in either periodic or constant struggle for years and still remain married; what the world does not know (because people don't often share) is how these stressful times affect their sexual relationships. Therefore the assumption usually is that their sex lives are OK.

It is striking that even in the clinical area one encounters the pervasive attitude that people are supposed to be able to separate their sex lives from what is going on in the overall relationship. This separation of sex can become a faucet syndrome—turned on and off. Patients labor under the assumption that they are supposed to learn to be able to leave the living room after an unresolved, angry, or painful interaction with their partners and walk into the bedroom feeling open, giving, and loving. The sexual relationship has been defined as an exchange of vulnerabilities. For most people, however, there are times in a relationship when things are so uncomfortable that one or both persons are unwilling to risk this vulnerability.

In our culture the overt and subtle socialization processes regarding sex and the meaning of sex differ for men and women. Women, more frequently than men, associate sex with love and with communicating feelings, especially those that are affectionate, warm, and positive. They are also more likely to report that one of the most valued components of sex, and therefore a significant incentive, is the physical closeness, the holding and comforting, that occurs. Conversely, the socialization that men undergo enables them to compartmentalize sex more easily and separate it from the rest of the relationship. They can, more easily than women, appreciate and enjoy passion and experience sexual arousal apart from other feelings they have about themselves, their lives, or their partners. It is easy to oversimplify these sex role stereotypes; there are no absolute boundaries. Many couples, however, find their different ways of approaching sex can create problems of varying severity and can have an influence in producing anger, pain, and conflict in the sexual relationship.

In *The New Sex Therapy* (1974) Kaplan discussed other factors nurses should be aware of and should include in their assessment of partner interaction: partner rejection, transferences, lack of trust, power struggles, contractual disappointments, sexual sabotage, and failure of communication. The nurse's feedback of information concerning partner interaction as a possible cause of the sexual concern or dysfunction may be a new realization for the patient and may serve as an intervention in itself. The nurse will then have the opportunity for additional intervention in dispelling myths and providing information about sexual relationships and the complex and psychophysiologic nature of the sexual response cycle, as discussed previously. The nurse also should be aware that a couple's responses to this assessment and intervention may cover a wide range. Some people welcome an offer of assistance in dealing with their relationship. They often feel that a professional's recognition of their pain legitimizes their need for help, and the feedback and encouragement enable them to confront the issues in their conflict. Others may respond with anger; they manifest frustration and avoidance; they have a sense of not being heard. They may disagree with the nurse's focus on the relationship, either before dealing with the sexual issues or concurrently, and they may choose to go elsewhere to attain help "for the sexual problem."

Attitudes and Values. In assessing the patient's need for information the nurse must have an idea of his attitudes and value system and the amount of investment he has in rigidly retaining and rationalizing his ideas. If the patient seems to be closed and self-limited as a result of his value system, the problem may be more serious than a lack of information. Sorting out and dealing with values may then have first priority. Sometimes the patient can rethink his values and be willing to look at new values; sometimes the nurse must settle for providing information that will shed new light on his current value structure. The latter approach is especially appropriate for those persons whose sexual attitudes and values have been formed within the framework of a specific religious doctrine. Assessment in such cases must focus on the degree of the person's current involvement in his religion and on his desire, need, or commitment to maintain values consistent with the tenets of his religion. Obviously a nurse would respond in different ways to persons who consider themselves inactive Catholics and to persons who view Catholicism as a vital part of their lives. The nurse must be sensitive to the person's religious commitment (especially when it is different from her own); she must respect the value boundaries of his commitment and work with him to arrive at alternatives that he can accept within his own framework.

A more specific type of value conflict arises when sexual issues involve cognitive dissonance. Cognitive dissonance arises when a person views a question one way on a rational or intellectual level but responds to the same question in a different way on an emotional level—the two areas are not consistent. People often assume that going through an intellectual process of accepting certain sexual attitudes and behaviors will change their feelings immediately. Indeed, the intellectual process is a beginning, but the difficult part is bringing the emotional reaction and the rational attitude into agreement. In this situation the nurse's intervention could be to assist the person to examine the development of the attitude. For example, with a patient who expresses concern about self-stimulation (masturbation) the nurse could consider the following:

1. What are the patient's current attitudes about self-stimulation?
2. Is this a change from former attitudes?
3. What is the patient's recollection of his earliest attitudes?
4. What has been the progression of attitudes throughout the patient's life experience?
5. What incidents and which people does the patient see as significant influences in the formation of his attitudes?
6. Does the patient think that his attitudes have affected his behavior? Have they restrained it or encouraged it?
7. Does the patient feel guilty or comfortable?
8. What kind of attitude does the patient wish to have?
9. What kind of behavior does the patient wish to have?
10. Are there any fantasies about future sexuality if this desired behavior becomes part of the patient's life?
11. If the patient were to adopt the desired behavior, would that change the way he sees himself?

Providing information is often a comfortable and easy response for the nurse, and it can be a helpful and appropriate response to sexual concerns. However, this intervention will be facilitated by at least some initial exploration of attitudes and values by biopsychosocial assessment. The three value positions (as previously outlined) can provide a guide and can be utilized as a framework in which to organize information gathered in the assessment. The process of eliciting values, however, may be difficult.

The patient may have minimal self-awareness of sexual attitudes and values and little understanding of their importance in his life. One helpful approach is to utilize the patient's environment; this encourages him to make comparisons, and in this process his individual feelings are clarified. For example, if the nurse is assessing a patient's concern that sex is boring, the value and attitude component of that assessment might begin in this way:

1. In what ways have you (and your partner) attempted to deal with this concern?
2. What were your parents' attitudes about sexuality? Were their attitudes influenced by their religion?
3. In what ways are your attitudes and values similar and in what ways are they dissimilar to those of your parents? Similarly, how do your values compare with those of your friends, your siblings, and your church?
4. Who are the most conservative and most liberal people you know, in terms of their sexual values? What values do you have in common with each of them? What aspects of their value systems do you find most unsettling?
5. Which of your own attitudes and values do you feel anxious or uncomfortable about?

Regardless of the nature of the sexual concern and regardless of whether it is resolved, the process of values clarification can be enormously helpful to the patient. The resultant increase in self-awareness, the experience of choosing, and the greater comfort with a large component of one's personality (attitudes and values) can create a sense of growth and increased self-esteem that is indeed a powerful intervention.

Fantasy. Another example of psychosocial conflict that involves a sexual issue is the realm of fantasy. The act of fantasizing (and it is most definitely an act, as it involves the expenditure of energy) is neither new nor unacceptable in this society. In fact, society strongly encourages it by continual fantasy-evoking stimulation. Books, movies, newspapers, television, and radio all offer tremendous opportunities for fantasy: exchange one's current life style, career, or situation for another that appears more glamorous, more exciting, or more rewarding. This fantasy, however, is independent of behavior, and it might be considered a healthy outlet in a rigidly organized society. Sexual fantasies, on the other hand, can be experienced as threatening and possibly destructive to one's self-image. This is probably because the most vivid sexual fantasies concern individuals who are close to us or behavior that is at least possible. In both cases, the fantasy is often socially unacceptable, and the fear exists that one will lose control and act on the fantasy. Remote fantasies, such as one concerning great and distant public figures, produce little or no anxiety because they seem clearly impossible, as do most general fantasies.

There are several possible interventions to deal with sexual fantasies. Initially, the listener (the nurse) has the responsibility to develop the trust that must be felt before an individual (particularly a woman) can share such an intimate secret. The nurse's responses, both verbal and nonverbal, are critical in two major ways:

1. To avoid being threatening and therefore unproductive the nurse must be completely nonjudgmental.
2. To help a person deal with fantasies the nurse must be supportive and convey the idea that fantasies are common and are a natural part of sexuality and sexual expression.

It will be helpful for the nurse to keep in mind the importance of conveying the message that sexual fantasies are basically no different from other fantasies; that is, what goes on in the mind does not have to be acted on in reality. Fantasy can serve as is (with no carryover into reality) to enhance pleasure during sexual activity. One can even learn to appreciate and cultivate fantasy for the sake of broadening and deepening sexual experience.

Referral Sexual Therapy (Level III)

Referral. After the nurse's extensive assessment the next step is to provide sensitive, thoughtful intervention. In sexual issues that are complex the nurse may choose to provide in-depth therapy or she may refer the patient to a more appropriate resource. The initial groundwork of assessment has been supported and facilitated with one or more of the possible basic interventions. The next step may be for the nurse to determine an appropriate referral.

Community resources often provide a wide range of options for referral. There are usually women's clinics, planned parenthood clinics, free clinics, and student health centers that provide various forms of medical care, and they often have progressive attitudes toward sexual concerns. Another option would be an institution that focuses more on counseling, such as an area mental health center, a university counseling center, family and marital counseling agencies, or a hospital outpatient psychiatric clinic. In smaller communities with more limited public resources the nurse may have to rely on professionals in private practice: psychosocial nurses, psychologists, psychiatrists, and social workers.

Sexual Therapy. Nurses providing level III intervention function in a variety of different roles and capacities. The treatment modalities that will be discussed are options for the client, and they are areas in which the nurse can be the provider of specific kinds of sexual treatment and therapy if she is appropriately prepared by education and clinical experience.

The basis of the initial treatment modality is the couple. One approach focuses primarily on the relationship and on developing and facilitating communication. This usually includes some discussion of the couple's sexual relationship and directions in that area. Another format is the behavioral approach developed by Masters and Johnson (1970). The structure is usually defined by the male–female therapy team, with primary focus on sexual interaction between partners. Emphasis on solving problems in other areas of the relationship is usually minimal, but this varies with the individual approach of the therapy team.

The second modality is directed at treating the individual alone. Some therapists are oriented toward dealing with significant intrapsychic conflicts over an extended period of time. Other therapists utilize intervention that is more crisis-oriented. They focus on developing coping mechanisms and reducing life stresses to enable the patient to deal more effectively with sexuality concerns. At the end of this short-term experience the patient with an ongoing sexual relationship will probably be referred for couple therapy when the individual issues are resolved. The person without an ongoing relationship or one whose partner refuses to be involved may be referred for group treatment.

One of the newer modalities is an expansion of the group treatment concept. One approach is a preorgasmic women's group, usually consisting of approximately 10 women and 2 female therapists. The focus is on sexual self-awareness and acceptance and self-stimulation techniques. The group interaction and sharing emphasize changes of attitudes and expansion of values by experiencing support from other women in a noncompetitive setting. A second approach is the couples group. The purpose of this group is enhancement of relationships through a sharing of communication skills and alternatives for problem solving with other couples. Depending on the approach of the therapist this experience may include desensitization in the form of massage and other body-awareness and self-awareness exercises.

Education, information, and human growth in sexuality form the basis of varieties of experiences. The more formal structure is a university or community college course or lecture, often didactic, concentrating on dispensing information. Another option is a short seminar or workshop (eg, a day or weekend) that may include any or all of the following: desensitization through explicit films and materials, values-clarifying exercises, small and large group sharing, and information on aspects of sexual functioning and various sexual life styles and behaviors.

SUMMARY

Nurses who value the approach of responding to the whole person can prepare themselves in the area of human sexuality and utilize the opportunities encountered to contribute to the health and well-being of their patients. A thorough knowledge of the physiologic aspects of the sexual system, including considerations relating to one's own body, sexual interaction, and self-stimulation, must be included along with an understanding of the sociocultural and psychosocial influences that affect human sexuality. The methods of assessment and intervention nurses use to respond to sexual concerns are dependent on the comfort and competence levels of each nurse. Some nurses will feel most comfortable providing information and acting as a role model, while others will feel competent to attempt clarification of sexual problems, often by taking a sexual history. The areas examined can include psychophysiologic aspects, partner interaction, attitudes and values, and sexual fantasies. Other nurses will feel prepared to engage in sexual therapy or will make appropriate referrals for such therapy.

Regardless of the level on which the nurse makes assessments and interventions, her responses will be important. Each response (or nonresponse) will provide the patient with new information and input into the way he sees himself and views the sexual issue. If the goal is to promote sexual health and provide sexual health care at each step of the patient's progress, each response must be valued and developed. For the patient to accept himself as a sexual being and develop satisfactory expressions of sexuality, assistance and encouragement are often required.

References

American Medical Association Committee on Human Sexuality: Human Sexuality. Chicago, AMA, 1972

University of Minnesota Medical School: Human Sexuality. Unpublished outline for InMD 5-233, Winter 1975

Friday N: My Secret Garden (Women's Sexual Fantasies). New York, Pocket Books, 1974

Hunt M: Sexual behavior in the 70's. Playboy 20:85–88, 1973

Jacobsen F: Illness and human sexuality. Nurs Outlook 22:52, 1974

Kaplan H: The New Sex Therapy. New York, Brunner/Mazel, 1974

Kaufman G, Krupka J: Integrating one's sexuality: Crisis and change. Int J Group Psychother 23:445–464, 1973

Levin R J: The end of the double standard? Redbook, October 1975

Masters W, Johnson V: Human Sexuality Inadequacy. Boston, Little, Brown, 1970

_____ Human Sexual Response. Boston, Little, Brown, 1966

_____ The Pleasure Bond. Boston, Little, Brown, 1975

_____ Treatment of sexual dysfunction. Unpublished notes from a seminar for professionals, St. Louis, June 1974

Mero R, Brown M A: Sexuality and health professionals. Address before women's health care nurse practitioners, Seattle, 1975

Mims F H: Sexual education and counseling. Nurs Clin North Am 10:526–527, September 1975

Vincent C E: Sexual and Marital Health. New York, McGraw-Hill, 1973

Woods N F, Mandetta A F: Human sexual response patterns. Nurs Clin North Am 10:529–538, September 1975

CHAPTER 7

LOSS: SOME ORIGINS AND NURSING IMPLICATIONS

Joan M. Baker
Lucille Kindely Kelley

Jim decided last night that because of his cough he must stop smoking. Alice and Tom have just moved into their dream house. Eight-year-old Peter overheard his father and the veterinarian talk of putting the aging family dog to sleep. Beth's husband left home last week; he moved into a singles apartment and filed for divorce. After 14 years as an executive secretary Trish became pregnant. What do these people have in common? Each one is facing a loss. A loss can be said to occur when a person is without something he formerly possessed. It is also possible that a person will experience a sense of loss when he only anticipates being without a given possession.

Of course it can be argued that giving up smoking, moving into a dream house, and having a baby are gains. Yet one would be hard put to identify any gain in life that has not grown out of a loss. For example, the gain of a dream house by Alice and Tom also means giving up their familiar surroundings and leaving behind one of the sources of their mutual involvement and commitment. Furthermore, the attainment of their dream means that the challenge of reaching that particular goal has been lost.

Admittedly, loss is an inevitable and inescapable human experience. Losses can be categorized in many ways, some of which are illustrated in Table 7.1. Loss can be a very complex phenomenon, and the categories of losses are not mutually exclusive. That is, a loss may fall into several categories. For example, an unexpected leg amputation necessitated by an automobile accident could be categorized as obvious, permanent, major, and overwhelming, according to the circumstances of the patient.

For another individual a leg amputation to stop a disease process might be categorized as positive, intentional, and manageable. Thus losses are categorized not only by the external event but also by a variety of other factors, not the least of which is the meaning of the event for each individual.

The majority of losses that most of us encounter on a day-to-day basis are neither threatening nor unmanageable. Rather, they are usual occurrences, and often they are not even labeled as loss but are viewed as something else, such as change, illness, stress, or even promotion. It is when a person feels very threatened or overwhelmed by his loss that help from an outside source may be needed.

On a daily basis nurses in every setting encounter patients who are experiencing some type of loss, many of whom could benefit from nursing intervention related to loss. Almost without exception patients in a hospital setting are undergoing some loss to their general health. Families of these patients, in turn, are affected directly or indirectly by these losses, in addition to experiencing their own losses. Compounding these more obvious losses, patients frequently experience a series of unavoidable concurrent losses: an expected friend fails to visit; the physician forgets to write the promised order; x-ray cancels the diagnostic test; the lawyer advises that the medical insurance will not cover this hospitalization.

Another loss that patients frequently must face is death, either their own or that of a loved one. Patients and family members may need help in facing this inevitable loss and its concomitant response of grief. Losses that are threatening to the patient or losses that accumulate without adequate resolution may cause energy depletion and leave the patient more vulnerable to psychophysiologic stress (Selye 1956).

Table 7.1. COMMON CATEGORIES OF LOSSES AS OPPOSING SETS

Object	Person
Situational	Maturational
Obvious	Subtle
Temporary	Permanent
Minor	Major
Positive	Negative
Intentional	Unintentional
Isolated	Cumulative
Preventable	Unpreventable
Reversible	Irreversible
Planned	Unplanned
Manageable	Overwhelming
Nonthreatening	Threatening
Usual	Unusual

Nurses need to be aware that each patient is experiencing some kind of loss. By providing the patient with an opportunity, if need be, to cope with the loss the nurse will be in a better position to facilitate healing from that loss, from other psychological injuries, and from any presenting physical pathology. This chapter is addressed to that end, and discussion will include the dynamics of the loss experience, resolution of loss, and nursing assessment and intervention.

DYNAMICS OF LOSS EXPERIENCES

We have all known the person who becomes distraught whenever a seemingly small thing does not go his way. On the other hand, most of us also know the individual who is able to weather great tragedy with dignity and composure. Then there are those whose reactions vacillate between the two extremes. What happens to a person experiencing a loss? Why do reactions to loss vary so greatly? The manner in which a person reacts to a given loss depends on a variety of factors: the way one learned to handle loss as a child; the significance one assigns the loss; the physical and emotional status of the individual; accumulated loss experiences throughout one's lifetime; and the perspective one has of the loss.

Learning about Loss as a Child

Initial experiences with loss usually occur within the context of the everyday happenings of childhood. The most common learning experiences center around situational losses, maturational losses, and learning by watching others.

Situational Losses. Most of us remember the Mother Goose rhyme describing the plight of the Three Little Kittens. When the kittens lost their mittens they dutifully reported their loss to their mother, who showed her disapproval through her response: "What? Lost your mittens, you naughty kittens! Then you shall have no pie." This rhyme illustrates a rather universal parental reaction to a situational type of loss common in childhood. From this adult reaction children learn very early in life that the loss of an object is undesirable and often punishable. The parents' disapproval over the loss gives rise to a feeling of anxiety in the child (Sullivan 1953). At the same time, the behavior of the parent may become increasingly anxiety-provoking for the child when the disapproval is followed by a stern command to "find it." If the parent fails to supplement the command by suggesting ways to find the object, the child's anxiety may increase. On the other hand, if the parent includes some specific directions on how to "find it" or offers other help, the child will feel better equipped for the task and hence will become less anxious.

As the experience of disapproval of loss is repeated a number of times the child will begin to feel anxious about loss of objects regardless of whether or not the parent is present. How the child learns to manage this anxiety (by taking constructive steps toward recouping or accepting the loss, by becoming immobilized by the anxiety, by striking out against others, or by becoming depressed) will have repercussions on his behavior in subsequent loss situations throughout his lifetime.

The initial behaviors learned in response to loss can be modified by a person's life experiences. For example, understanding and accepting nurses, teachers, neighbors, friends, and relatives can be instrumental in this resocialization process by providing different approval–disapproval reactions from those of the child's parents.

Studies have shown that young children are often unable to conceptualize the irreversibility of death (Nagy 1956, McIntire and associates 1972). Perhaps this inability is an extension of the child's experience with object loss. If parents insist that lost objects can and must be found or replaced, then it follows that the child will assume that people who are "lost" or dead can certainly be found or returned if one looks hard enough or hopes long enough. Nursing research in this area would seem timely.

Maturational Losses. In addition to the situational losses each of us experiences as a child, we must also learn to manage the anxieties related to losing past attachments as a result of growing up (Barlow 1974). Maturational losses may occur whether or not the person is physically or emotionally ready for them. This type of loss continues throughout one's life until the final loss—death. For the infant, weaning means loss of the breast or bottle. Adolescents must give up their dependence in order to achieve independence. The mother of grown children may need to find new resources to make her life meaningful after her children leave home. The retiree may need to modify his physical activities to correspond with declining stamina. As in the case of situational losses, early maturational losses and the manner in which one learns to handle them will affect the way future losses will be handled.

Learning by Watching Others. Children are great observers of other people's behavior. Much of the learning that takes place is the result of observing and then mimicking what others do. A few actions modeled by parents seem to have greater impact on a child's learning than a thousand words. Parents know this; witness the futile admonition "Do as I say, not as I do."

Parents who are reacting to their own losses are providing one source of behavior for their child to observe, to mimic, and hence to learn. By encouraging exploration and discussion of their own demonstrated behavior, and by pointing out differences of behaviors in a given situation, some parents enable their child to broaden his knowledge of the possibilities for dealing with anxiety in loss situations. On the other hand, some parents are unable to share their reactions to loss with their children. These parents may deliberately refuse to discuss a loss, such as death, when the subject is raised. They may even lie to the child about the loss event in order to hide their reaction to it, believing that they are protecting the child from the trauma of knowing about death (Wahl 1966). One mother of a preschool girl had the family's sick dog put to sleep. She thought her daughter would not understand the loss and might become frightened by it. She therefore told her daughter that the dog had been taken to a farm to live. For well over a year the daughter continued to search for the dog whenever she passed a farm or saw farm animals at a fair or was reminded of a farm in some other way. This child's anxiety was not alleviated as the mother had intended. Instead, since the child was deprived of the opportunity to deal with her anxieties over her missing dog, the learning possibilities within the situation were lost. The child's anxiety was prolonged, and the loss was not adequately resolved.

Television is another source of role modeling of loss behaviors within the home. This instrument provides a multitude of examples of how people deal with loss. Some of these examples give an accurate picture of loss, along with appropriate reactions to loss and ways of resolving it. Other programs are not as sensitive and realistic. Neither the resolution of grief over death on a half-hour television show nor the maintenance of composure during time-limited news coverage of a national hero's death nor the resurrection of a cartoon character after he has been totally annihilated depicts loss and loss reactions realistically, sensitively, or appropriately.

The child's ability to sort out the real from the unreal, to understand sometimes frightening and often conflicting feelings and reactions to loss, can be fostered by input from others. If parents or others are available to explain the ways in which television has depicted loss and to explore the child's questions and calm his fears by giving him facts about the loss, the child can grow in his understanding of the concept of loss. Without this interaction experience the child is left to wonder and sometimes worry, and is likely to fill in the information gaps with fantasy. These fantasies can be devastating to the child. More important, the absence of interaction around the experience of loss robs the child of a valuable opportunity to face and understand his own anxiety about loss.

Significance of Loss

Some other factors that affect the way one perceives and deals with loss include attitudes, values, and beliefs accumulated over a lifetime (Rokeach 1968). Emotional bonds both positive and negative, highly valued material objects, sentimental attachments, energy and interest investments, hopes and expectations—all give meaning and significance to the loss and affect the way it is perceived. The durability and intensity of these factors also help to determine the perception of the loss. For example, when Sandra's mother gave her the family heirloom clock, Sandra was thrilled. When the clock was smashed in moving, Sandra felt sad and guilty for not taking better care of it, and she cried periodically throughout the day. On the other hand, her husband, who had no sentimental attachment to the clock, had difficulty understanding Sandra's reaction; he wanted to throw the old thing out.

Physical and Emotional Status

Another important factor that affects the way one perceives and copes with a loss is the individual's physical and mental state of health. When some people are tired, in pain, or otherwise physically or emotionally ill, their ability to cope with a loss may be diminished (McGrath 1970). In addition to having diminished coping skills, a person who is under stress may also distort or exaggerate a loss. Stephen, for example, a 7-year-old boy hospitalized for a fractured pelvis, was unable to sleep during the night and complained all the following day of being unable to get into a comfortable position. During the evening he discovered that his favorite stuffed animal was missing. He yelled "Oh no, oh no, I've got to have him! What am I going to do? I can't sleep without him!" Stephen's crying and wailing was inconsolable. This was unusual behavior for Stephen, whose mother had described him as "an easy-going, mature boy." His reaction was probably exaggerated by his physical discomfort and lack of sleep. Both these factors lower the ability to utilize the usual coping skills.

Accumulated Loss Experiences

Resolution of previous losses is another factor to consider in understanding an individual's reaction to loss. If a person has resolved previous losses successfully, he is more likely to have attained some skill in managing his anxiety in loss situations. Therefore he will be more likely to resolve future losses with a degree of success. On the other hand, a person who has been unsuccessful in resolving previous losses may not have the skill and ability necessary to cope with subsequent losses. For example,

Becky always had trouble growing up. From the time she was a baby her mother decided when Becky should give up certain baby behaviors and "act like a big girl." When her mother took away her bottle at 8 months, Becky started to suck her thumb; she continued to do so for years, much to her mother's dismay. Becky's mother also toilet-trained her by 1 year of age; however, Becky had frequent accidents through the first grade. When Becky became a teenager her mother suddenly assigned her many responsibilities, such as preparing dinner every night, cleaning the house every day after school, and doing the grocery shopping. Instead of developing into the independent and responsible teenager her mother had hoped to mold, Becky didn't complete her tasks, often argued with her mother, and usually left the house in tears, leaving her work behind her.

Things were different for Kathy. When she was growing up her mother made an effort to allow Kathy to communicate her readiness for giving up her baby ways. Kathy's mother waited until Kathy gave an indication she no longer wanted the bottle before her mother put it away. Kathy's mother didn't feel her daughter was ready for toilet training until Kathy showed an interest in sitting on the potty chair. At that time, when Kathy was between 2 and 3 years old, her mother helped her learn to use the potty chair. After 2 days Kathy was completely toilet-trained and had no further accidents. When Kathy became a teenager her mother discussed with her the need for more help around the house. Kathy expressed an interest in helping with the yard work on Saturdays, keeping her room clean, and taking responsibility for doing the dinner dishes every night. Kathy not only recognized areas where she could be helpful but also took part in deciding what responsibilities she would assume, and she usually completed the tasks she had agreed to do.

Loss in Perspective

It is a fallacy to assume that every loss that occurs in a person's life is a problem. But what accounts for the difference between those losses that are problems and those that are not? One way of looking at this question is to consider all losses as events with the potential for becoming problems. Loss events can become problem events when the individual perceives the loss in some extreme fashion. The person who is overwhelmed by the importance of the loss or who feels devastatingly threatened by the loss is at greater risk of an emergent problem than the person whose appraisal of the situation is more realistic and less drastic. Another important determinant of risk of likelihood that a problem will emerge is the individual's coping skill. The greater one's level of coping skill and the greater the number of successful coping events completed, the greater the likelihood of successful coping in the future. It is also important to consider the availability of coping resources. For instance, if a person has available to him a network of others who are willing and able to assist him in a time of need, and if he utilizes that network, he has a better chance of managing the loss than his more unfortunate peer who lacks this resource. The nurse who is sensitive to the range of these considerations of loss events will be better able to appraise a person's condition of loss and make appropriate interventions.

Nursing Perspective on Loss

A condition that affects the nurse's ability to assess and intervene in a helpful manner is her degree of comfort with her own attitudes and feelings about loss, including death. A nurse who has not faced and resolved her own loss experiences runs the risk of having her own personal feelings interfere with her ability to help a patient (Baker and Sorensen 1973). She may find herself overreacting or even minimizing a patient's loss because of her own needs. When Ralph, a 20-year-old university student, was admitted to the hospital with a broken arm, the nurse made certain that Ralph had to reach for nothing. She frequently made comments about the terrible imposition the injury was for "poor Ralph." When Ralph initially broke his arm he began to make plans to recruit his friends for assistance so that he could continue with school. After listening to the nurse's emphasis on his helplessness for several days, Ralph decided he needed to drop out of school until the cast on his arm was removed.

On the other hand, the nurse who has more adequately resolved her own feelings about loss will be better equipped to help her patient with a loss experience. Such was the case in the following situation when the nurse decided that her most appropriate intervention was to be a learning reinforcer. Carol announced that she had just received word that her husband had been transferred by his employer and that they would be moving to another state on her discharge from the hospital. By exploring this loss event and the potential problems inherent in the move with Carol, the nurse determined that the loss was outweighed by the fact that for Carol this was a welcomed and long-awaited move. Furthermore, Carol had already utilized her existing network of support in arranging for care of her children and in planning some aspects of the move based on what she had learned from their last move. The nurse was able to point out Carol's assets in coping and to reinforce her potential for continued successful coping with similar losses.

LOSS RESOLUTION

Any loss involves disruption of the status quo. Many losses result in physical injury or emotional injury or both. The psychological reaction to injury may vary from a total lack of awareness to slight uneasiness to total bereavement. Subsequent to the injury the natural process of healing begins to take place (Colgrove and associates 1976). That is, a person experiencing loss takes steps to resolve that loss.

The healing process may be spontaneous or prolonged, depending on the importance of the loss to the individual and the ability to cope with the loss. If the healing is successful the person's ability to function may be restored or actually improved by the opportunity for growth inherent in the healing process. On the other hand, if healing is incomplete and the person is unable to accept and resolve the loss, then there may be a cumulative negative effect (Colgrove and associates 1976, Barlow 1974).

Successful resolution of loss is accomplished in various stages. Final resolution varies for each individual. It is considered successful when the patient has been able to work through the various stages with some degree of satisfaction and subsequently take further action directed at substitution or replacement of the loss. In order to achieve success in working through each stage, an individual simultaneously works on three tasks imposed by a loss: survival, healing, and growth. Discussion of loss resolution must begin by focusing on the stages of recovery.

Stages of Recovery

A person who experiences a threatening loss will progress through the following stages of recovery as he moves toward successful resolution of that loss: shock and denial, anger and depression, understanding and acceptance (Colgrove and associates 1976). These stages may vary in length, intensity, and scope according to the type of loss and the meaning it has for the individual. Although some degrees of these feelings usually occur in any loss situation, here we are concerned primarily with losses that are perceived as stressful or threatening.

Shock and Denial. The first stage has been identified as shock and denial (Colgrove and associates 1976). A person in this stage of loss is experiencing an initial state of disbelief. Patients' comments typify this stage: "You must be kidding." "I feel like this is happening to someone else." "I don't believe it." "Oh, no, not me!" Some people become physically immobilized, psychologically immobilized, or both, some may weep uncontrollably, others seem oblivious to their loss, some may deny the meaning of the loss by minimizing its significance, and still others may attempt to escape the loss by losing themselves in other activities or by refusing to acknowledge the facts.

Anger and Depression. The second stage that occurs during resolution of a loss is that of anger and depression (Colgrove and associates 1976). As the person begins to realize and admit that the loss has actually happened, it is not uncommon for him to feel angry and to strike out against others through such actions as blaming others for the loss or becoming argumentative or unduly or unfairly critical of others. Depression, the turning inward of anger, may also occur during this stage of recovery. The person feels sad over the loss; he may cry frequently, may feel guilty, and may even try to inflict self-punishment, the ultimate form of which is suicide. The depression may be accompanied by other painful feelings such as helplessness, hopelessness, fearfulness, loneliness, guilt, and despair.

Several different feelings about the loss may occur simultaneously, and they may reflect earlier conflicting attitudes toward the loss. A young woman who has just lost her alcoholic mother may be torn between feelings of love and hatred for the mother: the love for her mother's warmth, gentleness, and kindness; the hatred for her mother's degrading behavior caused by her alcoholism.

It is during these first two stages of recovery that a person may experience a feeling of fatigue that can show up in such behaviors as lack of energy to do everyday tasks, proneness to error, and slowing of speech and movement (Colgrove and associates 1976). The person may become more isolated than usual and may lack the energy for initiating contacts with others. Numerous physical symptoms may appear, thus adding to the person's distress and diminishing his energy reserve.

In addition, it is not uncommon for the person who has experienced loss to have trouble concentrating and to lack general motivation. There may also be a diminution in appetite or sexual drive or disruption of sleep patterns (Colgrove and associates 1976). It must be kept in mind that all of these reactions are relative. The presence or absence of a reaction, as well as its intensity or extent, will depend on the individual and on the circumstances of his current loss and his past losses that remain unresolved. Each person's loss experience is unique, and by no means are all reactions to loss obvious to an observer or even to the person experiencing the loss.

Understanding and Acceptance. The next stage of recovery involves understanding and acceptance (Colgrove and associates 1976). During this stage the person examines his loss in terms of its meaning and importance to him and his reactions to it. He reaches some sort of emotional armistice. He begins to feel an inner peace, and he feels ready to expand his thinking and to plan for a future without the loss. Both acceptance and understanding may ebb and flow with the other stages as the person moves toward resolution of the loss. This acceptance occurs in relation to existing circumstances; if circumstances change a new level of understanding and acceptance may have to be worked out. For example, Ann, a young woman in her early twenties, had reached a positive level of acceptance about her new body image following her mastectomy. Subsequent to achieving this acceptance Ann became engaged. She was then faced with the task of achieving a new understanding and acceptance about herself and her body in relation to her husband-to-be.

Beyond Understanding and Acceptance

Once a person has achieved some degree of understanding and acceptance related to the loss, the person needs to decide how his life shall go from now on. Some people stop at the point of acceptance, taking the loss for what it is, continuing to live in the absence of the lost object, and doing nothing further about it. Such people may feel that their life is satisfactory despite the loss, maintaining an underlying awareness of a void, but never trying to fill it in. A man who retires from an active work role to a sedentary role in his own home, never engaging in activities to fill the time void, typifies this sort of response. Another person may find it necessary to move beyond understanding and acceptance and may be driven to seek a substitute for the lost object or replace it in some other way. One school of thought is adamant that a loss has never been successfully resolved until such substitution or replacement is attempted (Peretz 1970). This replacement endeavor may involve revising one's life style, changing one's values, or redefining priorities. For the previous 10 years 78-year-old Mrs. Canfield had stayed at home to nurse her ill husband and tend to his every need. About a year after her husband's death Mrs. Canfield took a class in sculpting; she began visiting her old friends, and she joined a card group. She declared, "It's about time I began doing things again. You're never too old to change."

Along with experiencing the stages of recovery a person must accomplish three tasks related to loss: survival, healing, and growth. To a certain extent all three tasks occur at different levels during all three stages of recovery. That is, one must survive the shock of a loss and heal and grow as a result of it, at least to some extent. Likewise, one must survive one's anger and depression, as well as heal and grow from it. The resolution process, as well as the loss itself, is indeed complex. The stages are interrelated and the tasks are interrelated, and the two groupings are also interrelated.

Tasks Related to Loss

Survival, healing, and growth are the three tasks intimately involved in the resolution of a loss, especially a threatening one. The nurse is in a unique position to assist the patient experiencing a threatening loss in accomplishing these tasks. Some patients the nurse encounters will be facing the prospect of surviving a loss, while others will have progressed through survival and healing to a point of growth. Others may be experiencing regression back to old hurts, a behavior that is common with a loss. The nurse who is aware of the possible tasks facing her patient and who is able to intervene in a manner that is congruent with the patient's needs at the moment will be better able to assist the patient to work through his experience.

Survival. Surviving means to continue living in spite of the loss. In each stage of recovery survival may become a concern. During the stage of shock and denial the patient's survival may be threatened because he fails to eat and subsequently becomes ill. During the stage of anger and depression the patient's feelings may become violent and internalized to the point that he considers suicide, and survival is once again an issue. The patient who is working primarily at the understanding and acceptance stage of a loss may suddenly feel overcome by his new insight about the meaning of the loss. If this new insight generates feelings of guilt, remorse, and unhappiness, the patient may experience new or renewed depression, which in turn may threaten his survival.

The nurse's main challenge in relation to survival is to help the patient acknowledge his loss and explore his feelings in relation to the loss. The processes of acknowledging and exploring a loss prepare a patient to take steps later toward acknowledging the event more fully and subsequently working through the loss.

It should be noted that some people appear to survive their losses without every resolving their denial or anger. Such people may continue their denial of the significance of the loss of loved ones for the rest of their lives in an attempt to protect themselves from feelings that seem too painful to acknowledge. In some cases this denial suffices, although growth is stunted. In other cases denial is an effective self-protective mechanism until another loss occurs or until the denial is challenged; then the person's coping defenses are weakened or destroyed. In the event that the person's coping is not enhanced, survival once more becomes an issue. The nurse must keep in mind the patient's right to exercise denial, and she must carefully consider the implications involved in taking away the patient's self-protective mechanisms of denial

Healing. Loss is a type of wound, primarily psychological. As with a physical wound, a healing process is necessary to restore a condition of well-being (Peretz 1970). The task of healing involves achieving greater awareness of what is happening to oneself. It is a process of actively examining one's feelings about the loss in relation to one's life. Most healing takes place when denial begins to diminish and feelings related to the loss begin to emerge.

The helping role of the nurse at this point is to assist the patient in exploring those feelings and to encourage him to assign them a meaning. In addition, the patient needs an opportunity to examine his behavior and put it into perspective in relation to the loss experience.

People in the healing phase often have special needs. Some may find it difficult to accept the finality of their loss; they try to hold on to that loss. A person may refuse to accept advancing age and continue to wear the latest teenage fashions. Another person may try to alter his life style drastically, even to his own detriment: Mr. Fox, a middle-aged executive, made a series of unwise investments that resulted in the loss of his home, his savings, and ultimately his family. Feeling bereft, he joined a communal living group, where he started taking drugs; the result was his untimely death from an overdose.

Many people who are healing from a loss are vulnerable to others who desire to take advantage of them. For example, an 80-year-old widow signed up for a lifetime series of dance lessons soon after her husband's death. The lessons cost her all her savings.

Finally, there are those who throw themselves into a frenzy of activities and involvements subsequent to a loss, rather than taking time out for needed adjustments. Immediately following the death of her first-born child Paula plunged into many activities in her home and in the community. She thus had no time for herself, and she grew increasingly dissatisfied without knowing why.

A nurse who is sensitive to the special needs of people experiencing loss will be better able to recognize from a patient's behavior that he needs help in dealing with his loss. Once this need is recognized, the nurse can help the patient explore and evaluate his feelings and behaviors. The patient may then be in a better position to reappraise his life and decide more rationally which direction he wants to take.

The nurse must realize that if the challenges of survival and healing in a loss situation are not met they can lead to depression and suicide. If the patient perceives his loss as catastrophic, or if he feels totally helpless following his loss, he may begin to think that suicide is his only recourse. Losses that commonly lead to suicide include the death of a loved one, the diagnosis of a terminal illness, loss of financial security, and loss of a major life goal or value. Further discussion of assessment and intervention related to suicide is given in Chapter 9.

When a person is able to understand and manage his feelings, an air of self-confidence begins to develop. As healing accelerates, the person enters into a readiness for further growth that is evidenced by certain signals (Colgrove and associates 1976). The person may act stronger; he may say that he feels better able to cope with his situation. He may indicate an ability to take more responsibility by initiating a few well-thought-out changes in his life. He may report feeling happier, and he may actually provide evidence of this happiness in more open relationships with others.

Growth. Growth is an expansion of the healing process. In the growth phase the person demonstrates his awareness of healing by taking the action necessary to complete the resolution of his loss. For instance, the decision to acknowledge a loss during the stage of shock and denial marks the growth that allows a person to progress to the next stage of recovery.

Growth involves doing things at a level different from previously. Actions related to growth are more goal-directed and rational than former scattered, nondirected activity. Instead of trying to maintain involvement in five community projects, as she had done shortly after her husband's death, Clara grew to the point where she recognized the importance of focusing her energy on the one project that was most meaningful for her. George, an alcoholic, decided to stop drinking. Initially he didn't know what to do with himself, and he lay on the couch and watched television for 12 hours a day. He began to feel sorry for himself and to long for the days when he was drinking with his cronies. As he faced these feelings in his counseling sessions with the nurse, he realized he had to find something to do or he would probably resume drinking. He considered returning to his old job as a bartender, but he rejected this idea because of its constant temptation. Instead, the nurse assisted him to explore other alternatives, and as a result he enrolled in a course to prepare him to become an alcoholism counselor. George is now actively employed and his sobriety has continued for many years.

The main role of the nurse in helping the patient achieve his growth potential is to help him examine alternative actions for dealing with his feelings and achieve a new state of well-being. This problem-solving approach is an important step in working through a loss.

The process of working through a loss involves examination of the loss and its attending circumstances to the point that the patient can independently face and master the loss alone (Lee 1968). Generally, this working-through process between the nurse and the patient who has experienced loss consists of focusing on the loss, on his reactions to the loss, and on steps that will enable him to resolve the loss. This process of working through will be discussed and developed further in the next section.

NURSING ASSESSMENT AND INTERVENTION

In order to begin her assessment of the loss experience for a given patient, the nurse can focus attention on three areas: the current behavior of the patient, what has happened to the patient, and what the patient says or avoids saying about his situation. A nurse may hypothesize that a patient is experiencing loss and needs help in resolving that loss if the patient exhibits any of the behaviors or any combination of the behaviors discussed in the previous sections. The following are a few examples:

The patient has trouble concentrating.
The patient tries to become involved in myriad activities.
The patient consistently finds fault with his family or himself.
The patient cries often or seems to be on the brink of tears.
The patient appears to be helpless and seems unable to become involved in any constructive activity without assistance and encouragement.
The patient closes himself off from contact with others, except when contact is absolutely necessary.

Any assessment the nurse makes must also take into consideration what has happened to the patient. The nurse may need to determine the following:

What has happened to the patient that he requires health care services?
Is the patient being kept fully informed of his progress, or is he at a loss concerning his condition?
Is the loss of health that the patient is experiencing a reversible or irreversible state?
Does the patient have a support system, such as friends and relatives who visit him?
Are other things going on in the patient's life that add further stress to his situation?

For additional clues to his readiness or reluctance to discuss his situation, the nurse also needs to listen to what the patient says or avoids saying. She might consider these factors:

Does the patient ask numerous questions about what is happening to him or about his condition?
Does he talk about how difficult it is for him to believe that his illness (or other experience) is happening to him?
Does he talk of feeling depressed, lonely, angry, irritated, or upset in some other way?
Does he respond as if nothing extraordinary is happening to him, even though he may be experiencing a very threatening situation?

When the nurse decides that the patient may be experiencing loss, the next step is to invite him to discuss that loss. Such a discussion should take into account which stage of recovery the patient is experiencing; this information will be used by the nurse in determining the next step in the helping process.

The nurse can invite the patient to discuss his loss by making a comment about one or more of her initial observations and then exploring that observation further. The nurse knows that Jack has ostensibly been reading, but he hasn't turned a page for half an hour. She might say something like this: "I notice that you have been reading that same page in your magazine for the past half hour." Then she could follow that up with an exploratory question: "Is something bothering you today?"

"Would you like to talk for a while?" "Are you having difficulty concentrating?" "Have you got something on your mind that you would like to talk about?"

The patient may initially refuse to discuss his situation. When that happens the nurse can consider several possible actions. Whatever she chooses to do, the nurse's actions need to be guided by the open-door principle. That is, a patient is more likely to talk about his concerns if the nurse provides frequent opportunity for discussion whenever the patient is ready, rather than when it is most convenient for the nurse. If the nurse misinterprets the patient's initial refusal to discuss his concerns and responds as if his refusal is a personal rejection, she may prematurely close the door on any future discussion and imply disinterest in the patient. Such premature closure is demonstrated when a nurse informs a patient that "It's all right with me if you don't want to talk." Premature closure can even be compounded further if the nurse makes the mistake of trying to reassure the patient by telling him that the subject need never be brought up again. On the other hand, the nurse who insists that the patient discuss his concerns immediately, whether he wants to or not, also runs the risk of prematurely closing the door to helpful communication. To ensure that a discussion about the patient's loss will eventually occur, the nurse must provide continual opportunity for the patient to talk about his concerns. Such an approach is usually better than either avoiding the subject or coercing the patient to talk before he is ready.

In order to maintain this open door when the patient has initially refused to discuss his concerns, the nurse might consider several options. For example, the nurse can wait for the next opportunity to talk about loss. At that time she can once again verbalize her observations and invite the patient to discuss his concerns. Another way of keeping the door open is for the nurse to demonstrate to the patient that she will spend time with him whether he chooses to talk about his concerns or not. By indicating her availability the nurse demonstrates her acceptance of the patient's stand, neither forcing him to abandon his stand nor reinforcing it.

When the patient chooses to accept the nurse's invitation to discuss his concerns he may be in any of the stages of recovery from loss, as previously described, or he may be experiencing aspects of more than one stage. If the patient's responses indicate shock and disbelief, one of the most helpful things the nurse can do is offer moral support. One way she can do this is to let the patient know she can empathize with him by reflecting back to him some of the thoughts and feelings he is experiencing. Such a response on the nurse's part can also assist the patient in identifying his feelings more clearly, and it can help the nurse and the patient decide how to work together.

The following interaction, which occurred between a nurse and Jack, a 22-year-old patient, illustrates several of the above points:

N: Are you having difficulty concentrating?	
J: Yes, I am. I keep trying to convince myself that I'm really here in the hospital.	Expresses disbelief.
N: Go on.	
J: Well, yesterday I was up walking around and today I'm totally helpless—a broken arm and two broken legs. I can't walk, I can't comb my hair, I can't even eat without help.	
N: Yes, your automobile accident certainly changed things for you. Yesday you were independent and today you feel helpless.	The nurse is helping Jack to interrelate his loss with the precipitating event and his subsequent feelings.
J: The worst part is that I don't remember much about the accident. I wish I knew what really happened.	Jack shares more information with the nurse about his present concerns.
N: I was on duty when you were admitted. Perhaps I can answer some of your questions.	The nurse recognizes his need for information and responds with a suggestion for an appropriate course of action.
J: Oh, good! I want to know everything.	Jack agrees to work with the nurse in the way the nurse suggests.

In this interaction the nurse encourages the patient to lead the conversation. She reflects back to him some of his feelings about his current situation. She does not insist that he accept his condition and "face reality." Instead, by listening to him, she learns further about his concerns and about how she might help him begin to deal with those concerns by finding out some of the circumstances related to his loss experiences.

Survival does not seem to be a problem for Jack at this time. Instead, he seems to be working on the task of healing, since he is taking the initiative to seek more information about what has happened to him. The nurse must keep in mind that survival, healing, and growth are not mutually exclusive tasks. Jack is working on healing, but this does not mean that survival as a task is completed, nor does it mean that growth has not begun. Future nursing assessments of Jack's recovery status will have to be made in order to keep pace with his changing needs.

In the above situation the nurse helps Jack to become better aware of his loss circumstances. Although Jack says he wants to know everything, the nurse should keep in mind that Jack is physically debilitated, upset, and feeling helpless and frustrated. Too much information at such a time may overwhelm a patient and leave him feeling even more helpless and more threatened by his loss. The nurse who understands the factors that influence loss and its resolution will temper her nursing care according to clues from the patient about what he wants and according to her knowledge of what any patient needs.

N: So you want to know everything?	The nurse begins exploration by following up clues the patient has given about what he wants.
J: I think I do.	Jack seems to be becoming more realistic and less global.
N: Where do you think you would like to start?	The nurse helps Jack to focus. She does not allow him to become overwhelmed by telling him everything.
J: Was I driving? Did someone hit me?	
N: Two questions at once. I'll start with your first one. Yes, you were driving. Do you remember getting into the car?	The nurse focuses the interaction and explores further an issue introduced by the patient.
J: No, I don't.	
N: What had you been doing last evening, before the accident?	The nurse asks a question that is meant to help the patient recall more about the events leading up to his accident.
J: Well, to tell you the truth, I don't remember much about last night. My buddy and I went to this party given by some friends of his. We started drinking about 4 o'clock in the afternoon. We'd just finished an exam in math and wanted to celebrate.	Jack is able to recall and describe some of the events preceding the accident.
N: So you were drinking and celebrating?	The nurse summarizes in order to encourage the patient to continue.
J: Yeah. We just kept drinking and telling jokes. I remember asking what time it was, and Bob, my buddy, told me it was 7:30 P.M. The next thing I remember is being in here. What time was the accident?	Jack cannot account for much of the evening, and he seeks information from the nurse to fill in the gaps.
N: The accident occurred at 1:30 A.M., and you were admitted to the hospital at 1:45 A.M.	
J: That's 6 hours of time I can't remember. That's scary. That's happened to me before.	
N: What has happened to you before?	Clarification.
J: Not being able to remember. It's awful. Somebody told me it's because I drink too much sometimes. Was anyone else hurt in the accident?	Jack gives a clue about his drinking but does not seem to connect his drinking with the accident.
N: Yes, your buddy, Bob, was also admitted. He was put into the intensive care unit because of a head injury, but he is feeling better now. You may visit him later if you like.	
J: (With anguish.) Oh no! A head injury. Poor Bob. How about the other guy?	
N: What other guy?	

J: (Angry.) The one who's responsible for all this! The guy who ran into us.	The angry affect and the blame of another person may mean that Jack is moving into the anger and depression stage.
N: As far as I know there was no one else involved. The police report said it was a one-car accident.	The nurse casts doubt about someone else being at fault. She bases this doubt on additional facts available to her through records, and she shares this information with Jack.
J: That's impossible. If I was driving. . . . It's impossible. I've never had an accident in my life. No. Someone must have hit us or forced us off the road. Some nut!	Denial.
N: In other words, you think the accident must have been someone else's fault?	The nurse interprets the meaning of Jack's previous statements so that Jack has the opportunity to think further about his part in the accident.
J: Yeah. I hope it was. How's Bob doing?	Jack is no longer adamant that he was not at fault. He indicates that he wishes he were not at fault and then changes the subject.
N: He told me earlier that he will be moved to this unit tomorrow.	
J: What's for dinner?	Jack indicates that he can no longer tolerate discussion of the accident and his part in it at this time.

In this interaction the patient vacillates between shock and denial and anger and depression. The nurse's comments are supportive in that she avoids making any judgments about the patient's behavior and instead seeks to help him communicate more clearly about his concerns. She is open and honest in responding to his questions. She does not reinforce his denial, nor does she agree with it. Instead, she reflects back the meaning of his statements of denial, which helps him to begin to heal. The healing takes the form of lessening denial on Jack's part of his responsibility for the accident. The nurse is able to discriminate between Jack's desires (wanting to know everything) and his needs (limited information until he is ready).

Several days later, as Jack learned more about the circumstances of the accident from talks with Bob and others, he fully acknowledged his responsibility as a drunken driver. He experienced a great deal of remorse, especially in relation to the injuries suffered by Bob, and he apologized to Bob often. At one point during this recovery period, as his feelings of guilt increased, his survival was threatened. Jack expressed suicidal ideas to the nurse and to his family. On one occasion he told the nurse, "Sometimes I really feel I should kill myself for what I've done to Bob." On another occasion he told his wife, "What's the use of living? I can't stand myself for what I did to my best friend."

During this painful time of self-blame Jack was able to discuss his feelings with various members of the staff, including the nurse. He was helped to become more aware of his feelings, to analyze them, and to put the accident into a different perspective. He was helped to look at his pattern of drinking. He recognized that his heavy drinking had contributed to his irresponsible driving and the subsequent accident.

It was at this point that Jack came to understand his role in the accident and the reason for it more clearly. He no longer denied his responsibility. He realized that he could continue to punish himself or that he could put his guilt aside and take constructive action. He chose the latter course. Jack decided to talk with the hospital's alcoholism counselor in order to get accurate information about drinking and to evaluate his own drinking habits. Jack confessed that he had worried about his drinking for a number of years, and he felt relieved that he was finally going to do something about it. Another decision that Jack made about his drinking was that he would avoid consuming alcohol on those occasions when he was driving. Although Jack knew that his decision would not be the right decision for everyone, he thought it was a decision essential for his own peace of mind. He also concluded that he needed to stop apologizing so much to Bob and begin discussing their accident experience on a different level. Jack wanted to know Bob's reactions to the accident. He also thought it was important to talk with Bob about how the accident had affected their long friendship.

Jack, in planning these actions, and in feeling good about them, demonstrated growth. He achieved a high level of understanding and acceptance of his responsibility for the losses he and Bob suffered. Jack used his understanding and acceptance as motivation for continued growth, despite the painfulness of that growth.

Although Jack worked through his loss, the memory of the accident will linger on. He may experience occasional feelings of guilt and remorse about the accident throughout his lifetime, although such feelings will no doubt diminish as time passes. By using the loss as a learning experience, Jack grew because of the accident as well as in spite of it.

As Jack grew stronger physically the time drew near for him to leave the hospital. The nurse with whom he had been working knew that she and Jack would soon need to face another loss situation — the ending of their working relationship. On several previous occasions Jack and the nurse had discussed the fact that he would eventually be leaving the hospital and would no longer have counseling sessions with her. The nurse planned for the final counseling sessions to be focused more specifically on the termination of their relationship:

N: We will be meeting for three more times before you leave.	
J: Oh, we'll still see each other.	Jack is trying to avoid facing separation from the nurse.

N: You don't want our relationship to end?	Reflection on the meaning of Jack's comment.
J: No, I'll come up to visit Bob and the other guys. Can't we say hello, too?	Jack is still trying to hold on to his relationship with the nurse.
N: I will probably be here, and of course I'll say hello to you. But our relationship will be different.	
J: Won't you talk with me anymore?	
N: What do you think you might like to talk with me about when you come to visit Bob and the other guys?	
J: Well, problems — like we do now.	Jack is still trying to hold on to his relationship with the nurse.
N: Sounds like you still feel you need someone to talk things over with.	Nurse reflects on meaning of Jack's statement again.
J: Yeah, and I'm used to talking with you. Why can't I keep on?	
N: You're wondering who you can talk to when I'm not available?	
J: Right. I don't have any family, except for my wife.	
N: What would happen if you talked with her?	
J: Well, Marie is always complaining that I don't talk to her enough. I don't know if she could take it if I told her some of my real feelings.	

The nurse continued discussing Jack's ideas and feelings about talking with his wife. He recognized that he did need to talk more with Marie; he also recognized that he would still be involved in outpatient sessions with the alcoholism counselor.

During Jack's final session with the nurse the following interaction took place:

J: I guess what you're saying is that I've got to find someone other than you to talk to.	Jack recognizes his need to replace the nurse with someone else.
N: Yes, that is what I'm saying.	The nurse validates with clarity.
J: I guess you're right. I can't come running to you with my problems. But I do want you to know you've helped me a lot.	
N: (Warmly.) I'm glad to know that.	In this instance the nurse accepts Jack's gratitude and chooses not to explore it. Exploration could open a new area for discussion and could be counterproductive to her termination with Jack.

SUMMARY

The interactions between Jack and the nurse illustrate the stages and tasks of loss resolution and the helping role of the nurse. Nursing assessment and intervention begin with the nurse's observations of the current behaviors of the patient that are indicative of loss. By sharing these observations with the patient the nurse initiates an exploration and discussion of the loss event.

As the nurse and the patient work together to clarify the patient's thoughts and feelings about the loss, the patient will be assisted to put the experience into a more realistic perspective. The nurse thereby helps the patient to pass through the various stages of loss resolution and to accomplish the tasks that challenge him. Hence the overwhelming loss can become more manageable, and the threat of a loss can be diminished. Furthermore, the nurse can assist the patient to terminate his relationship with her by further utilizing the skills he has developed for dealing with loss. Thus the nurse encourages continued growth.

References

Baker J M, Sorensen K C: A patient's concern with death. In Roe A, Sherwood M (eds): Nursing in the Seventies. New York, Wiley, 1973

Barlow J M: Loss and mourning: Some implications for psychotherapy. J Tenn Med Assoc 67:834, 1974

Colgrove M, Bloomfield H H, McWilliams P: How to Survive the Loss of a Love. New York, Leo Press, 1976

Lee J M: Working through—A conceptual framework for nursing. In Zderad L T, Belcher H C (eds): Developing Behavioral Concepts in Nursing. Atlanta, Southern Regional Education Board, 1968

McGrath J E: Major substantive issues: Time, setting and the coping process. In McGrath J E (ed): Social and Psychosocial Factors in Stress. New York, Holt, Rinehart and Winston, 1970

McIntire M S, Angle C, Struempler L: The concept of death in midwestern children and youth. Am Dis Child 123:527–532, 1972

Nagy M: The child's view of death. In Feifel H (ed): The Meaning of Death. New York, Harcourt, Brace and World, 1965, pp 79–98

Peretz D: Reaction to loss. In Schoenberg B et al (eds): Loss and Grief. New York, Columbia Univ Press, 1970

Rokeach M: Beliefs, Attitudes and Values. San Francisco, Jossey-Bass Behavioral Science, 1968

Selye H: The Stress of Life. New York, McGraw-Hill, 1956

Sullivan H S: The Interpersonal Theory of Psychiatry. New York, WW Norton, 1953

Wahl C W: The fear of death. In Feifel H (ed): The Meaning of Death. New York, McGraw-Hill, 1965

CHAPTER

8

PERSPECTIVES ON ALCOHOLISM

Nada J. Estes
M. Edith Heinemann

Alcoholism has been called our nation's most treatable untreated illness. It is a health problem of major significance. The lives of an estimated 10 million people have been adversely affected by the use of alcohol, and countless others such as family members and employers are directly or indirectly affected by alcoholism (USDHEW 1974). The scope of this problem is so immense that every person in a health profession is likely to encounter many clients with alcohol-related problems.

Professional nurses have the potential to make an important contribution in dealing with the problem of alcoholism. To be successful in intervening and preventing this disease, nurses must have knowledge about alcoholism and skills in dealing effectively with alcoholic people. The purpose of this chapter is to provide a perspective on facts, trends, and definitions in alcoholism, ways to assess alcoholic manifestations, and means of intervention.

FACTS, TRENDS, AND DEFINITIONS

Alcoholism is the number-one drug problem in the United States. It is a progressive illness, usually developing over a period of 5 to 20 years. Moreover, persons close to someone with an alcohol-related problem usually endure the problem for a long time. In over half of such instances family members have delayed seeking help for at least 10 years (USDHEW 1971).

Alcoholism is prevalent in all segments of our society. It tends to occur most frequently among those 35 to 55 years of age (Plaut 1967); however, in recent years there has been an increase in problem drinking and alcoholism among teenagers as well. The number of women with alcoholism is also increasing. Whereas the ratio of women alcoholics to men alcoholics formerly was estimated at 1:5, recent statistics show a 1:3 distribution. Alcoholism is more prevalent among persons in higher economic groups who are well educated and employed. Only 3 to 5 percent of alcoholic persons are in the skid-row category (Alcohol and Alcoholism, Problems, Programs and Progress 1972). Another subculture within our society is even more severely affected: that of the native American. Among American Indians alcoholism is virtually epidemic.

Recent federal legislation has had an impact on alcoholism through the establishment of the National Institute on Alcohol Abuse and Alcoholism (NIAAA) and the adoption of the Uniform Alcoholism and Intoxication Treatment Act. The aims of NIAAA, which was established in 1971, are to find new approaches to treatment and rehabilitation, to establish effective modes of prevention, to train more personnel in the field of alcoholism, and to erase public misconceptions about the nature of the ailment (Chafetz 1973). In the same year (1971) the Uniform Alcoholism and Intoxication Treatment Act was approved and recommended for adoption by all states. This legislation provides that alcoholics and intoxicated persons may not be subjected to criminal prosecution because of their consumption of alcoholic beverages, but rather shall be afforded a continuum of treatment in order that they may lead normal lives as productive members of society (USDHEW 1971).

Alcoholism has been difficult to define, most likely because it is not a single illness with a specific etiology, a known course, and a proven response to treatment. Rather, alcoholism takes different forms in different individuals, and it is the result of complex interacting forces. One definition of alcoholism is that of the World Health Organization (1952):

> Alcoholics are those excessive drinkers whose dependence upon alcohol has attained such a degree that it shows a noticeable mental disturbance or an interference with their bodily and mental health, their interpersonal relations, and their smooth social and economic functioning; or who show the prodromal signs of such developments.

One of the first scientists to define alcoholism as a disease that was progressive in nature was Jellinek (1952). He described four phases of alcohol addiction: (1) the prealcoholic symptomatic phase, in which the person experiences considerable reward from drinking; (2) the prodromal phase, characterized by the occurrence of blackouts* and preoccupation with drinking; (3) the crucial or basic phase, wherein loss of control over alcohol occurs, along with social withdrawal; (4) the chronic phase, which is heralded by the onset of the first bender and leads into psychologic and

**Partial amnesia without loss of consciousness.*

physiologic deterioration. It must be recognized that the symptoms described represent merely a sampling of all those described by Jellinek under the various phases.

A definition by Plaut (1967) that was built on Jellinek's work emphasizes a loss of control over alcohol: "Alcoholism is a condition in which an individual has lost control over his alcohol intake in the sense that he is consistently unable to refrain from drinking, or to stop drinking, before getting intoxicated" (Plaut 1967, p. 39).

Perhaps the most significant recent contribution in defining alcoholism was made by the Criteria Committee of the National Council on Alcoholism (1972). This group of medical authorities published the article "Criteria for the Diagnosis of Alcoholism" to establish guidelines for the proper diagnosis and evaluation of the disease. The committee viewed these criteria as a means of promoting early detection, providing a uniform nomenclature, and preventing overdiagnosis. Three diagnostic levels are identified that make it possible to arrive at a definite diagnosis, a probable diagnosis, or a potential diagnosis of alcoholism.

It is necessary for the nurse to have a clear understanding of what constitutes alcoholism in order to accurately assess alcoholic patients. Assessment, the initial step in providing patient care, has been defined by McCain (1965, p. 82) as an orderly and precise method of collecting information about the physiologic, psychologic, and social behavior of a patient. Accurate assessment of the alcoholic patient involves making careful observations about the patient and interpreting these observations on the basis of knowledge and practice. The prevalent physiologic and psychologic manifestations of alcoholism and the screening methods useful in assessing patients will be described.

PHYSIOLOGIC MANIFESTATIONS OF ALCOHOLISM

Alcoholism has been implicated as a primary or related causal factor in a large number of pathologic conditions. It is often associated with nutritional and mental disorders, diseases of the neurologic and digestive systems, and diseases of the heart, muscles, blood, and blood-forming organs. Moreover, alcoholics who are not successfully treated are subject to exceptionally high rates of mortality, with life spans being reduced by as much as 10 to 12 years (USDHEW 1971).

Alcohol directly affects the functioning of the central nervous system. Although the exact pharmacologic actions are unknown, it is known that the behavioral and depressant effects are dependent on dosage. The rapidity with which alcohol causes altered function of the central nervous system is related to such factors as its rate of absorption from the stomach and small intestine and the drinking history of the individual.

The rate of metabolism of alcohol in man is fairly constant at about 1 g/10 kg body weight per hour. In other words, an average 150-lb adult male who is not addicted to alcohol will under ordinary circumstances metabolize approximately 0.6 ounce of straight whiskey, 4 ounces of wine, or 16 ounces of beer in 1 hour (Manual on Alcoholism 1968). If a person drinks at a rate faster than the alcohol can be metabolized, the drug accumulates in the body, resulting in higher and higher concentrations of alcohol in the blood. Three major phenomena that result from the effects of alcohol on the central nervous system are alcohol intoxication, tolerance to alcohol, and physical dependence.

Alcohol intoxication is characterized by a range of symptom that increase in severity as the level of alcohol in the blood rises. In the average-size nonalcoholic person 2 or 3 ounces of whiskey in the body will raise the alcohol level of the blood to 0.05 percent, causing depression of the functions of the uppermost levels of the brain. Judgment, inhibition, and restraint are diminished, and the drinker may impulsively take many personal and social liberties. Five or 6 ounces of whiskey in the body result in a concentration of 0.10 percent alcohol in the blood. This concentration causes dulling of the lower motor area, resulting in slurring of speech and staggering gait. (A blood alcohol level of 0.10 percent is legal evidence of intoxication in most states.) Ten ounces of whiskey in the body cause a blood alcohol concentration of 0.20 percent. At this stage the entire motor area of the brain is affected, and the individual usually needs assistance to walk or dress. At 0.30 percent alcohol, which can result from 1 pint of whiskey in the body, the drinker has little comprehension of what he sees, hears, or feels. Coma ensues at higher levels, and at a level of 0.60 or 0.70 percent death may result because of inability of the lower brain centers to control breathing and other vital processes (Roebuck and Kessler 1972).

Tolerance is defined as adaptation or reduced sensitivity of the central nervous system to the effects of alcohol. It is a phenomenon common with chronic use of all addictive drugs, and it is believed to be one basis of addiction or dependence. It is this phenomenon that enables the alcohol-dependent person to consume up to a quart of whiskey a day without signs of gross inebriation. Such a person can accurately perform a series of complex tasks at blood alcohol levels several times as great as those that would lead to behavioral impairment in moderate and heavy drinkers (USDHEW 1971). According to the "Criteria for the Diagnosis of Alcoholism," evidence of tolerance, manifested by blood alcohol levels of 0.15 percent without gross evidence of intoxication, makes a diagnosis of alcoholism obligatory.

Tolerance permits large quantities of alcohol to circulate in the body, thereby permitting the development of physical dependence. Physical dependence involves cell adaptation to the presence of alcohol, which leads to the onset of symptoms of withdrawal when alcohol is abruptly removed. The alcohol withdrawal syndrome has been described as occurring in two major phases. The early phase, or minor withdrawal, makes its appearance 6 to 8 hours following cessation of drinking and is characterized by tremor and diaphoresis and in some instances by hallucinations or convulsions or both. A relatively small number of patients go on to experience the major syndrome, known as delirium tremens or DTs, which begins about 60 to 80 hours following cessation of drinking. It is characterized by increased psychomotor activity, gross tremor, profuse sweating, hallucinations, an absence of convulsions, and profound disorientation (Wolfe and Victor 1970).

Other disorders caused by the effects of alcohol on the nervous system include Wernicke's syndrome and Korsakoff's psychosis. Wernicke's syndrome is characterized by clouding of consciousness and paralysis of eye nerves and is associated with an acute severe deficiency of vitamin B_1. It responds well to prompt treatment with thiamine. Korsakoff's psychosis is characterized by disorientation, failure of memory, and a tendency to make up for the defect by substituting imagined occurrences. It sometimes follows on the symptoms of Wernicke's syndrome. Thiamine deficiency is also suspected in the causation of Korsakoff's psychosis (USDHEW 1971).

Another system frequently affected by chronic alcohol intake is the digestive system. Most of the harm done to this system occurs after alcohol is absorbed; however, when strong alcoholic beverages are consumed the irritating effect may cause direct local injury. The possible sites of such injury are the mouth, esophagus, stomach, and intestines. Ill-effects include inflammation, ulcerations, and malabsorption of various substances, the latter often leading to nutritional deficiencies and blood dyscrasias.

The liver is the organ most significantly involved with processing alcohol in the body, and at the same time it is most seriously affected by heavy drinking and alcohol abuse. Alcohol is implicated in producing fatty liver, alcoholic hepatitis, and alcoholic cirrhosis (Fenster 1969). The disorder of fatty liver is generally entirely reversible when alcohol abuse is terminated. Alcoholic hepatitis, not to be confused with viral or drug-induced hepatitis, usually subsides when drinking is stopped. The reversibility of alcoholic hepatitis is variable, depending on severity and chronicity. It is a potentially lethal condition, and some patients may die in hepatic failure despite discontinuing alcohol intake. Alcoholic cirrhosis, which is generally irreversible, is estimated to occur in about 10 percent of all alcoholic persons. It is characterized by diffuse scarring of the liver, and it correlates with the duration and amount of alcohol consumption.

The phenomena discussed above represent major pathologic disorders accompanying alcoholism. For a more comprehensive discourse on the pathologic complications of alcoholism, other references are available (Kissin and Begleiter 1974; Seixas and associates 1975).

PSYCHOLOGIC MANIFESTATIONS OF ALCOHOLISM

In addition to causing physiologic impairment, alcoholism has a great impact on a person's psychologic well-being. A wide range of behavioral and personality deviations have been attributed to alcoholism. One authority summarized the major psychologic problems of alcoholism as the three Ds: dependence, denial, and depression (Blane 1968).

Dependence has been viewed in different ways: some say it contributes to drinking problems, and others say it results from irresponsible drinking. A person who is unable to satisfy his dependence needs because of societal prohibitions against their expression may turn to alcohol to relieve the painful experience. On the other hand, the person who has developed alcoholism becomes less adequate in managing life situations and may as a result become overly dependent on others.

Three possible solutions have been identified that can occur as a person attempts to resolve the conflict that invariably accompanies unmet dependence needs: open dependence, counterdependence, and alternators. Each of these solutions results in a different set of observable behaviors.

Openly dependent persons have surrendered to dependence needs; they rely heavily on others for care. The person with alcoholism who expresses his dependence needs with openly dependent behaviors may freely admit to alcoholism in order to procure the attention of health care personnel. The counterdependent person submerges his wishes to be dependent from his awareness and acts in an overly independent manner. Such persons with alcoholism may come to the attention of health care personnel only because of some alcohol-related disorder, such as pneumonia or a fracture. The behavior of the alternator fluctuates between denying and displaying dependence needs according to circumstances and current life situations.

As a general rule it is better to support and reinforce the alcoholic's solution to conflict about dependence rather than to try to change it. This is especially true in early stage of sobriety when the person is involved in establishing a life without alcohol.

Denial has been described as "perhaps the most salient psychologic symptom of alcoholism" (Bailey 1972, p 6). It may be defined as the negation of reality by means of fantasy (Paredes 1974). The use of denial is prevalent among alcoholic people for several reasons. They often believe that alcoholism is shameful and should not occur. Extreme guilt about his behavior while intoxicated, the need to protect his falling self-esteem, and the false belief that he can stop drinking whenever he wishes, in spite of overwhelming evidence to the contrary, are additional reasons for the alcoholic's use of denial.

The use of denial occurs on a continuum. Psychotic denial, on the one extreme, is present when no amount of reason can sway a fixed idea. Normal denial, on the opposite end, does not involve a blanket, unqualified ignoring of reality, and rational thought can break through it.

Behaviors that fall between normal and psychotic are particularly observable in alcoholism. Alcoholic people sway between wish and reality. When the wish to drink dominates, denial is intense. When reality dominates, such as following a citation for drunk driving or when a spouse threatens divorce, denial is weak. Usually when alcoholic people are seen in treatment settings, some crisis has occurred in their lives. At this point denial is often minimal, and they are at that time more likely to accept intervention into their alcohol problems.

Depression is the most common psychologic disorder associated with alcoholism (Cadoret and Winokur 1974). It involves the lowering of self-esteem, which leads to feelings of worthlessness, helplessness, and hopelessness.

Alcoholics frequently experience disappointment and failure in living up to their own expectations, as well as the expectations of others, and this partly explains why they are prone to depression. In an effort to obliterate the pain of their depression many patients self-medicate with alcohol. This is initially effective, in that it temporarily dulls the pain, but continued intake eventually leads to deepening depression and the possibility of suicide.

The alcoholic population is considered a high-risk group for suicidal behavior. Many suicide attempts are made while drinking, as the potentially suicidal person may be able to make the transition from thought to action while drinking. Of all those who attempt suicide the alcoholic person has a much higher rate of success (Benensohn and Resnik 1974).

SCREENING FOR ALCOHOL PROBLEMS

Familiarity with the physiologic and psychologic manifestations of alcoholism is necessary for accurate screening and assessment of patients. The use of screening questions to determine the presence of alcohol problems needs to become a part of all routine intake information wherever patients are seen. When alcohol problems are identified by means of gross screening, more rigorous assessment should follow. There are instruments available to aid in the identification of alcoholism. One such tool, presented in Table 8.1 is the questionnaire of the National

Table 8.1. WHAT ARE THE SIGNS OF ALCOHOLISM?*

The following questions will help a person learn if he has some of the symptoms of alcoholism. He might use the questionnaire as a rough checklist to determine whether he or a member of his family may need help.

	YES	NO
1. Do you occasionally drink heavily after a disappointment, a quarrel, or when the boss gives you a hard time?	______	______
2. When you have trouble or feel under pressure, do you always drink more heavily than usual?	______	______
3. Have you noticed that you are able to handle more liquor than you did when you were first drinking?	______	______
4. Did you ever wake up on the "morning after" and discover that you could not remember part of the evening before, even though your friends tell you that you did not "pass out"?	______	______
5. When drinking with other people, do you try to have a few extra drinks when others will not know it?	______	______
6. Are there certain occasions when you feel uncomfortable if alcohol is not available?	______	______
7. Have you recently noticed that when you begin drinking you are in more of a hurry to get the first drink than you used to be?	______	______
8. Do you sometimes feel a little guilty about your drinking?	______	______
9. Are you secretly irritated when your family or friends discuss your drinking?	______	______
10. Have you recently noticed an increase in the frequency of your memory "blackout"?	______	______
11. Do you often find that you wish to continue drinking after your friends say they have had enough?	______	______
12. Do you usually have a reason for the occasions when you drink heavily?	______	______
13. When you are sober, do you often regret things you have done or said while drinking?	______	______
14. Have you tried switching brands or following different plans for controlling your drinking?	______	______
15. Have you often failed to keep the promise you have made to yourself about controlling or cutting down on your drinking?	______	______
16. Have you ever tried to control your drinking by making a change in jobs, or moving to a new location?	______	______
17. Do you try to avoid family or close friends while you are drinking?	______	______
18. Are you having an increasing number of financial and work problems?	______	______
19. Do more people seem to be treating you unfairly without good reason?	______	______
20. Do you eat very little or irregularly when you are drinking?	______	______
21. Do you sometimes have the "shakes" in the morning and find that it helps to have a little drink?	______	______
22. Have you recently noticed that you cannot drink as much as you once did?	______	______
23. Do you sometimes stay drunk for several days at a time?	______	______
24. Do you sometimes feel very depressed and wonder whether life is worth living?	______	______
25. Sometimes after periods of drinking, do you see or hear things that aren't there?	______	______
26. Do you get terribly frightened after you have been drinking heavily?	______	______

If you answered "Yes" to any of the questions, you have some of the symptoms that may indicate alcoholism. "Yes" answers to several of the questions indicate the following stages of alcoholism: questions 1–8, early stage; questions 9–21, middle stage; questions 22–26, the beginning of final stage.

**Reprinted by permission of the National Council on Alcoholism, 733 3rd Ave., New York, N.Y. 10017.*

Council on Alcoholism. It is a rough checklist to help a person determine whether he has a problem with alcoholism. It further enables him to determine if the symptom pattern being experienced fits the early, middle, or final stage of alcoholism.

A second tool useful in the identification of alcohol problems is the Short Michigan Alcoholism Screening Test (SMAST) presented in Table 8.2 (Selzer and associates 1975). This is considered to be a reliable and valid tool for diagnosing alcoholism.

Another means of eliciting information about alcohol problems is to use a set of direct questions requiring factual responses. The nurse can begin by asking such questions as these: "Has anyone ever said that drinking might be causing a problem for you? Has your wife ever complained about your drinking? How much do you drink on the average? Have you ever had to consider cutting down on your drinking?" (Weinberg 1974, p 109).

The specific screening instruments or questions used, although important, are of less significance than the patient's style and quality of response to the questions asked. The nurse should pay close attention to the way the patient reacts to the questions. Individuals who give matter-of-fact responses and who show no evidence of difficulty with alcohol can most likely be regarded as nonalcoholic. A second group of individuals includes

Table 8.2. SHORT MICHIGAN ALCOHOLISM SCREENING TEST*

1. Do you feel you are a normal drinker? (By normal we mean you drink less than or as much as most other people.)	No
2. Does your wife, husband, a parent, or other near relative ever worry or complain about your drinking?	Yes
3. Do you ever feel guilty about your drinking?	Yes
4. Do friends or relatives think you are a normal drinker?	No
5. Are you able to stop drinking when you want to?	No
6. Have you ever attended a meeting of Alcoholics Anonymous?	Yes
7. Has drinking ever created problems between you and your wife, husband, a parent, or other near relative?	Yes
8. Have you ever gotten into trouble at work because of drinking?	Yes
9. Have you ever neglected your obligations, your family, or your work for two or more days in a row because you were drinking?	Yes
10. Have you ever gone to anyone for help about your drinking?	Yes
11. Have you ever been in a hospital because of drinking?	Yes
12. Have you ever been arrested for drunken driving, driving while intoxicated, or driving under the influence of alcoholic beverages?	Yes
13. Have you ever been arrested, even for a few hours, because of other drunken behavior?	Yes

**Reprinted by permission from Selzer M L, Vinokur A, van Rooijen L: A self-administered Short Michigan Alcoholism Screening Test. J Stud Alcohol 36:117, 1975.*

Note: Scoring the SMAST involves assigning 1 point for each alcoholism-indicating response. Subjects scoring 0–1 are considered nonalcoholic; those with 2 points, possibly alcoholic; those with 3 or more points, alcoholic. The alcoholism-indicating responses are given at the right.

those who also respond in a straightforward manner to questions about alcohol but who express concern about their drinking. These individuals may be in the early stage of alcoholism and may be quite responsive to a discussion about the symptoms and progressive nature of alcoholism and the desirability of abstaining from alcohol. A third group includes those individuals who give responses that are aimed at convincing the history-taker that the person has no problem with alcohol. These individuals are most likely alcoholic; they reflect the denial system that is symptomatic of alcoholism. A more thorough drinking history should be taken with this group, along with questions to determine how alcohol has affected the person's physical and psychosocial health (Weinberg 1974).

A final group consists of late-stage alcoholic people who have been in and out of health care facilities for many years because of their alcoholism. These people's lives revolve around alcohol. When questioned about use of alcohol they readily admit to problems, often with a sad defeated affect. Some of these people may be experiencing severe depression and may be suicidal because the cycle of events surrounding their use of alcohol seems so futile and hopeless. A screening device to help determine the lethality (the likelihood of a person taking his life) of such people is an important aspect of assessment (see Chapter 9).

In addition to making direct inquiry, the nurse can be alert to clues that may indicate alcoholism. Clues mentioned in Table 8.3 (Estes and Hanson 1976) are those manifestations that can be readily observed or conveyed in conversation; this listing is not considered exhaustive.

After the brief gross screening, patients in whom alcoholism cannot be ruled out require more detailed assessment. Here reference is made to the nursing history for use with patients with alcohol problems, as presented in Table 8.4 (Heinemann and Estes 1976). This tool is designed to focus on those aspects that frequently cause problems in alcoholic patients. Major content areas cover information about drinking history, symptoms related to damage-prone systems, psychosocial status, and use of other drugs. Questions related to emergency conditions and impending withdrawal symptoms are marked with an asterisk, while the remaining questions are for acquiring information from patients who have completed the drying-out or withdrawal period.

When the data obtained from the nursing history interview are combined with information from other sources, such as physical assessment, laboratory findings, and past health records, it is possible to design a plan of care that is comprehensive and responsive to the patient's needs. The quality of the data gathered in the assessment process is dependent on the nurse's interviewing skills and knowledge about alcoholism. The nursing history serves primarily as a guide, and the nurse should strive for ingenuity in its use.

Table 8.3. CLUES IN ASSESSMENT OF ALCOHOL-RELATED PROBLEMS*

PHYSICAL	BEHAVIORAL
Multiple bruises of different ages, most frequently at table-top height, or oven burns of different ages on arms, particularly in women (both caused by psychomotor incoordination during intoxication)	Coming to a scheduled appointment with alcohol on breath
Numerous scars on hands and face from falling when drunk or when in fights.	Failure to report for medical attention following an injury until several hours or days have passed; such delay can result from the fact that pain is masked by the anesthetic properties of alcohol or from the individual's reluctance to be seen intoxicated.
Healed or unhealed slashmarks across wrists, reflecting the high rate of suicide attempts in alcoholic persons	Frequent Monday morning absences from work for minor illness that in reality is a hangover
Flushed face caused by vasodilation effects of alcohol	Employment choices that facilitate drinking, such as those where a person can function independently or those that encourage business conducted over a three-martini luncheon
Periorbital edema and pretibial edema due to retention of fluid following a drunk	Frequent major or minor auto accidents, with vague explanations as to cause
Appearing older than stated age because of the debilitating effects of prolonged excessive use of alcohol	Frequent changes of residence for poorly defined reasons, reflecting attempts to seek geographic cure
	Frequent references to alcohol or alcohol use indicating the importance of alcohol in the individual's life

**Adapted from Estes N J, Hanson K J: Perspectives for the Nurse Practitioner 1:125, 1976.*

INTERVENING IN ALCOHOLISM

Alcoholism is a treatable illness from which as many as two-thirds of those afflicted can recover. When the alcoholic person is still living in an intact family unit and holding a job, the outlook for recovery with appropriate treatment is quite optimistic. Complete abstinence, which is only one measure of recovery, is more difficult to attain for the majority of alcoholic people. However, if one accepts as measures of rehabilitation the reestablishment of a good family life, a satisfactory work record, a respectable position in the community, and the ability to control drinking most of the time, a successful outcome can be expected in 60 to 80 percent of treated individuals (Alcohol and Alcoholism, Problems, Programs and Progress 1972).

Table 8.4. NURSING HISTORY TOOL FOR USE WITH PATIENTS WITH ALCOHOL PROBLEMS*

1. For what reason did you come to this agency?
2. What do you most want help with at the present time?

DRINKING HISTORY

3. How old were you when you started drinking alcohol regularly?
4. How long have you had problems with alcohol?
5. How often do you drink alcoholic beverages?
6. What kinds of alcoholic beverages do you drink?
7. How much of each alcoholic beverage do you drink?

†8. When did you have your last drink?
†9. When did you start your last drinking bout?
†10. What have you been drinking during this last drinking episode?
†11. How much alcohol did you consume each day during your last drinking episode?
†12. Has your drinking created problems for you in any of the following areas?

with spouse ______ on the job ______
with family ______ with children ______
with friends ______ ____________

13. Have you ever been injured because of drinking? Yes ______ No ______
in fights ______ accidental fall ______
auto accident ______ other ______
14. Have you ever been arrested because of drinking? Yes ______ No ______ On what charge:
DWI ______ fights ______
drunk in public ______ other (specify) ______
15. Have your ever been in prison or jail because of drinking? Yes ______ No ______
16. What previous treatments have you had for alcohol problems?

Date	**Place**
____________	____________
____________	____________

SYMPTOMS RELATED TO GASTROINTESTINAL SYSTEM

†17. What have you been eating during this most recent drinking bout?
†18. What is your usual eating pattern?
(a) When not drinking:
(b) When drinking:

19. Have you had recent changes in appetite?
20. Have you had any recent weight changes?
21. Are you on a special diet?
22. What fluids do you drink other than alcohol?
Kind of fluid and amount per day.
regular coffee ______ tea ______ water ______
decaffeinated coffee ______ juices ______ milk ______
23. Do you have frequent irritation of your mouth and throat?
24. Are you having pain in your stomach?
25. Are you bothered by heartburn or gas?

†26. Are you nauseated?
†27. Are you vomiting or having dry heaves?
†28. Have you ever vomited blood? If yes, when?
†29. Have you ever had stomach ulcers or other stomach problems?

30. How frequently and for what reason do you use aspirin?

Table 8.4, cont.

31. What medications do you use to relieve stomach pain?
32. Are you having pain in your abdomen?
33. Are you having diarrhea or constipation?
34. Do you have hemorrhoids?
35. Have you had bleeding from your bowels?
36. Have you noted a change in the color of your stool?
    clay colored ______ black ______ bright red ______
37. What problems have you had in the past with your bowels?
38. What medications do you use to relieve abdominal or bowel pains?
39. Have you ever had problems with your pancreas?

†40. Has your skin or the white of your eyes ever turned yellow?
†41. Have you ever had problems with your liver?
†42. Do you have diabetes? If yes, what medication do you take?

SYMPTOMS RELATING TO NEUROLOGICAL SYSTEM

43. Have you noticed any change in the amount of alcohol it takes to get the effect you desire? If yes, describe the change.

†44. What reactions occur when you stop drinking?

tremors	____________	d.t.'s	____________
seizures	____________	other	____________
hear or see things	____________		____________

†45. Have you ever taken Dilantin or any other drug for seizures?
46. Have you ever experienced a period of time you don't remember when drinking?
47. Have you experienced tingling, pain, or numbness in hands or feet?
48. Have you experienced muscle pain in your legs or arms?

†49. Are you experiencing any difficulty in keeping your balance?
†50. Are you experiencing any difficulty with your vision?
51. Do you have problems with your sleep? If yes, describe.
52. How many hours do you usually sleep? ______________________________
    When sober ______________________________
    When drinking ______________________________
53. Do you feel rested after a night's sleep?
54. What do you do when you are unable to sleep?
55. Have you noticed any recent changes in your sex life? If yes, describe.

SYMPTOMS RELATING TO CARDIOVASCULAR AND PULMONARY SYSTEM

†56. Do you have heart trouble? If yes, describe.
†57. Do you have swelling of the hands and feet?
†58. Do you have shortness of breath?
†59. Do you have chest pain?
†60. Are you taking any medication for heart disease?
61. Have you had pneumonia?
62. Have you ever had tuberculosis? If yes, are you taking any medication for it?
63. Do you have frequent infections? (e.g., colds, flu, boils, sores that don't heal quickly).
64. Do you have a chronic cough? If yes, describe.
65. Have you ever coughed up blood or phlegm?
66. Describe any other lung problems you have had.
67. Do you smoke? If yes, how many packs a day?

PSYCHOSOCIAL STATUS

68. What is your marital status?
69. With whom do you live?

(Continued)

Table 8.4., cont.

70. Does this person have alcoholism or use alcohol regularly? Yes ______ No ______
71. To whom do you feel close?
72. Do your neighbors, relatives, and/or friends use alcohol regularly?
    Yes ______ No ______
73. How many children do you have?
74. How often do you see your children?
75. Describe the place you live.
    type of residence (ie, house, apartment, room, etc)
    cooking facilities
    number of stairs
    availability and type of transportation
76. Have you had mental or emotional problems?

depression	______	suicidal attempt	______
nervousness (anxiety)	______	other	______
loneliness	______	____________________	

77. Are you currently involved in a counseling program?

†78. Are you currently taking medication for emotional problems? If yes, describe.

79. Are you actively affiliated with a religious group?
80. What is your current employment status?
81. Do you have some special job skills?
82. If employed, how does this period of treatment affect your employment?
83. If unemployed, what is your current source of income?
84. What hobbies or special interests do you have?
85. How do you spend a typical day at home?

DRUG TAKING OTHER THAN ALCOHOL

†86. What drugs do you take that you haven't mentioned?
    prescribed drugs ____________________
    over-the-counter drugs ____________________
    drugs obtained on the street ____________________

†87. What is your usual manner of taking drugs?
    as directed____________________
    more than directed ____________________
    less than directed____________________

†88. Are you allergic to any drugs?

FINAL QUESTIONS

89. What are your ideas for managing your drinking when you leave this agency?
90. Are there any further comments you would like to make?
91. Are there any questions you would like to ask?

Write a summary of the nursing history interview.

1. Describe your overall impressions of the client (mood, attitude, intelligence, ability to relate, social skills, general physical and emotional health, level of orientation, reliability of information given).
2. List all the problems identified in order of priority.
3. Suggest a plan of action for each problem identified.

**From Heinemann E, Estes N: Am J Nurs 76:5, 785–789, 1976, with permission.*

†Indicates questions providing important information for a quick survey of intoxicated patients.

Treatment interventions for alcoholic persons can be successful primarily at times of acute intoxication, during withdrawal, when health problems associated with alcoholism become evident, and when the person desires to alter long-term destructive drinking patterns. While the latter goal of altering destructive drinking patterns is best accomplished in settings where specialized treatment for alcoholism is provided, the former situations usually require intensive care in a hospital environment.

Communities typically offer a variety of services for the person with alcohol-related problems: community alcohol centers, alcohol inpatient treatment centers, outpatient clinical services, and Alcoholics Anonymous.

The community alcohol center is an agency where anyone may receive information about the disease of alcoholism. Primarily it is a place where the needs of persons with alcohol-related problems are assessed; when it is appropriate, these clients may be referred to an alcoholism treatment program. To ensure the success of the referral the client must play an active role in deciding on an appropriate treatment plan.

An alcoholism inpatient treatment center offers comprehensive intensive care to alcoholic persons who require periods of continuous inpatient care, usually lasting from 3 weeks to 3 months. Professional and paraprofessional personnel offer a number of basic services, including evaluation and diagnosis, education about alcohol and alcoholism, individual and group counseling, referral to specialized resources in the community following release, and orientation to Alcoholics Anonymous. In addition, many such centers offer family counseling and a follow-up program after discharge. Some patients may require a longer treatment program in an alcoholism facility where vocational, recreational, and social rehabilitation services can be added to the patient's treatment plan.

Outpatient clinics for alcoholic clients provide the customary diagnostic and evaluative service, along with individual, group, and family therapy. Therapy is provided for the problem drinker and the alcoholic person and members of their families.

The best known self-help organization for alcoholic persons is the voluntary organization known as Alcoholics Anonymous (AA). AA was formed in the 1930s; the sole purpose of this fellowship of alcoholic individuals is to help themselves and each other to get sober and stay sober. AA claims to offer its members a way back to life and a design for living. It is estimated that perhaps 450,000 to 500,000 alcoholic men and women participate in AA around the world. Despite its breadth, AA reaches only a small percentage of the estimated 10 million alcoholic people and problem drinkers who need help.

Not only does an alcoholic person's drinking have deleterious personal effects, but also it profoundly affects close family members. Another organization, Al-Anon, has been established to help wives and husbands of alcoholic persons, using techniques similar to those of AA. Alateen is a program devoted to aiding the children of alcoholic parents to understand and cope with their parents' problems.

It has been noted that the general population of alcoholic persons includes different types who do better in different kinds of treatment. Tailoring the treatment approach to meet individual needs yields the greatest benefits for alcoholic persons. Treatment techniques that have met with success for various alcoholic persons who have progressed beyond the acute stages of intoxication and withdrawal include psychotherapy, hypnosis, aversion therapy, and use of deterrent agents.

Psychotherapeutic approaches for alcoholic persons tend to be more actively directed than therapy for general psychiatric patients, focusing on the immediate situation and on the person's drinking problem. In counseling alcoholic persons, whether individually or in groups, it is essential to break through the person's denial of a drinking problem. This process is often complex. Its goal is to enable alcoholic persons to recognize the pivotal role of alcohol as the destructive force in their lives. When the reality of the problem has been confronted, the person needs assistance in rebuilding a life without reliance on alcohol. This entails a search for new meanings and goals in life, a journey that may require prolonged intensive effort but one that can be rewarding in terms of evolving maturity.

Hypnosis can be used to explore feelings and memories that are not readily available to conscious experience but that play an important role in precipitating drinking episodes. Posthypnotic suggestion can be given to make abstinence seem desirable and drinking unpleasant (USDHEW 1971).

Aversion therapy consists of administering an alcoholic beverage at the same time as an aversive stimulus, such as electric shock or an emetic drug. Repeated treatments with such a combination are intended to develop a conditioned reflex loathing for alcohol in any form (Alcohol and Alcoholism, Problems, Programs and Progress 1972).

Two commonly used deterrent agents are disulfiram (Antabuse) and citrated calcium carbimide (Temposil). The alcoholic patient regularly taking one of these compounds will find that if alcohol is taken in any form a pounding headache, flushing, and usually violent nausea, vomiting, and other unpleasant symptoms will result (Fox 1967). In no instance is the use of aversion methods or deterrent agents considered a total therapy in itself. The drug simply helps the alcoholic person maintain sobriety long enough to permit involvement in a deeper form of therapy necessary to arrest the disease.

Many challenges remain in the alcoholism field, even though a great deal of progress has been made in recent years in understanding and treating the alcoholic person. It is now possible to view the alcoholic person with real hope. It is very timely for nurses to prepare themselves to participate in therapeutic interventions in alcoholism.

SUMMARY

Facts, trends, and definitions relating to alcoholism have been presented. Ways of assessing manifestations of alcoholism and some means of intervention have been discussed to better enable nurses to deal effectively with alcoholic people.

References

Alcohol and Alcoholism, Problems, Programs and Progress. National Institute of Mental Health, National Institute on Alcohol Abuse and Alcoholism, Washington DC, US Government Printing Office, 1972

Bailey M B: Alcoholism and Family Casework: Theory and Practice. New York, Community Council of Greater New York, 1972

Benensohn H S, Resnik H L P: A jigger of alcohol, a dash of depression, and bitters. A suicidal mix. Ann NY Acad Sci 233:15–21, 1974

Blane H T: The Personality of the Alcoholic: Guises of Dependency. New York, Harper & Row, 1968

Cadoret R, Winokur G: Depression in alcoholism. Ann NY Acad Sci 233:35–39, 1974

Chafetz M: An Interview with Dr. Morris Chafetz. Alcohol Health and Research World 1:2, Spring 1973

Criteria Committee, National Council on Alcoholism: Criteria for the diagnosis of alcoholism. Ann Intern Med 77:249–258, 1972

Estes N J, Hanson K J: Alcoholism in the family. Perspectives for the Nurse Practitioner 1:125, January-February 1976

Fenster F L: The spectrum of alcoholic liver disease. Bulletin of the Mason Clinic March 1969, pp 24–32

Fox R: Disulfiram (Antabuse) as an adjunct in the treatment of alcoholism. In Fox R (ed): Alcoholism. New York, Springer, 1967

Heinemann E, Estes N: Assessing alcoholic patients. Am J Nurs 76:5, 785–789, May 1976

Jellinek E M: Phases of alcohol addiction. Q J Stud Alcohol 13:673–684, December 1952

Kissin B, Begleiter H: The Biology of Alcoholism, Vol 3: Clinical Pathology. New York, Plenum, 1974

Manual on Alcoholism. Chicago, AMA 1968

McCain F: Nursing by assessment—not intuition. Am J Nurs 65:82–84, 1965

Plaut T F A: Alcohol Problems—A Report to the National Cooperative Commission on the Study of Alcoholism. New York, Oxford Univ Press, 1967

Paredes A: Denial, deception maneuvers, and consistency in the behavior of alcoholics. Ann NY Acad Sci 233:23–33, 1974

Roebuck J B, Kessler R G: The Etiology of Alcoholism. Springfield, Ill, Charles C Thomas, 1972

Seixas F A, Williams K, Eggleston S: Medical consequences of alcoholism. Ann NY Acad Sci 252:152, 1975

Selzer M L, Vinokur A, van Rooijen L: A self-administered Short Michigan Alcoholism Screening Test. J Stud Alcohol 36:117–126, 1975

United States Department of Health, Education and Welfare. First Special Report to the U.S. Congress on Alcohol and Health from the Secretary of Health, Education and Welfare. DHEW publication (HSM) 73-9031. Washington DC, US Government Printing Office, 1971

United States Department of Health, Education and Welfare. Second Special Report to the U.S. Congress on Alcohol and Health from the Secretary of Health, Education and Welfare, DHEW publication (ADM) 74-124. Washington DC, US Government Printing Office, 1974

Weinberg J: Interview Techniques for Diagnosing Alcoholism. Am Fam Physician 9:107–115, 1974

What are the signs of alcoholism? National Council on Alcoholism, New York

Wolfe M, Victor M: The physiological basis of the alcohol withdrawal syndrome. In Mello N, Mendelson J (eds): Recent Advances in Studies on Alcohol. Rockville, Md, NIMH, NIAAA, 1970, pp 188–199

World Health Organization, Expert Committee on Mental Health, Alcoholism Subcommittee: Second report. WHO Tech Rep Ser No. 48, August, 1952

CHAPTER

9

VIOLENT BEHAVIORS

Margaret L. Larson

Violence has been defined as "the exercise of physical force so as to inflict injury or damage to persons or property" (Gunn 1973, p 14). It is destructive aggression. Whether violence is turned outward to affect those around a person or inward to threaten his own existence, violent behavior is antithetical to our value system and a threat to our society. Suicide and homicide flaunt that which we hold in highest regard: human life.

Professionals working with the homicidal or suicidal person need to be acutely aware of their own feelings and values, for their anxieties about the crucial issues of life and death influence the decisions they make. Probably no situations require more self-understanding and introspection on the part of the professional than those associated with disturbed behaviors where life is threatened. Many nurses may never have to deal with such situations, but those who do will probably feel intense anxiety and doubt their ability to handle the situation. Understanding the dynamics of violent behavior can help the nurse to formulate an effective plan of action for intervening.

This chapter has been developed to provide the nurse with a better understanding of the dynamics of disturbed behaviors. Guidelines for assessing destructive behaviors are offered, with suggestions for interventions. Both aggression directed inward (suicide) and aggression directed outward (the threat to harm or kill a person or destroy property) are included. Measures related to the prevention of violence are also presented.

DESTRUCTIVE AGGRESSION TURNED INWARD: SUICIDE

Self-destructive behaviors have been studied extensively by many behavioral scientists. Their studies offer nurses who work with suicidal patients some understanding of the phenomenon and a rational basis for intervening. Profiles have been developed for identifying high-risk populations and assessing suicidal potential. This is important information for everyone working in the health care field; it is of paramount importance to those who have the primary responsibility for assessing patients and initiating interventions (Diran 1976). This might be the nurse in the emergency room, the nurse in a general hospital unit, or the nurse in the community.

Populations at Risk

Statistics reveal that suicide occurs with greatest frequency among middle-aged men who have experienced recent life crises and who live alone in urban areas. Depression is frequently a precursor to the decision to kill oneself. Drug and alcohol abuse increase the likelihood of suicide, as does a history of life crisis events: recent illness or terminal illness, intractable pain, a significant loss such as loss of a job, death of a spouse, or loss of a pet, a history of previous suicide attempts, or a suicide of a family member. Although more women attempt suicide, more men succeed, because they tend to select more lethal means (Shader 1975).

Each individual's total situation must be considered, for self-destruction can accompany the clinical patterns of the adolescent in turmoil, the middle-aged woman, and the elderly person who has abandoned hope. It is a possible choice that is considered by many psychotics of all ages who despair of ever living a normal life (Diran 1976).

Threat of Suicide

A telephone call from a desperate friend or relative or from a stranger contemplating self-destruction may be your first involvement with the problem of suicide. Farberow and associates (1970) have identified the steps in handling such a call; these guidelines are based on the experiences of the Los Angeles Suicide Prevention Center, and they have become basic to most crisis services.

Maintain Contact with the Caller. The call is an opportunity to obtain information and establish a relationship. You will want to get as much information as possible, such as the caller's name, telephone number, address, and any possible resources (friends or relatives). Ask direct, specific questions about suicidal feelings even if the person does not mention suicide. For example: "Have you thought of killing yourself?" "Are you thinking of suicide?"

Identify the Major Problem. Frequently the suicidal person is confused and overwhelmed by his situation and his feelings. An objective outsider can often assist in sorting out the problems and validating the feelings. Acceptance of the person, without challenge or criticism of his verbalizations, is important in conveying one's respect and gaining his trust.

Determine Whether the Caller Is Likely to Take Specific Action. Review the high-risk factors such as the person's age, sex, and life style. Suicide potential increases with age and with instability as evidenced in a poor work record, poor family relationships, and prior suicide attempts. Ask him if he has a plan; the lethality of the method, the availability of means, and the specificity of detail increase the potential for suicide. Explore the responses of significant others to the caller's suicidal behavior. A total breakdown of all communication with others is reason for alarm, because this cuts off potential rescuers. Rejection or withdrawal of those close to the person, or their denial that his suicide threat is serious, conveys to him the impression that help is not available or that his situation is hopeless, and this intensifies his desperate feelings.

Assess His Strengths and Resources. Evidence of success in past endeavors, response by the caller to your suggestions or directions, improvement in mood during the call, or even ability to focus on the conversation may be considered strengths. Any other people near the caller are resources you can consider involving in a plan of intervention.

Develop a Plan of Action. A plan of action may include mobilization of emergency resources such as police or an outreach team if the situation warrants this. More frequently, urging the caller to go to a hospital emergency room or arranging an appointment for him to meet with someone at a mental health center the following day, along with supportive listening during his call, will get him through his immediate crisis. Contact should be maintained with the caller until a plan is worked out and some change has occurred in his mood and tone or the situation is otherwise altered (Farberow and associates 1970).

An example of assessment of the seriousness of a suicide threat occurred in an emergency room. A nurse received a call from a man who spoke with slurred speech; he announced that he was going to "blow his head off" because his wife had left him. The nurse's opinion was that he sounded upset and desperate. He said he had been drinking to get up the nerve to kill himself. She inquired whether he had a gun and whether it was loaded. He did not have one, but he planned to purchase one the following day. The nurse explored the situation in greater detail and eventually made a referral so that he could receive help in working on his marital problems. Had the man been holding a loaded gun, the plan would have been to get his address and then alert police and the outreach team to help; the nurse would have had to try to keep him on the telephone until this was accomplished. The support she provided in talking with him and her ability to give him a specific time and place for getting additional help were sufficient in this instance.

> There has been a tendency recently for mild suicidal attempts to become an almost fashionable means of coping with crises among immature individuals, occasionally with fatal results and certainly with increased demands on medical and social services. Some cases of suicidal behavior are quite trivial and manipulative episodes, while in others the patient may possess considerable determination to kill himself (Bridges 1971, p 85).

Suicide Attempt

A deliberate act to end one's life is called a suicide attempt. In one instance a 22-year-old woman was admitted to an emergency room accompanied by her husband. He reported that she had gone to the bathroom and gulped a handful of sleeping pills (four times the lethal dose). Then she went to the den where he was studying and told him what she had done. Following gastric lavage she was permitted to return home. The couple were willing to talk about their frustrations and anger with each other, and they agreed to seek help. The woman's behavior was considered a form of communication, and it had already brought about some changes in the relationship so that she was no longer at high risk.

Stengel (1974) calls this the appeal effect, since some response from others in the person's environment is usually forthcoming. Every suicide attempt has an appeal function; it is a cry for help, even when there may be little conscious awareness of this fact. It is necessary to discriminate between a serious attempt and what may be called a suicide gesture. Stengel (1974, p 83) has defined the effort to end one's life as a deliberate act of self-damage that the person committing the act cannot be sure he will survive. The seriousness of the act can be evaluated on the basis of four factors: (1) the risk taken, or the degree of danger to his life that the individual believed his act involved; (2) the hazard that actually was involved; (3) the actual damage the individual suffered, such as injury or level of consciousness when found; (4) the social situation at the time of the act, which includes the degree of probability that no one would intervene or rescue the person.

If there is a high rating on any two of these factors the attempt can be considered as potentially fatal and indeed serious. Only if the person clearly took no subjective risk (ie, he knew the act was not risky) should the attempt be considered a gesture. The jilted adolescent who cuts her wrists when someone is nearby is at less risk than the woman who reveals her plan to wait until her husband leaves on a business trip and then take all the pills in her possession.

Assessment of Intent

Beck and associates (1974) developed a scale to measure suicidal intent. Although this is a research tool, it identifies major areas for a practitioner to explore in determining the seriousness of an individual's self-destructive attempt.

When the person is cooperative and responsive the nurse can obtain by interview much of the information needed to assess the gravity of the attempt. The patient's chart may provide some facts if the person has been admitted to the hospital. It is well for the nurse to familiarize herself with whatever facts are available. Friends and relatives of the person may be helpful in offering additional details.

The circumstances related to the suicide attempt can be assessed by reviewing six factors. These constitute a continuum that measures the degree of the individual's intention, from gravely serious intent to extreme ambivalence (Beck and associates 1974, pp 54–56):

1. *Timing and isolation.* If no one was nearby or was in contact with the person, intervention was highly unlikely; at the other extreme on the continuum, if someone was present or was within easy reach intervention was to be expected.
2. *Precautions against discovery.* Extensive precautions were taken to prevent discovery versus nothing was done to avoid discovery.
3. *Attempt to get help.* The person made no effort to contact someone for help; alternatively, an effort was made to obtain help after the attempt was made.
4. *Plans for attempt.* Elaborate plans were made, including making out a will or taking out insurance; at the other end of the continuum the person made no plans and acted on impulse.
5. *Communication of intent.* An unequivocal message of intent, written or verbal, was given; at the opposite extreme there was no note or other communication regarding the act.
6. *Purpose of attempt.* The person intended to remove himself from his environment; on the other hand, he merely wanted to effect changes or manipulate his environment.

The intent scale also includes subjective information from the person regarding the suicide act. The following points of information reveal the person's perception of his behavior regarding the attempt on a continuum (Beck and associates 1974, pp 54–56):

1. *Expectations of fatality.* Either the individual believed death was certain or he did not consider death or did less damage than he knew to be necessary for death.
2. *Perception of seriousness.* Either the individual considered the act a serious attempt to end his life or he did not think that it was.
3. *Ambivalence toward living.* Either he specifically wanted to die or he did not.

4. *Reversibility of attempt.* Either the individual did not believe medical attention could save him or he thought death unlikely if he was given medical attention.
5. *Degree of planning.* Either he thought about the act for more than 3 hours or he gave it no thought and acted on impulse.

Exploration of each point gives a more complete picture of the person's behavior than assuming that the act was just an accident or that it was a manipulative gesture. Exploring these aspects of his behavior may also lead the person to accept responsibility for his behavior, rather than deny it or minimize the seriousness of what he has done. Confronting the person with the fact that his self-destructive efforts are taken seriously has been called crisis maintenance and is aimed at encouraging the suicidal person to recognize his need for more effective ways of coping with his situation and to seek help after the crisis subsides (Blaker 1969).

The need for continued close observation arises when the attempt has been deemed serious and there are minimal resources to draw on after the rescue. A 60-year-old widower was admitted to a psychiatric unit following an attempt to use carbon monoxide poisoning. He was brought to the hospital by a concerned friend who described the man's increasing despondence following retirement for health reasons 6 months earlier. Although the patient protested that he had been foolish and had learned his lesson, he was admitted for treatment because he showed symptoms of severe depression and he lived alone.

Management of Suicidal Patients

An attitude of acceptance, hope, and encouragement must be conveyed to the self-destructive person to offset the hopelessness and despair that he is experiencing. Treatment of depression by medication may be indicated. Hostility and anger frequently are expressed following an attempt. Accepting these feelings and exploring them are important parts of assisting the suicidal person to find better ways of dealing with his aggression. This is an important responsibility because the unpleasantness of his anger and depression succeeds in driving so many people away from him, further confirming his belief that he has no value (Floyd 1975).

The nurse must establish communication and attend fully to what the person is saying and how he says it. This is an ongoing process that keeps her in touch with his mood and conveys her availability and her acceptance of the person. She can restore the individual's self-esteem by letting him know that she cares. She can encourage involvement with others and discourage isolation, because suicide is a solitary act. Having people near him and involving him in interactions lessens his opportunity and reduces his need for self-destruction as an alternative.

Confidentiality is not a concern when the patient's life is at stake. The nurse must not collaborate in keeping suicidal ideas or plans a secret. She must involve other people, such as family and friends, and when the patient is in a treatment program his fellow patients can also be involved. The more secret and devious the communication remains around suicide, the more possible self-destruction becomes.

A depressed teenager in a day-treatment program sought out a student nurse and confided that she thought that only the student nurse really understood her. The patient said that she had something important to tell but it must be kept a secret. The student agreed to this, only to have the patient reveal her plans to kill herself. Alarmed, the student pointed out that this could not be kept confidential; the patient had to share it with staff members and other patients in the program. With the student's support and assistance the patient discussed her suicidal ideas in the group meeting that followed.

Talking with a suicidal person about his ideas on suicide helps him to gain some understanding of why he wants to die and what would make life worth living. The nurse should help him set some goals; however short-term or small they may be, they represent the first step toward planning for the future. The shift to less observation and protection of the suicidal person is a crucial risk that must be taken eventually. The decision should be based on his improvement, as evidenced by his mood, his involvement with others, and an indication that he is oriented to the future (Shader 1975).

The suicidal person who should be managed on an outpatient basis usually is at low risk, or if he is at high risk, he usually has a number of people around him who are involved with him and can provide some protection. Treatment frequently involves establishing a contract or agreement with the person to the effect that he will not attempt to harm himself but rather will get in touch with the therapist or a clinic when he is distressed, so that they can talk about his problem. A three-way conference between the therapist, a significant other, and the suicidal person is recommended in which approaches to helping him when he is upset can be discussed. The three-way conference provides on-the-spot evidence of how those around him are responding to his threat of suicide (Balsam and Balsam 1974).

The question of a person's right to die by his own hand if he so chooses has been raised with increasing frequency in the past few years. Given the suicidal person's ambivalence about dying and the fact that the person who is intent on self-destruction is usually depressed when he makes the attempt, it seems reasonable to try to intervene. The desire to live is often restored when the person realizes that someone cares about him, and the depression is usually a temporary condition that can be treated (Fawcett 1974).

> No matter how thoughtful or responsible we are in caring for people who are self-destructive, there will be people who commit suicide. We may listen carefully and try to understand, but it is not possible to help everybody. The important point is to try (Balsam and Balsam 1974, p 187).

There are those who find life so empty and so distressing that the chance presented by being rescued from suicide is only the chance to try suicide again, rather than the chance to live and overcome the disappointments of life (Shader 1975).

DESTRUCTIVE AGGRESSION TURNED OUTWARD: HARMING OTHERS

While guilt is the major feeling evoked by another person's suicide, fear is our reaction to the threat of homicide. There is fear for the intended victim and fear for one's own life. Less has been written about homicidal behavior than about suicidal behavior in the psychiatric literature because once definite steps are taken to kill or to harm another person it becomes a legal matter. However, there are incidents in psychiatric treatment settings and in the community where overt aggression requires intervention, and the nurse may be called on to intervene. A recent study indicates that more patients who are impulsive and violent are being seen for psychiatric treatment than ever before (Whitman and associates 1976).

The threat to harm others requires evaluation, just as does the threat of suicide. Although less research has been done on the topic, there are guidelines available.

Populations at Risk

Who are the people most likely to act out their destructive and hostile feelings? What are the characteristics of the violent person? In what situations is violence more likely to erupt? Research indicates that men are more likely to resort to violence than women. The men who are involved in overt aggression are usually between 20 and 40 years of age. They are often members of ethnic minorities who live in social and economic deprivation (Tupin 1975).

The early history of the violent person frequently reveals severe emotional deprivation and rejection in childhood; the pattern often includes the triad of enuresis, setting fires, and cruelty to animals or other children. People who resort to violence often have been exposed to brutality and violence at home by parental beatings, or they may have witnessed other violent behaviors of adults (MacDonald 1963).

Other findings that have been associated with violent persons include a history of blackouts or other dissociative and trancelike states. Previous assaults are frequently reported, indicating low frustration tolerance and a lifetime of poor impulse control. In fact, it is not unusual to discover that such a person has killed before, although it may have been legitimate, such as on guard duty or in battle (Menninger and Modlin 1971).

Dynamics of Violence

The potential for violence exists in everyone, for fantasies of murder and destruction are a part of the human psychologic makeup. The problem is in predicting when someone will act on these ideas. Statistics reveal that the homicide victim more often than not is known to the assailant; ie, the victim is usually a family member, a close friend, or a neighbor. It is not the intensity of hatred of the victim that is the major factor; rather, the situation around the relationship contributes to escalating feelings into murderous proportions.

Feelings of helplessness and powerlessness when one is threatened by outside forces that are real or imaginary are the basic cause of violent behavior. Loss of control over one's impulses or over the situation can precipitate overwhelming anxiety, and the response can be the choice of fighting, fleeing, or freezing (Penningroth 1975, p 607).

Aggression as a form of expression is carefully repressed and regulated in our society. Aggression and hostility are difficult to control; they are more easily kept completely in check than controlled once they have been aroused (Flynn 1969). Thus we find people who store anger and resentment until they reach their limit of tolerance or boiling point, at which time they explode in violent behavior. Megargee (1966) calls this overcontrolled violence, because the person is usually described as a good person, quiet and conforming. He passively accepts a chronically frustrating situation, then suddenly blows up and directs his rage at the people who have thwarted him. Occasionally this includes strangers.

Undercontrolled violence is usually evident from an early age. It occurs in the person who is considered to have a chip on his shoulder. He is easily provoked, and people around him may try to avoid the confrontations and showdowns that he frequently seeks. After an episode he offers a plausible explanation for his behavior and is unconcerned about the uproar it created. Such behavior is considered to be sociopathic (Tupin 1975, pp 125–126).

One important factor that predisposes an individual to violent behavior is life experience in which conquest by force is culturally sanctioned. Those members of our society who are discriminated against, who are constantly frustrated, and who see little hope for change in the future readily accept violence as a way of resolving conflicts. The relationship of racial hatred, intolerance, and poverty to violence is clear. Saul (1972, p 1579) said that the emotional patterns of hate and hostility generated and shaped within individuals by harmful treatment at the hands of others, and specifically including those patterns taking the form of hostile acting out against others, are the chief causes of violence.

Emergencies of Disturbed Behavior

Tupin (1975) classified the situations that arise when disturbed behavior erupts as acute, subacute, or chronic quiescent. The acute category requires immediate intervention, for it involves the combative or assaultive individual who is not willing to cooperate. The subacute situation involves the person who is severely agitated and is threatening harm but has not resorted to violent action. Cooperation may or may not be possible. The third category, chronic quiescent, involves the recurrently violent person who is in control but who requires care to prevent disturbed behavior. He may or may not be cooperative when he becomes upset.

Both the acute and subacute situations require immediate action to prevent injury to the individual or to others. Control must be instituted as rapidly and as humanely as possible. Verbal intervention may be tried, but it frequently is ineffective in a situation where the person already is out of control. If force is necessary to restrain a potentially dangerous individual, there must be enough people available to overpower him without injury. The usual procedure is to assign one person to each of his extremities, since four adults are usually able to control a violent person (Zusman 1975, Bridges 1971).

When it is clear to the person that he cannot win the struggle, surrender is more likely. During or immediately after restraining him the nurse can explain to him specifically what is happening: "We cannot let you hurt yourself and others. We are going to give you medication by injection that will help you control yourself." Prolonged struggle should be avoided because it increases the risk of injury to the patient and the staff and creates anxiety and guilt in both (Zusman 1975).

In responding to the subacute situation, where the threat of harm exists but where no action has been taken, verbal intervention can be used. A willingness to understand the person, an attempt to offer reassurances, and an attitude of respect for him will usually accomplish more than a punitive authoritarian approach (Bridges 1971).

Outbursts of disturbed behavior can be frightening to the staff and to other patients in a treatment unit. It is essential to review the circumstances surrounding any disturbance and explore the causative factors and the feelings evoked (Penningroth 1975). Staff meetings and community meetings where staff and patients meet together are the usual arenas where this occurs in a psychiatric treatment facility. Disturbed behavior is more apt to recur when there is no provision for such meetings.

Violent patients rapidly acquire a reputation, and this can cause a cycle wherein the staff expects trouble and the patient fulfills the expectation. In one instance police brought an extremely agitated Oriental youth to an emergency room following a disturbance between the young man and a neighbor. On admission to the psychiatric unit he terrified everyone by bragging about his expertise in karate and judo. He shouted in a menacing manner and attacked anyone who came too close to him. Rumors of his prowess circulated throughout the hospital. When the patient's intense fear was recognized, his violent behavior subsided. He required medications to maintain control of his behavior, but he became more cooperative when the escalating spiral of his fear and staff anxiety was acknowledged and discussed.

Assessing Threats of Violence

When someone threatens to kill, the threat should be taken as seriously as a threat of suicide. Denial has been identified as the most common defense against the anxiety aroused by physical assaultiveness. For members of a treatment team this may take the form of failing to gather relevant information related to violence (Lion and Pasternak 1973). Total rejection of the violent patient is another response that may be observed on the part of nursing staff members. Disturbed and disturbing behaviors are upsetting to hospital routine, and the immediate reaction may be to attempt to transfer responsibility for the patient to some other professional or some other agency as quickly as possible. There are some basic facts that the nurse needs to know when she is involved with a patient who threatens to kill or harm others; the degree of disturbance can be assessed by exploring the following areas:

1. Determine whether he is under the influence of drugs or alcohol.
2. Note what level of anger he is displaying.
3. Determine whether he is fearful of attack and whether his fear is based on reality or on fantasy.
4. Determine whether the object of his wrath is available to him.
5. Determine whether he has a weapon and how easily he can get one.
6. Determine whether his circumstances seem to have him trapped.
7. Review his situation to see whether his self-esteem is threatened (Balsam and Balsam 1974, pp 210–211).

The more of these points that pertain, the greater the potential for actual harm. The circumstances around the crisis situation may dictate the nurse's response to it; the safety of all persons involved is the major concern.

Intervention and Management of Violent Behavior

Seek additional help if necessary. The fundamental rule is to be sure there is adequate assistance before dealing with a seriously disturbed patient. If the nurse is frightened of the patient she should not see him alone but should involve others in the encounter so that she will feel secure. Relatives or friends can be included, or a staff member or policeman may remain nearby while the nurse talks with the patient.

Avoid physical entrapment. Leaving the office door open can help to alleviate the terrified person's feeling of being closed in or of being too near people he cannot trust.

Do not humiliate a disturbed person. The dynamics of his disturbance are apt to include low self-esteem and feelings of powerlessness.

Keep words simple, concise, and clear. Destructive behavior and his threat of violence indicate that the person may be in a state of panic or close to it.

Be direct and frank. For example: "I can see that you want to hit me; that is not necessary. I will do what I can."

Avoid a power struggle. The conflict should be kept as public as possible; hazardous or heroic measures should not be attempted.

Do not threaten. The nurse must strive to establish a sense of trust and respect.

Keep communication open. The nurse must continue efforts to hold the patient's attention and maintain involvement. If telephone calls are to be made to obtain information or to make arrangements for care, it is best to do this in the presence of the patient and keep him informed of the rationale and the alternatives. If he is given options and an opportunity to participate in the decisions, his anger may subside, thus permitting cooperation or surrender (Kuehn and Burton 1969).

Alert the intended victim. As with the threat of suicide, the threat of homicide is not bound by confidentiality. The nurse's responsibility is to let the person know that a threat has been made to harm him.

Whitman and associates have suggested that therapists need to increase their repertoire of responses to crisis situations such as are presented by the assaultive patient. Role-playing different interventions is recommended as a way of preparing for more innovative and therapeutic modes of handling disturbed people. Playing the role of the assaultive person can also provide insight into the feelings and impulses of such people and their responses to various therapeutic techniques (Whitman and associates 1976, p 429).

The management of violent behaviors with medications requires a thorough understanding of the effects and side effects of psychiatric drugs. Intravenous medications, or more often intramuscular injections, are used in situations where the patient must be controlled as quickly as possible. Physical restraint should end as soon as the medication takes over. Because of the time lag when medications are given by mouth, titration of the proper dosage to help the patient control his behavior and still function is best accomplished by starting with intramuscular administration. Close observation of the patient is indicated whenever medication is administered to control an acute disturbance.

Violence in Conjunction with Intoxication

Alcohol or a combination of alcohol and drugs can cause disturbing behaviors, such as aggression and belligerence or the psychotic manifestations of hallucinations, paranoia, and confusion. People often resort to alcohol or drugs in an effort to cope with the distress they experience with psychotic symptoms. The effect can be to mask or to intensify the symptoms.

When working with a disturbed patient who is intoxicated, the nurse should follow these guidelines: (1) don't try to handle the situation alone; (2) be cautious when you approach him, and explain what you plan to do before you touch him; (3) try to get an adequate estimate of what substances and how much he has taken, both alcohol and drugs.

The use of medications to control disturbed behavior in these situations is to be considered only if absolutely necessary. The best course of action is to allow the patient to sleep off the effects of what he has taken. Close observation is imperative, especially if medications are administered to calm him.

The combination of intoxication and depression is sometimes encountered. The patient may be verbally abusive and threatening; then he may rapidly shift to maudlin crying and threats of self-destruction. His suicidal threats must be considered seriously, for one of the effects of alcohol is to lower inhibitions; it may be that he has gotten drunk seeking the courage to carry through with his suicidal ideas. All of the precautions regarding the suicidal person then apply (Ottenberg and associates 1975).

Legal Considerations

Since the late 1960s, when the patients' rights movement became more vigorous, there has been increasing attention paid to the implications of any measures that are taken without the consent of the patient, including involuntary hospitalization and administration of medications without the patient's consent (Thorner 1976).

Infringement of civil rights is a matter of serious concern to all professionals who work with disturbed people. The actual use of force as well as threats to use force are criminal acts unless extenuating circumstances warrant it. Failure to use force in a situation that culminates in injury can also leave personnel and institutions open to legal action and criticism. There must be clear evidence of disturbed behavior; one must not act on rumor or suspicion. The nurse must be aware of the laws and procedures regarding detention and commitment of people in the state where she practices, because the laws vary from state to state (Parad and associates 1975).

There are three basic criteria that pertain to holding a person against his will: (1) he is thought to be dangerous to himself or others; (2) he is in need of treatment and care; and (3) in some states the detention must be in the best interest of the patient and society (Parad and associates 1975). Changes in many state commitment laws have been made to assure that whoever is hospitalized without his consent is afforded safeguards protecting his civil rights.

The nurse's best protection from lawsuit is knowledge of the commitment laws and documentation of what she observes and what she does. She should keep an accurate record of her objective findings and information and avoid speculations not based on specific facts (Parad and associates 1975). She should be informed regarding the nursing practice act in her state. This includes an awareness of its limitations and its content. The specifics regarding administration of medications are particularly relevant. Also important will be any new legal decisions affecting nursing practice (Thorner 1976).

Prevention of Violence

The implications of effective parenting as primary prevention of violent behavior are obvious. Programs that help to reduce child abuse make a significant contribution by decreasing the number of children subjected to violence. Crisis prevention services are another specific resource that a community can provide. Suicide prevention centers have been in operation in Europe and in this country for decades, and recently many of these have defined their goals in broader terms to include other crises in addition to suicide. Thus they can include violence prevention programs that are responsive to a broad spectrum of aggressive behaviors.

Newspapers tend to headline tragic incidents of desperation, such as the case of a man who is unable to find employment or obtain welfare and feels driven to take a hostage and threaten to murder unless his demands are met. Innocent workers in welfare offices have been assaulted when the bureaucratic system has not been responsive to clients trapped in a dismal spiral of poverty, frustration, and powerlessness. In most major cities there is need for an ombudsman-type resource that can assist the troubled, the aged, and the disadvantaged through the maze of bureaucratic jungle (Resnik 1969, p 138). If such assistance is readily available, especially to groups and subcultures on our society's fringes, there can be constructive alternatives; the causes of much of the violent action that people take to dramatize their circumstances can be removed. Hearing the cry for help and responding to it would be the most effective prevention of violence.

SUMMARY

Aggression directed inward and aggression directed outward have been explored in terms of behavioral dynamics and some of the situational determinants. Criteria for assessment, guidelines for intervention, and major factors in prevention have been presented.

References

Balsam R M, Balsam A: Becoming a psychotherapist. Boston, Little, Brown, 1974

Beck A T, Dean S, Herman I: Development of suicidal intent scales. In Beck A T, Resnik H L P, Lettieri D J (eds): The Prediction of Suicide. Bowie, Md, Charles Press, 1974, chap 3

Blaker K: Crisis maintenance. Nurs Forum 8:42–49, 1969

Bridges P K: Psychiatric Emergencies: Diagnosis and Management. Springfield, Ill, Charles C Thomas, 1971

Diran M O: You can prevent suicide. Nursing '76 6:60–63, January 1976

Farberow N L, Heilig S M, Litman R E: Evaluation and management of suicidal persons. In Schneideman E S, Farberow N L, Litman R E (eds): The Psychology of Suicide. New York, Science House, 1970, chap 15

Farberow N, Litman R E: Suicide prevention in emergency psychiatric care. In Resnik H L P, Ruben H L (eds): Emergency Psychiatric Care. Bowie, Md, Charles Press, chap 6

Fawcett J: Clinical assessment of suicide risk. Postgrad Med 55:85–89, 1974

Floyd G J: Nursing management of the suicidal patient. J Psychiatr Nurs 13:23 March-April 1975

Flynn E: Hostility in a mad, mad world. Perspect Psychiatr Care 7:153–158, July-August 1969

Gunn, J: Violence. New York, Praeger, 1973

Kuehn J L, Burton J: Management of the college student with homicidal impulses—the "Whitman syndrome." Am J Psychiatry 125:1594–1599, 1969

Lion J R, Pasternak S A: Countertransference reactions to violent patients. Am J Psychiatry 130:207–209, 1973

MacDonald J M: The threat to kill. Am J Psychiatry 120:125–30, 1963

Megargee E I: Undercontrolled and overcontrolled personality types in extreme antisocial aggression. Psychol Monogr 80:1–29, 1966

Menninger R W, Modlin H C: Individual violence: Prevention in the violence threatening patient. In Fawcett J (ed): The Dynamics of Violence. Chicago, AMA, 1971, pp 71–78

Ottenberg D J, Rosen A, Fox V: Acute alcoholic emergencies. In Resnik H L P, Ruben H L (eds): Concepts and Principles in Emergency Psychiatric Care. Bowie, Md, Charles Press, 1975, pp 63–77

Parad H J, Resnik H L P, Ruben H L, Zusman J, Ruben D D: Crisis intervention and emergency mental health care. In Resnik H L P, Ruben H L (eds): Concepts and Principles in Emergency Psychiatric Care. Bowie, Md, Charles Press, 1975, chap 1

Penningroth P E: Control of violence in a mental health setting. Am J Nurs 75: 606, April 1975

Resnik H L P: Urban problems and suicide prevention. Am J Psychiatry 125:137–138, 1969

Saul L J: Personal and social psychopathology of the primary prevention of violence. Am J Psychiatry 128:1578–1581, 1972

Shader R I: Assessment of suicide risk. In Shader R I (ed): Manual of Psychiatric Therapeutics. Boston, Little, Brown, 1975

Stengel E: Suicide and attempted suicide. New York, Jason Aronson, 1974

Thorner N: Nurses violate their patients' rights. J Psychiatr Nurs 14:7–12, January 1976

Tupin J: Management of violent patients. In Shader R I (ed): Manual of Psychiatric Therapeutics. Boston, Little, Brown, 1975, chap 7

Whitman R M, Armao B B, Dent O B: Assault on the therapist. Am J of Psychiatry 133:426–429, 1976

Zusman J: Recognition and management of psychiatric emergencies in emergency psychiatric care. In Resnik H L P, Ruben H L (eds): Emergency Psychiatric Care. Bowie, Md, Charles Press, 1975, chap 3

CHAPTER

10

CRISIS INTERVENTION

Reg Arthur Williams

All of us experience periodic crises in our lives. These crises vary widely, from losing a job to delivering an infant prematurely. Usually each individual has a method of coping with such situations. However, if an individual finds himself temporarily overwhelmed and unable to cope, crisis intervention may be indicated as an effective short-term treatment.

Parad and Resnik (1975, p 3) emphasized that "the word 'crisis' is part of our national way of life: the energy crisis, the food crisis, the population crisis, the political crisis, and crises associated with disasters like tornadoes and floods." Indeed, we confront such crises every day in addition to the personal crises we experience.

The nurse is often in the most strategic position to do crisis intervention. A high percentage of the patients and families nurses encounter in the hospital setting could qualify for crisis intervention. It is by no means uncommon for a nurse to walk into a hospital room and find that a patient has just been informed that he has an incurable disease. Nurses must frequently console family members who have just lost a loved one. These are the more dramatic examples of crisis situations; there are equally real crises when a young child becomes hysterical because his parents are late for their visit and when a demanding patient screams for attention.

This chapter will provide an overview of the process of crisis intervention. Sections are concerned with the meaning of crisis, the feelings associated with crisis, the crisis sequence, the classification of crises, the generic and individual approaches, an assessment scale for an individual in crisis, and crisis intervention techniques.

THE MEANING OF CRISIS

Whenever an individual confronts a problem situation the attack is begun with customary problem-solving methods. When a person is faced with a situation that threatens his life goals, he may feel helpless and ineffective in facing the problem; he may see the problem as insoluble. When this occurs the person finds himself in disequilibrium. His anxiety increases as he makes many abortive attempts to solve his problem (Barrell 1974, Caplan 1961).

Although the terms crisis and emergency are often used interchangeably, Getz and associates (1974, p 21) indicated that a crisis state includes "such features as a sudden onset of problems with marked behavior changes, accompanied by feelings of helplessness and defeat. The person perceives himself to be in a unique situation and often experiences generalized physical tension."

Holmes and Rahe developed the Schedule of Recent Experience that serves as a significant indicator of illness onset (see Chapter 4). If an individual has a cluster of life change events within a 1-year period, as described in Chapter 4, he may encounter a life crisis ranging in severity from mild to major. This scale has been found to be a very useful assessment tool for patients encountering crises in their lives. Many of the events listed on the scale can evoke a state of crisis; others are life situations the client must deal with in order to resolve the crisis.

Crisis is believed to be self-limiting, lasting from several days to 4 to 6 weeks (Aguilera and Messick 1974). Without intervention the crisis episode will run its course, but the danger of psychologic vulnerability is increased if the person experiences a crisis alone. However, working through a crisis with a helping person can provide an opportunity for personality growth, as this increases the likelihood that the crisis will be resolved in the most productive way possible.

One point that must be remembered is that the individual himself defines whether or not he is in a crisis. Grace (1974, p 2) commented on this as follows:

> . . . it is dangerous to assume that all individuals respond to stressful experiences as though they constituted crisis situations. An individual may cope with major stressful events without being in crisis. Conversely, a situation that to the nurse appears minor may prove to be an insurmountable problem to a particular individual. What is important is that the nurse be alert to the patient's cues that he is in need of help and be able to respond appropriately.

FEELINGS ASSOCIATED WITH CRISIS

When an individual experiences a crisis he often attempts to use a problem-solving process to regain equilibrium. When he perceives the problem as overwhelming and his available coping skills do not help, he is very likely to experience these feelings: (1) anxiety, (2) helplessness, (3) guilt or shame, (4) anger, and (5) ambivalence (Berg 1970).

Anxiety is the most nearly universal of these reactions. At a reasonable level anxiety can help mobilize the individual's resources against a threatening situation; however, in excess it can produce confusion, distortion, poor judgment, questionable decisions, and self-defeating behavior (Berg 1970). The patient might describe the manifestations of his anxiety as tightness in the chest, dry mouth, rapid heartbeat, perspiration, or dizziness. In more severe forms of anxiety he might describe the feeling that everything is going wrong and that he is unable to identify what is going to happen (see Chapter 5).

Helplessness is a feeling often experienced by the person in crisis. If he finds that his usual coping skills do not work, he may make more unsuccessful attempts to solve the problem. At some point the person may begin to feel helpless. He may feel as if there is nothing he can do to change his circumstances.

A feeling closely associated with helplessness is depression. Zusman (1975, p 40) described depression in its milder forms as a "persistent pessimism and a tendency to cry easily at emotion-provoking events." Feelings of hopelessness and worthlessness are expressed in their more severe forms. The person may become emotionally labile; he may lose his ability to concentrate and have difficulty functioning at work or at home. In some ways depression is a natural defense for the individual in crisis who needs to ward off feelings of inadequacy to cope with the problem. If the depression interferes with the individual's ability to deal with the crisis, measures must be taken to manage the depression.

Guilt and shame are other feelings that may be experienced by an individual in crisis. We are taught at an early age that we must be self-reliant, independent, and competent. It is easy to see why one might feel guilt or shame when unable to solve a crisis situation.

Anger is another feeling that frequently is seen in the crisis patient. Anger may be expressed toward another person, or it may be directed inward at oneself. The patient may react by becoming easily hurt and upset by minor events that usually would be passed over without notice. In the more severe form the patient may interpret certain actions by others to be direct put-downs; he may feel that they are challenging him to battle. Anger can be expressed in violent temper outbursts, and the intensity is usually out of proportion to the situation. If the patient expresses anger toward the nurse he may quickly become apologetic or attempt to justify his explosive behavior (Zusman 1975). The important thing to remember is that the patient has a multitude of pent-up feelings and will need support in learning to express them appropriately.

The last feeling frequently associated with crisis is ambivalence. Ambivalence is seen as two opposing feelings, desires, or drives that coexist and are directed toward a person, object, or specific goal. Ambivalence can be conscious or partly unconscious (Psychiatric Glossary 1969). The individual in crisis is struggling to be self-reliant even while he requires support and assistance from others. He may be attempting to stay in control of his feelings and behaviors, yet feeling as if he is losing control. Frequently the nurse will see ambivalence in its most insidious form when engaging in problem-solving around a specific issue. The patient will often block a solution before it is even tried; he may state that he has already tried it unsuccessfully or that it just won't work. The nurse must be careful not to misinterpret ambivalence and then act on that misinterpretation. It is all too easy to give in to sentiment such as this: "I've suggested a number of solutions and you've turned every one down. Don't you want to help yourself?"

CRISIS SEQUENCE

A crisis sequence was described by Parad and Resnik (1975) as involving three time periods: the precrisis period, the crisis or upset state, and the postcrisis period (Fig. 10.1). During the precrisis period the individual is operating at a level that meets most of his needs. In other words, he may be relatively free of emotional and physical stresses. If the individual experiences a change-producing event that has special significance for him, he may move into the crisis period (upset state). It is important to understand that the precipitating or stressful event can have a wide range, from the sudden death of a loved one (unexpected stress) to the fear of losing one's job because of financial problems within the employing company (more or less expected stress). If the individual sees the event as stressful and feels that he is unable to cope with the situation, he is in a crisis (perception of threat/hazard). This does not imply that all stressful events put a person in crisis. If the person views an event as threatening to his life goals* and feels that it is overtaxing his current coping mechanisms, he is experiencing a crisis state.

When a person finds himself in a crisis, he faces a period of disorganization. At such a time he expresses feelings such as anxiety and helplessness. In an attempt to deal with the feelings of discomfort he is experiencing, he will make attempts to resolve the crisis. Crisis resolution refers to the development of effective adaptive and coping mechanisms, either from the patient's own resources or with the assistance of health care professionals, family members, and significant others (Parad and Resnik 1975). The crisis period generally lasts from several days to about 4 to 6 weeks. With appropriate intervention the patient can actually obtain a

**Life goals include "such basic security needs as love or affectional ties, a sense of identity, or most important of all, body integrity, one's very existence" (Parad and Resnik 1975, p 6).*

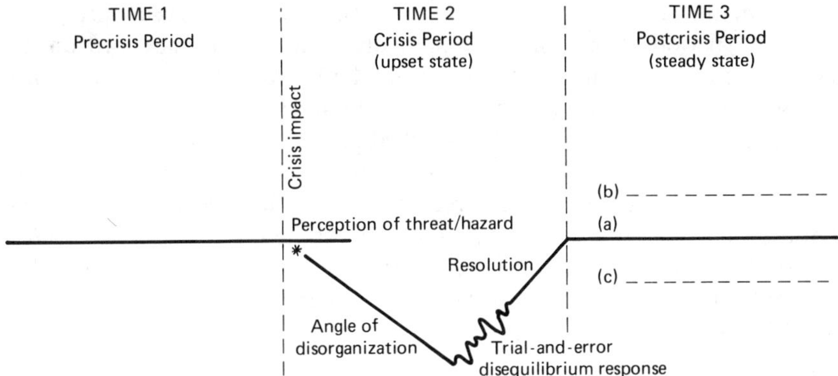

FIG. 10.1. Crisis sequence diagram. Asterisk indicates onset of crisis period, which occurs directly after crisis impact. An angle of disorganization develops during the crisis period and may vary from steep to gradual. This variance also occurs during the resolution (recovery or reorganization) phase. During time period 3 (postcrisis period) the level of functioning may be about the same as during time period 1 (precrisis period), or it may be higher or lower, depending on the nature of the stress, available resources, and whether the crisis resolution is adaptive or maladaptive. (From Parad H J, Resnik H L P: In Resnik H L P, Ruben H L (eds): Emergency Psychiatric Care, 1975. Courtesy of The Charles Press.)

higher level of functioning than he had in the precrisis period. He may learn new coping behaviors and problem-solving skills that he did not have previously. If he receives inadequate support from friends and relatives and resolves the crisis in a maladaptive manner, he may actually be at a lower level of functioning.

CLASSIFICATION OF CRISES

Crises may be divided into two categories: situational crises and maturational crises. A situational crisis usually is preceded by an identifiable external event. Murray and Zentner (1975, p 209) defined a situational crisis as "an external event or situation, one not necessarily a part of normal living, often sudden, unexpected, and unfortunate, which looms larger than the person's immediate resources or ability to cope and which demands a change in behavior." Examples are the death of a loved one, a natural disaster such as an earthquake or tornado, and hospitalization for mental illness.

Maturational crises, on the other hand, "are transition points, the periods that every person experiences in the process of biopsychosocial growth and development and that are accompanied by changes in thoughts, feelings, and abilities" (Murray and Zentner 1975, pp 208–209). Maturational crises are described as developmental phenomena; we all experience them in the process of growing up. Freud's psychosexual development and Erickson's developmental stages are fundamental in understanding this type of crisis.

In a maturational crisis disorganized behavior is observed during the transition periods from one developmental stage to the next. In an attempt to cope with this period of upset, the person will often recall the solution that worked in the previous developmental stage and apply it to the current stage. However, what worked at one stage may not be an appropriate coping skill for the next. As a person matures, new and increasingly complex behaviors are required to deal with life events. Examples of maturational crises are "entry into school, puberty, leaving home, engagement, marriage, pregnancy, childbirth, middle age, menopause, retirement, and facing death of others and of the self" (Murray and Zentner 1975, p 209).

Another system for classifying crises is centered around the family unit. The categories within this system are dismemberment, accession, and demoralization. This classification system was first suggested by Eliot and expanded by Hill (1965). Dismemberment refers to the loss of a family member. Examples might be the death of a spouse or the hospitalization of a member of the family. Accession, on the other hand, refers to an unexpected addition to the family. An unwanted pregnancy may occur, or a stepfather, mother, or an aged grandparent may come to live with the family. Demoralization includes those situations that reflect discredit on the family and cause a loss of morale and unity. Examples might be alcoholism, drug addiction, infidelity, or delinquency. Professionals obviously must take into consideration the cultural values and mores of the individual and the family before applying this classification. As with other aspects of a crisis, if the family views the situation as demoralizing, it can be labeled as such.

A family can experience the combination of dismemberment with accession or demoralization. An example of accession and demoralization might be a birth out of wedlock. Dismemberment combined with demoralization would include suicide, homicide, divorce, and runaways. Institutionalization for mental illness would be a combination of dismemberment and demoralization; when the individual returns to the family, this might create a crisis of accession and demoralization. Hill (1965, p 38) emphasized that most crises of dismemberment, accession, and crippling illness sooner or later involve demoralization, since the family's role patterns are always sharply disturbed. Dismemberment engenders a reallocation of roles within the family structure, and this creates a period of confusion while the family members learn these new roles. This model helps to explain why a family might be in crisis when the father becomes critically ill and is hospitalized. The mother and children must readjust their role functions, meaning that the children and the mother will be required to assume many of the father's functions. Another crisis can ensue when the father returns from the hospital after an extended stay; roles must again be reallocated.

The primary purpose of classifying crises is to give the nurse a better understanding of the meaning a particular crisis has for the patient. It can also be valuable in assessing the distressing events the patient has encountered and determining the interventions to be used to help him develop additional coping skills for his specific situation.

GENERIC AND INDIVIDUAL APPROACHES

The two approaches to crisis intervention are the generic approach and the individual approach. They are considered to be complementary. In using the generic approach the nurse assumes that there are certain recognizable patterns of behavior in most crises (Aguilera and Messick 1974). These patterns are thought to be universal for all members in a specific group. Kubler-Ross (1969) stated that when a person is confronted with death he will work through five stages to eventual resolution: (1) denial and isolation, (2) anger, (3) bargaining, (4) depression, and (5) acceptance. These stages constitute a basic pattern in our culture, and most people will move through these stages when confronted with the crisis of death. Another example would be Maslow's hierarchy of needs.

For the individual approach to crisis intervention Aguilera and Messick (1974) have emphasized assessment by a professional of the interpersonal and intrapsychic processes of the person in crisis. This modality is designed to assess the unique needs of an individual in crisis. The nurse does not expect that the patient will respond with a set pattern of behaviors. The goal is to help the patient reach a solution for the particular circumstances that precipitated the crisis. The following was designed as an individual approach for assessment of a person in crisis.

ASSESSMENT SCALE FOR CRISIS INTERVENTION

The scale in Fig. 10.2 was developed by Williams, based on the paradigm of Aguilera and Messick (1974), for assessing the effects of balancing factors in a stressful event. The scale will be discussed in relation to the distressing events leading to crises and the balancing forces moving toward crisis resolution.

Distressing Events

In the arrow to the left of the assessment scale the distressing events identified by the patient can be listed. The number of events is not an indicator of the degree of crisis; what is important is how serious the patient considers each event. In other words, the patient may view one event as being quite distressing, with the other events listed having only moderate significance. As can be seen, this will tip the scale to the left; if these events go unattended the patient is likely to experience a crisis.

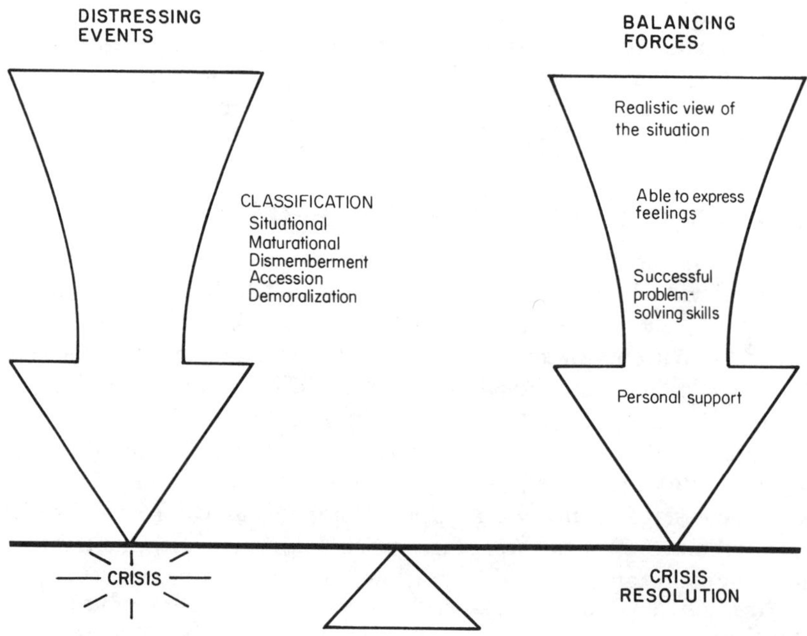

FIG. 10.2. The assessment scale for crisis intervention.

Much of the first session with the patient will be spent in determining the specific distressing events that brought him to seek help. The nurse must attempt to get the patient to be as specific as possible about the events in his life that created his discomfort. The nurse can ask what behavioral changes have occurred in the patient and whether these behavioral changes have been observed by other people as well as the patient (see Chapters 1 and 2 for specific methods of approach). An appropriate thing to ask the patient when he first appears is the nature of the precipitating event: What happened today that prompted you to come in for help? (Aguilera and Messick 1974, p 58). Often the patient will have experienced some difficulty the day he arrives, such as a family argument or loss of his job. In a medical setting the question is still appropriate; the patient may have experienced something very upsetting the day of the crisis, such as being told that he requires surgery.

The task of identifying the actual events that precipitated the crisis is not always easy. The patient may begin by citing situations or experiences that are troubling him, but these may be only symptoms of the real event or events precipitating the crisis. An example of this is a patient who described having difficulty sleeping and concentrating, which was affecting his work. On exploration it was found that the real event causing his disorganization was that his wife had threatened to leave him just before these symptoms began.

Another question that must be assessed is whether the problem can be solved in the immediate future. Even though the nurse may be able to alleviate the immediate anxiety and discomfort the patient is experiencing, the problem may be so extensive that long-term psychotherapy is required.

The crisis then must be classified. Is it a situational or maturational crisis? Is the patient experiencing dismemberment, accession, or demoralization in his family? If the individual is in a maturational crisis, the nurse must consider those phases he has already worked through in his growth and development. It is important for the nurse to know how he worked through these phases and what difficulties he encountered in the process.

Balancing Forces

The items in the arrow to the right side of the scale in Fig. 10.2 are those parameters the nurse will need to assess to determine if the individual has personal and situational resources to deal with the crisis.

Realistic View of the Situation. When asking the patient what caused him to seek help, the nurse has an opportunity to determine if he has a realistic view of the crisis situation. Because of the feelings the patient may be experiencing, he may have a distorted view. Recall the effect that anxiety has on the way we perceive specific events and what we focus on. There may also be an element of subjectivity on the part of the nurse involved in assessing the patient's view of the situation. Several methods can be utilized to assess whether he has a realistic view of the crisis. The nurse can ask him if he has all the facts about the situation. Often a patient will make a number of assumptions about a situation before he has checked them out with others. Another method involves contrast of the nurse's view with the patient's view: "I would be thinking the boss meant that I would be the only one discharged if we didn't get the new contract. Would you be thinking that?"

The nurse must be very careful in making her assessment, because her judgment is affected by her own culture, values, and life experiences. As an example, consider the crisis of rape (Williams and Williams 1973, Burgess and Holmstrom 1974). If those interviewing the victim were of the old school that believed that a woman could not be raped, this attitude would subtly or overtly be communicated to the victim, thus further compounding the rape victim's crisis. Supervision or consultation from an experienced professional can be very useful in helping to determine if the patient is viewing the situation in perspective. If one is unsure, it is essential to secure a second opinion.

In making the assessment the nurse can determine what issues need to be worked on with the patient. If the nurse determines that the patient has a distorted view of the situation, this will warrant work in the therapeutic situation. On the other hand, if the nurse determines that the patient's perception is a particular strength, she can point this out to the patient to enhance his self-esteem.

Able to Express Feelings. As noted previously, the person in crisis is likely to feel anxious, helpless, guilty, shameful, angry, and ambivalent. In addition, he may find himself depressed over his situation. When the nurse is assessing the feelings of the patient, she should consider these questions: Does the patient express what he is feeling? Can he identify the feelings he is experiencing?

Any individual in crisis can have difficulty identifying what he feels. Feelings can be denied, ignored, or somatized. He may be afraid to express his feelings for fear of losing control. He may not be given the opportunity by significant others to express himself. The nurse is often the first person to whom he can express these feelings and not feel incompetent or abnormal. The person in crisis may need to hear that the feelings he is experiencing are not abnormal. Helping the patient to express himself gives him a better perspective on both the situation and himself.

Successful Problem-Solving Skills. Any patient has experienced and dealt with other distressing events in his life, and the nurse should determine how he is handling his current crisis as well as how he dealt with similar circumstances in the past. He then may be aided in connecting past events and problem-solving methods with the situation he is currently experiencing. It is also beneficial to assist him in examining his problem-solving approach. Aguilera and Messick (1974, p 64) described the use of coping mechanisms to deal with crises:

> Available coping mechanisms are what people usually do when they have a problem. They may sit down and try to think it out or talk it out with a friend. Some cry it out or try to get rid of their feelings of anger and hostility by swearing, kicking a chair, or slamming doors. Others may get into verbal battles with friends. Some may react by temporarily withdrawing from the situation in order to reassess the problem. These are just a few of the many coping methods people use to relieve their tension and anxiety when faced with a problem.

Although the patient may have handled distressing events in his past effectively, his current crisis may be an overwhelming threat to some life goal. We know that it is common for people to have suicidal thoughts during crises, and the patient may feel that his current situation is so hopeless that suicide is the only way out. However, some patients are unable to discuss their suicidal ideations. Instead, they may talk ambiguously of wanting to sleep forever, passing on, leaving, or forgetting it all.

The nurse should ask for clarification; she should directly question the patient about suicide: "Do you feel so down that you are thinking of killing yourself?" Some patients find it a relief that a nurse will discuss the issue openly with them. (See Chapter 9 for more specific ways of assessing the suicidal patient.)

If the patient has relatively ineffective or inadequate coping mechanisms, the nurse will need to help him learn new ways of dealing with his current crisis. The nurse should reinforce adequate coping mechanisms used in the past and point out how they might be used in the current situation.

Personal Support. Although people like to think of themselves as independent, they are dependent on others to validate their self-worth. If an individual lacks personal support because of a loss, a threatened loss, or feelings of inadequacy in a significant relationship, he may experience a state of disequilibrium that can lead to a crisis (Aguilera and Messick 1974). Personal support is provided by those individuals in the patient's immediate environment who are dependable, available, and willing to help solve his problem. Frequently the individual providing support can listen to the patient, give supportive reassurance, and actually help with the problem. This support system might include parents, friends, spouse, pastor, and the nurse. It is usually advisable for the patient to enlist as much support from significant others as possible. The nurse should determine just how much situational support the patient has and help him reestablish supportive networks where possible. (See Chapter 14 for information on assessing social networks.)

EXAMPLES OF CRISIS INTERVENTION

Two examples will illustrate the use of the assessment scale for crisis intervention (Fig. 10.2). The first example concerns a woman involved in an automobile accident.

CLINICAL EXAMPLE I

Judith, a 32-year-old woman, was admitted to the emergency room following an automobile accident. She had sustained a mild concussion; following examination she was to be released. When the nurse entered her room to check on the arrangements for her transportation home, Judith was found to be breathing rapidly, trembling, and crying softly. When the nurse asked her what was going on, she explained the situation. She said she had been driving home from work and had been preoccupied with many things going on in her life. The automobile in front of her had stopped quickly, and she had run into it. Her only injury had been sustained in hitting her head on the steering wheel.

The nurse questioned Judith further about what had been on her mind just before the accident occurred. Judith explained that she and her husband had recently separated and that he had filed for divorce. She said that the marriage had been fine until she got a job about a year ago. Her husband was upset because she had a better job with higher pay than he had. Judith was able to express her anger over her husband's unreasonableness about the job situation. She also described feelings of failure, in that she was not able to make her marriage work. She felt that she should have quit her job before the marriage failed.

When the nurse asked how she had handled other distressing events in the past, Judith indicated that she usually withdrew and became depressed. She had not been able to sleep well at night since the divorce proceedings began. In addition to her feelings of increasing depression, she had had dreams about committing suicide. The nurse asked her directly if she was thinking of suicide. Judith affirmed that she had considered it. She emphasized that she could not give it serious thought because she had two small children who needed her. The next part of the assessment process was to ask Judith about her situational support. She reported that she had several friends who were willing to help her and that she could rely on her parents, who cared greatly about her and the children.

Figure 10.3 illustrates Judith's situation on the crisis scale. The distressing events identified were the automobile accident and the divorce. Since Judith viewed the divorce as entirely her fault, the nurse would help her gain a more realistic view of the situation. As an example, the nurse could help her to examine the interpersonal marriage relationship and see that she and her husband share responsibility for what happened. Emphasis should also be placed on the sequence she perceives: the job preceded the difficulties in her marriage. Through this interaction the nurse can continue to support Judith and aid her expression of feelings.

Judith described having had dreams in which she committed suicide. Although she claimed that she would not go so far as to kill herself, the nurse should carefully assess this question with Judith and take precautionary steps if necessary.

Since Judith indicated that she tends to withdraw and become depressed in a crisis, the nurse could help her identify more productive coping skills, such as talking with someone rather than withdrawing. She could be given assistance in developing new methods of dealing with distressing events. It is essential to explore with Judith the new skills she has acquired and reinforce the problem-solving methods used in the current situation.

Judith's experience can be classified as a situational crisis. It is possible to determine specific events, such as the automobile accident, that precipitated her problem. In addition, it is possible to classify Judith's family situation as dismemberment and demoralization. Changes in role responsibilities occurred when the father left the family system. The divorce will be demoralizing, especially with Judith blaming herself for failure of the marriage.

The personal support available to Judith is one of the brighter aspects of her situation. Since she has friends and parents to provide emotional support, the nurse can help her mobilize these resources.

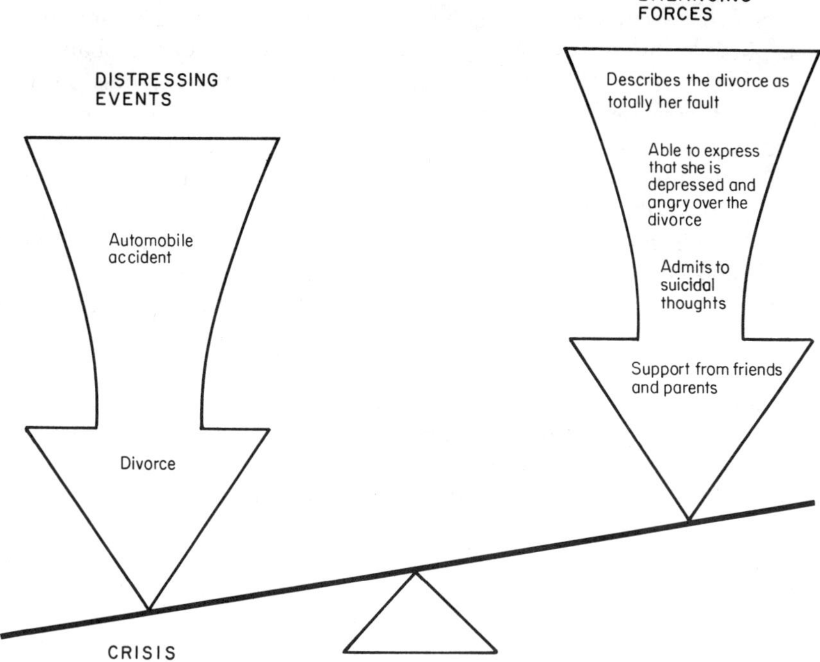

FIG. 10.3. Case example of Judith.

CLINICAL EXAMPLE II

John was a 55-year-old successful business executive who suffered a massive myocardial infarction. He was married and had three adolescent children. Although he had a large income, he also had a mortgage on an expensive home. At one time John had had the opportunity to take out insurance to cover lost income in the event of illness, but at that time he thought it unnecessary. He had always viewed himself as being very healthy. John was making a satisfactory recovery in the hospital until his boss visited him. The boss implied that he might have to "let John go" because it appeared that he would be unable to work for quite a while. The boss suggested early retirement. Shortly after this visit John became very restless and irritable. When the nurse asked him about the visit, John indicated that his return to work was anticipated by his boss. He also emphasized how important he was to the company and that his job was waiting for him.

John's wife told the nurse that a mortgage payment on the house was due soon. She wasn't sure how it could be paid, since they had no savings: "We always lived high on the hog. John said you could never take it with you, so we spent it on us and the kids."

Whenever the nurse brought up these crisis issues with John, he became anxious; he maintained that everything was fine. John indicated that in dealing with distressing events in the past he had usually weighed all the available alternatives and made a decision after discussing the situation with his wife. However, during his hospitalization, although his wife visited frequently, John would not discuss these problems with her.

Figure 10.4 illustrates the crisis situation experienced by John. The distressing events were identified as his hospitalization for myocardial infarction, possible loss of his job, and financial problems. John probably did not have a realistic view of the situation. Because of his illness and his feelings of powerlessness, he was denying the problems. The nurse observed that John was very anxious and restless, but he was not able to identify the source of his anxiety. However, he was able to describe effective methods of problem-solving he used in past crises. The threat inherent in his current situation created much disorganization, and because of the denial he was experiencing, his usual coping skills were not being employed. The nurse encouraged communication between John and his wife and provided him the opportunity to discuss his situation whenever he was able.

Although John's experience could be classified as a situational crisis, the loss of his job and the necessary change in life style could be considered to constitute a maturational crisis. If his physical limitations should force his early retirement, he would be in a transition period from middle age to retirement. This would necessitate a great deal of support from the

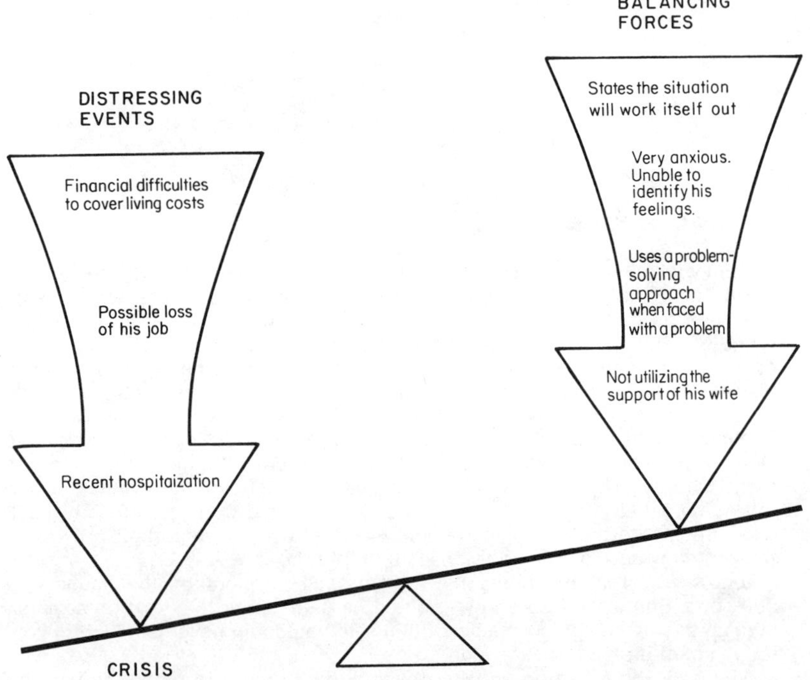

FIG. 10.4. Case example of John.

nurse to enable him to accept the physical limitations imposed on him by his illness. Both John and his wife would require assessment of their crisis situation, because his hospitalization could represent dismemberment of the family.

These two examples have been used to illustrate the assessment process in crisis situations. The remainder of this chapter will be devoted to general intervention techniques that can be used by the nurse when working with a patient in crisis.

CRISIS INTERVENTION TECHNIQUES

The following intervention techniques can be used by the psychosocial nurse when working with the patient in crisis. The only limits on the number and types of techniques used are the nurse's imagination and experience.

Take an active and directive approach. It can benefit the patient for the nurse to take an active role, rather than being passive or reflective about his problems. We know that many individuals in crisis are open to suggestion, especially the guidance the nurse might offer; therefore she can often help in finding appropriate alternatives to specific problems. The choice of which approach to use, of course, remains with the patient.

Enhance the patient's strengths. Because the patient feels incompetent to resolve his situation, his self-esteem is lowered. The nurse can best enhance his self-esteem through appropriate support and reinforcement, such as pointing out the times he has successfully solved other problems in the past.

Assist the patient in exploring alternatives. Because of the high degree of anxiety often experienced in crisis situations, it is not unusual for a patient to have tunnel vision regarding his situation and what to do about it. If the nurse talks with the patient and helps him decrease his anxiety, he may find effective and appropriate plans for crisis resolution.

Allow the patient an opportunity to express his feelings. The nurse can provide assistance in exploring feelings and helping the patient label these feelings. When the patient can appropriately label a feeling, the nurse can point out this strength to him. In addition, the nurse should be aware that her feelings are being communicated, directly or indirectly, to the patient, and she should consider the effect this can have on him.

For some people an expression of feelings is often accomplished through crying. If the nurse sees that the patient may cry, it may be helpful to offer him a Kleenex. This gesture often serves to give the patient permission to cry. In some cases, often with men, the nurse may need to say, "You look like you want to cry. It really is OK to cry." The nurse should bear in mind the struggle the patient is facing: needing to be self-reliant, yet needing to be dependent. The therapist who works with patients in crises must be prepared for a range of emotional responses. This means becoming comfortable dealing with anger, anxiety, fear, and tears.

Identify the methods the patient uses when faced with a problem. The nurse can help the patient determine why his usual coping mechanisms may or may not be effective in the current situation.

Involve significant others. It is important to assist the patient in relating his needs to supportive individuals who are important to him. They may include friends, spouse, parents, or the nurse. If he has no other person in his support system, the nurse might assist him outside the therapy sessions. This expanded role necessitates establishing a contract with the patient concerning how available the nurse will be. For example, if the nurse gives the patient her telephone number, the patient may feel more secure knowing that he has round-the-clock access to his therapist. On the other hand, the nurse must consider whether she wishes to be available on a 24-hour basis.

Demonstrate interest, hope, patience, self-assurance, and knowledge. When a patient is in crisis, he is most likely to be responsive to a nurse who shows him genuine concern (see Chapter 2).

Help the patient identify means of coping other than self-destructive behaviors. If the patient has suicidal thoughts, it is important to help him identify appropriate alternatives. Helping him to develop a strong and effective support system can give the patient's life purpose and meaning.

Help the patient obtain medication if needed. Some degree of anxiety may be helpful to the patient in working out his problem, but if the anxiety is severe and the patient is near panic, he may need some medication to help him cope with the situation. Lieb and associates (1973) have suggested that the psychotic patient first be assessed for medical or psychiatric contraindications to the use of drugs. If there are no contraindications, appropriate antipsychotic medication can be prescribed to effect a rapid change in the patient's behavior, thinking, and feelings. However, it must be remembered that medication will not remove all the psychotic patient's symptomatology.

Help the patient narrow the problem. After assessment of the crisis has been completed, it can be helpful to make a list of the possible approaches to his problem. The patient can then order these approaches into two categories: approaches he will consider trying and approaches he will not consider. The nurse can help him explore the advantages and disadvantages of those he is willing to consider. Using this method the patient should be able to find the best approach for his particular problem area.

If the patient needs resources which the nurse cannot provide, referral is necessary. Some services such as job placement, housing, financial assistance, and transportation may be appropriate referrals for some patients; others may need the help of a professional social worker. Parad and Resnik (1975, p 32) stated that "we must start to help the person build a new 'support system' for himself when we note important psychosocial deficiencies contributing to his health emergency." The support system can serve as a social network to sustain and strengthen the patient. It can enable the patient to cope with his everyday stresses and find new sources of security, recognition, and practical help (Parad and Resnick 1975).

Establish a nursing care plan. A wider range of resources can be provided for the patient if the responsibility is shared with others. For instance, if a patient needs to ventilate his feelings, a nursing care plan can alert the nursing staff and physicians that he needs assistance in this area.

Help the patient manage his depression. The nurse needs to focus attention on the individual's state of depression. Depression can easily interfere with his daily living and his ability to use his energy in problem-solving. If a patient is not getting enough sleep, the nurse might suggest that he organize his day so that he is able to get at least 8 hours of sleep. If a patient's nutritional intake is poor, the nurse can point out the importance of eating three well-balanced meals, or at least five or six snacks, during the day.

Often a patient's appearance reflects his inner mood. If his personal grooming needs attention the nurse can point this out and suggest that he may feel better if his outward appearance improves.

Sometimes depression may be so severe that it requires referral for medication.

Help the patient find appropriate outlets for the time he spends alone. The nurse should explore with the patient what he will do after he leaves the mental health center or hospital, and help him structure the time he has alone. The nurse can ask questions: "What will you do this evening?" "Do you have anyone you can talk with this weekend?" Those in his personal support system will often be willing to stay with him. But what will happen when his support eventually leaves? Can he utilize his time to think constructively or do things for himself that he will enjoy? If the patient only broods about his problems he is likely to lose his perspective of the situation, and his anxiety will increase.

Even if the patient has support from significant others, the nurse can give him instructions for contacting a crisis worker if necessary. Many communities now have 24-hour crisis hot lines. It is usually wise to write the number down on a piece of paper and suggest that he keep it with him.

Crisis resolution is usually self-evident. The patient and the nurse can usually agree when progress has been made and the problem is under control. The patient usually reports that he feels relieved, has a more positive attitude, and feels in control of the situation. The nurse usually observes behavioral changes indicating that the patient is involved in active problem-solving.

Review the process of crisis resolution. The nurse can explore the problem-solving process that the patient used to resolve his crisis. This may prove useful when the patient is confronted with a similar situation in the future. Aguilera and Messick (1974, p 21) have described this anticipatory planning.

SUMMARY

The possibilities for crisis intervention are limited only by the nurse's imagination and experience. This chapter has considered the process of crisis intervention from the perspective of what crisis means, the feelings associated with crises, and the sequential development of a crisis. Crises may be classified as situational and maturational crises. In addition, the family classification system of dismemberment, accession, and demoralization has been explored.

When the nurse approaches the patient in crisis, she can utilize a generic or individual approach, or both. An assessment scale for crisis intervention has been developed to aid the nurse in assessing the patient's strengths and coping mechanisms for managing his crisis situation. Examples have been given to illustrate the use of the scale as an assessment instrument. In addition, some intervention techniques have been suggested.

References

Aguilera D C, Messick J M: Crisis Intervention: Theory and Methodology. St Louis, Mosby, 1974

Barrell L M: Crisis intervention: Partnership in problem-solving. Nurs Clin North Am 00:5, March 1974

Berg D E: Crisis intervention concepts for emergency telephone services. Crisis Intervention 2:11, 1970

Burgess A W, Holmstrom L L: Rape: Victims of Crisis. Bowie, Md, Brady Press 1974

Caplan G: An Approach to Community Mental Health. New York, Grune & Stratton, 1961, p 18

Getz W, Wiesen A E, Sue S, et al: Fundamentals of Crisis Counseling. Lexington, Ky, Lexington Books, 1974

Grace H K: Symposium on crisis intervention. Nurs Clin North Am 00:1–3, March 1974

Hill R: Generic features of families under stress. In Parad H J (ed): Crisis Intervention: Selected Readings. New York, Family Service Association of America, 1965, pp 32–52

Holmes T H, Masuda M: Life change and illness susceptibility. In Scott J P, Senay E C (eds): Symposium on Separation and Depression. AAAS Publication 94. Washington DC, American Association for the Advancement of Science, 1973, pp 161–186

Kubler-Ross E: On Death and Dying. New York, Macmillan, 1969

Lieb J, Lipsitch I I, Slaby A E: The Crisis Team. New York, Harper & Row, 1973

Murray R, Zentner J: Nursing Concepts for Health Promotion. Englewood Cliffs, Prentice-Hall, 1975

Parad H J, Resnick H L P: A crisis intervention framework. In Resnik H L P, Ruben H L (eds): Emergency Psychiatric Care. Bowie, Md, Charles Press, 1975, pp 3–7

______ The practice of crisis intervention in emergency care. In Resnik H L P, Ruben H L (eds): Emergency Psychiatric Care. Bowie, Md, Charles Press, 1975, pp 25–34

Psychiatric Glossary. Washington DC, American Psychiatric Association, 1969, p 9

Williams C C, Williams R A: Rape: A plea for help in the hospital emergency room. Nurs Forum 12:388–401, 1973

Zusman J: Recognition and management of psychiatric emergencies. In Resnik H L P, Ruben H L (eds): Emergency Psychiatric Care. Bowie, Md, Charles Press, 1975, pp 35–60

CHAPTER

11

UNDERSTANDING GROUP PROCESSES

Margaret L. Larson
Reg Arthur Williams

Participation in various groups is an important part of living in our society. At work, at play, and in a number of other activities we find ourselves participating as members of some group. It has been estimated that the average person belongs to five or six different groups at any given time (Mills 1967). The interface between the individual and society occurs in these associations. How constructive a person is in any group setting depends on two things: his understanding of how a group influences individual behavior and his understanding of the forces that operate in any group.

Certainly it is incumbent on all professionals involved in human services to become knowledgeable about group functioning, because much of the planning for and actual delivery of services is accomplished through group action. Whatever its goal, a group can be a potent force for change, both constructive and destructive.

This chapter has been developed to promote better understanding of what happens when more than three people get together to accomplish a common goal. The approach is to describe the general characteristics of group behavior which occur when any group interacts, whether it be a committee meeting or a therapy session. The chapter begins by considering the relevance of the family to the individual's behavior in groups. The next section focuses on what makes a therapy group different from other collective endeavors. Another section considers how a group operates. The things that leaders can do to encourage member participation and foster positive, supporting behaviors as a group evolves are also explored. The last half of the chapter is devoted to behaviors frequently occurring in groups and some ideas for leader responses.

Although some of these behaviors may seem more likely to occur in the therapy setting, they are not infrequently observed in other groups as well.

FAMILY AS ORIGINAL GROUP

The family is the first and perhaps the most important group, for here the individual is socialized and given a sense of identity and a set of values. The family provides the nurturance, affection, and protection necessary for survival. Through intimate and sustained relationships with family members the child learns how to relate to others and how to behave to ensure that his needs are met. There is a tendency for an individual to respond in other groups as if he were still among his family: leaders and authority figures occupy the places of parents; peers within the group are like siblings and may be seen as rivals and competitors. Behaviors that were successful or behaviors that at least provided comfort within the family unit tend to be repeated over again in other groups.

As the child moves out from the home and becomes involved in school, church, and recreational activities (eg, Boy Scouts, Little League, Campfire Girls), group participation continues to be an important part of living and learning. Group projects and other shared responsibilities in the classroom are the preparation for work in the committees and other task-oriented groups of adult life. It is not unusual to see individuals move from one group to another, deeply involved but unaware of the dynamic forces that make these experiences rewarding or frustrating, pleasant or unpleasant. Unfortunately they may be equally oblivious of their own behaviors that impede or facilitate the progress of a group toward its goal.

WHAT MAKES A GROUP?

What is the difference between a collection of individuals and a group? Often one may see three or four patients in a four-bed unit sharing common space and mutual experiences, but with minimal communication and with no sense of identifying with each other. The next occupants of the unit may be interacting with each other and referring to themselves as the Three Musketeers or the Fearless Foursome. Staff members demonstrate similar group behaviors. The members of one team may go about their tasks with little socialization, restricting communications to the essentials necessary for carrying out the job, having little concern for the feelings of the other team members. Another group may spend considerable time, both on the job and off, in socializing with each other. They may be keenly aware of the tensions and conflicts that arise, and they may make a concerted effort to resolve them to preserve the integrity of their group. What are the forces that bring people together to make a cohesive group?

The reasons people voluntarily join groups have become a topic of interest to behavioral scientists. Cartwright and Zander (1968) have identified the major factors that seem to be involved: (1) interpersonal attraction, or the desire to be with the members of the group; (2) the activities of the group are attractive; (3) the group's goals are valued by the individual; and (4) group membership itself, which is called affiliation need or the wish to belong.

Generally speaking, to be a member of a group is to find acceptance and receive the recognition and respect of the other members; there is a sense of belonging. The individual identifies with the group that offers a communal feeling and a climate of trust. Small groups with opportunity for face-to-face contact and personal knowledge of each other are essential in counteracting the alienation inherent in a complex society. We all have a need to belong, and it is in various groups that we can find acceptance that is basic to our social existence.

TYPES OF GROUPS

Two major aspects of group functioning have been identified: the work orientation (socio) and the emotional dimension (psyche). Most groups tend to function in both spheres simultaneously. There are purely social groups, such as a bridge club or a coffee klatch, that meet regularly and endure solely because of the satisfaction the members get from participating with friends. Such groups are voluntary, and since they tend to be comprised of people with much in common, they are called homogeneous groups.

Work groups meet to carry out designated tasks; they include committees, staff workers assigned to a specific area, and other such task-oriented groups. They usually have a more diverse membership (heterogeneous), for it is the task that brings them together rather than mutual affinity for each other. Success in the work group is measured primarily by the work the group accomplishes. However, the emotional component frequently is an essential ingredient for an effective work force, for it determines the interest and morale of the members and their degree of involvement in accomplishing the group's goal. Many workers are dissatisfied if they do not find a warm social dimension in their work setting. Corporations and businesses have shown increasing interest in this fact, and they make an effort to structure their organization such that compatible work groups can evolve. They also may provide recreational facilities and sponsor activities such as a bowling team to further encourage the workers' involvement and identification with each other and with the firm.

Many different groups are therapeutic for their individual members without being therapy groups per se. Self-help groups such as Weight Watchers and the consciousness-raising groups made up of peers who get together to share their frustrations, concerns, and strivings benefit from the acceptance and sense of identity afforded. Alcoholics Anonymous is a good example of this type of group; it has been able to assist many people to maintain sobriety when other attempts to accomplish this have failed. These are known as supportive groups because they bolster the member's self-image. If members wish to change their behaviors or go into extensive exploration of crucial personal issues, professional assistance may be sought.

A therapy group has certain distinguishing characteristics. Its major purpose is to treat or help alleviate what the patient defines as a problem. The primary goal is to expand the individual's ability to cope with problems. This usually entails a discussion of the individual's life history and his unresolved difficulties in interpersonal relationships. A wide range of groups, from psychoanalytic groups to groups employing such treatment modalities as transactional analysis and Gestalt or reality therapy, are included in the category known as group psychotherapy.

Therapy within the group requires the same basic elements as individual therapy: (1) the structure of the situation, such as time and place; (2) clarification of the goal or purpose of the group; (3) the therapist's commitment to follow through on the treatment plans and bring professional judgment to bear on the encounters as they occur; and (4) a group of members who have identified a problem or problems.

The leader of a therapy group must have preparation for that role. At one time therapy was more narrowly defined as requiring a psychiatrist or psychologist. Today a variety of mental health workers have undergone professional preparation and supervision in group work and are involved in group therapy. It is important to note that achieving proficiency as a therapist requires training, professional supervision, and years of practice.

STAGES IN GROUP DEVELOPMENT

When different groups are observed, no matter what the setting, there are certain features that are seen to be reasonably consistent. One of these features is the developmental sequence of the group. It is proposed that every group moves through five stages of development.

The first stage of group development is called the RELIANCE STAGE. The formation and orientation of the group occur primarily in this first stage. The usual questions arise: What are we doing here? What is our purpose?

If the group is task-oriented, time is spent identifying the specific task or tasks to be accomplished. In addition, groups often experience the swivel phenomenon in the reliance stage: when a group member speaks all eyes focus on that person; when the next person speaks every head swivels to the individual talking and then back to observe how the leader reacts.

One predominant feature of this stage is great reliance on the leader, who is often viewed as almost omnipotent. It is common for the group to expect this person to do all the leading and provide all the structure.

The second phase of group development is called the WAR STAGE. The group moves from a social chit-chat communication pattern to general intragroup conflict. Tuckman (1965, p 386) found that group members became hostile toward one another and toward the leader. This phenomenon frequently is "a means of expressing their individuality and resisting the formation of group structure." This hostility can at times be very open, with verbal anger expressed toward group members or toward the leader. However, the war stage can also be more covert, with half-serious–half-joking messages, passivity, or passive-aggressive acts within the group. Tuckman described this stage as storming. He found that this stage was characterized by conflict and polarization of interpersonal issues. Many members would respond emotionally to the task the group was working on.

The third stage of development is the WE STAGE. If the members are able to express frustration and anger effectively with each other and with the leader, they will move toward a feeling of togetherness, a sense of purpose; the group will begin to demonstrate cohesion. Jones (1973, p 129) called this phase the stage of cohesion: "They begin sharing ideas, feelings, giving feedback to each other, soliciting feedback, exploring actions related to the task, and sharing information related to the task." During this stage the group can briefly abandon the task and have a period of play to enjoy the cohesion being experienced (Jones 1973). On the other hand, Tuckman (1965) defined this as the stage of norming. In addition to developing cohesion, the group will set new standards, take new roles, and adopt new rules.

It has been found that groups even do renorming. In other words, the norms and rules that were established with the formation of the group, whether they were spoken or not, are reexamined by the members. If they see these norms as important, they usually restate them. They may change some norms or even discard others.

In the PERFORMANCE STAGE, the fourth phase, the group demonstrates its efficacy. The task is worked on, and problems that have been encountered are resolved. In general, problem-solving is a predominant trait. This stage is marked by interdependence, and group members can work singly or in subgroups, or they can return to function as a total unit (Jones 1973).

Many authors have suggested that a group's development concludes with the performance stage. However, in groups that have been together for some time we have seen a fifth stage, TERMINATION. In this phase the group is likely to resort to old behaviors or styles of interaction. If the group spent a considerable amount of time in the war stage, the members might go back to fighting and expressing anger with each other. Very often the group members are unaware that they are demonstrating these behaviors; it is usually because of their unwillingness to say goodbye. It is especially difficult to depart from a group that has taken considerable time in developing and in which members have had good feelings about the experience. However, the group members will profit if they are able to terminate with each other effectively and review the progress they have made both as a group and individually.

Although the stages in group development follow a predictable pattern, the amount of time spent in any stage is not predictable; no group will spend a 2-week period in the reliance stage and another 2 weeks in the war stage and so on. It is not uncommon to see a group move through the reliance stage, the war stage, the we stage, and the performance stage in one meeting and then return to the reliance stage at the end of the meeting. On occasion, a group with a well-defined and accepted task may even bypass some of the stages.

ASSESSMENT OF GROUP FUNCTIONING

In a committee meeting, in group therapy, or in a rap session with friends we are interested in what people are saying. In other words, we tend to focus on the content of the group. Another aspect of groups that probably affords more interesting material is the process of the group meeting. Group process is "concerned with what is happening between and to group members while the group is working; . . . it deals with such items as morale, feeling tone, atmosphere, influence, participation, styles of influence, leadership struggles, conflict, competition, cooperation, etc" (Hanson 1972, p 21).

For an active participant in a group it can be difficult to identify the process, for it is much easier to follow the content of the meeting. However, if one takes the time to identify and monitor the following factors, the dynamics and process will become evident.

Group Goals

Groups may have short-term and long-term goals, as well as primary and secondary goals. The goals or purposes of the group provide a road map of the group and its functions. Shaw (1976, p 92) stated that "in many ways it is difficult to separate the activities of a group from its goals, and individuals may be attracted to a group because they enjoy its activities and also value its goals or purposes." Frequently the goal that is stated or implied in the early sessions of the group may change as the group develops. Some individuals in the group may have their own goals that differ from the goals of the majority and from the group goals; these make up what is called the hidden agenda.

If a student group is assigned a project, the group goal is development of the project. The majority of the group may establish the following goals: (1) completing the project by a specific date, (2) sharing in the work load, and (3) receiving an A grade. However, one or two members might not be so concerned with the A grade or with doing their share of the work; their hidden agenda is to get the other members to do most of the work.

Group Norms

The norms of a group are established for the purpose of controlling the behavioral consistency of the group (Shaw 1976). Hanson (1972, p 24) determined that "norms usually express the beliefs or desires of the majority of the group members as to what behaviors *should* or *should not* take place in the group." Norms can be very formal, such as Robert's Rules of Order in a business meeting. However, in the small group they are implied, unspoken; they may not be clarified until they are violated. When this happens the guilty member is quickly reprimanded for his deviant behavior. The usual norm of being kind and considerate appears in the early phase of a group. When the norm of being nice has been established, members will be seen readily agreeing with each other, and expression of anger will not occur.

If a member should become angry during this phase, he will probably be reprimanded by the leader or by another member. He may be given the message that this is not the time for expression of feelings and that he should control himself.

Another example is the norm of starting and ending on time. Members will become irritated with those who continually come late to meetings; however, they will usually demonstrate their irritation to the latecomers in a circuitous fashion.

Hanson (1972) suggested that it may be easier to identify the norms of the group by looking at certain areas that are avoided by the group: sex, religion, talking about current feelings, or discussing the behavior of the leader.

Major Themes of the Group

The theme of a group is the thread of content that can be found running throughout the meeting. As with many of the aspects of the group process, one must look beyond the obvious. In a formal group the themes are usually identified by the agenda of the meeting. Again, these are the obvious themes; the underlying themes may be quite different. It can be useful to keep a record of the major themes that have surfaced in each meeting. If a theme keeps recurring, it is an indication that the group should discuss the theme and attempt to resolve the issues involved.

For example, in one group meeting the major theme appeared to be obvious: the coffee fund, and the fact that members must pay if they want it served at each meeting. However, the real theme was that the members were trying to avoid discussing an issue that was emotion-laden and upsetting to all: their anger with the group leader because he wasn't telling them what they should do. Identifying the major themes in a group may be difficult; it takes experience and evaluative skill. If a leader or a member of a group begins to feel confused about what is going on in the group, he should pause to identify the themes that are in operation.

Feeling Tone of the Group

As is the case in any human interaction, group discussion will generate some form of feeling in its members. "These feelings, however, are seldom talked about. Observers may have to make guesses based on tone of voice, facial expressions, gestures, and many other forms of non-verbal cues" (Hanson 1972, pp 23–24). Identifying the feeling tone enables the leader to allow or encourage the group to express feelings of anger, frustration, competitiveness, love, or excitement.

Types of Participation in a Group

Common types of participation in groups have been described in terms of roles or functions performed by the members (Benne and Sheats 1948, Knowles and Knowles 1972, Lassey 1976). Group maintenance functions are concerned with emotional forces, such as building relationships and cohesion, while group task functions facilitate the accomplishment of the work to be done.

Group Maintenance. Behaviors that promote group development include the following: *Encouraging,* as the name suggests, involves helping another person to express his thoughts or feelings. *Giving support* is observed when a member recognizes and endorses another member's ideas and creativity. *Gatekeeping* occurs when one member facilitates participation by other members: "Wait! We haven't heard from everyone yet." A gatekeeper frequently will remind the group when it is straying off course. *Mediating* moves the group toward harmony, for it encompasses efforts to bring about compromise or to reconcile the divergent ideas expressed.

Relieving tension is a useful function that often takes the form of joking or appropriately diverting attention from uncomfortable discussion to more neutral ground. *Following* is an important function of both the leader and the members; it includes going along with decisions and accepting the ideas of others.

Task Functions. Introducing ideas and suggestions that promote the group's work is called *initiating. Seeking information, giving information,* and *offering opinions,* especially when of a positive nature and relevant to the topic, are vital functions that encourage full exploration of the subject under consideration. *Clarifying* includes the members' efforts to make communications more understandable. Building on the contributions of others and adding to the ideas expressed is called *elaborating. Evaluating* entails checking out the group members to see if they are ready to take some action or make a decision. *Summarizing* reviews what has been accomplished so that the next step can be taken by the group.

Nonfunctional Behaviors. Nonfunctional behaviors interfere with accomplishment of the group's task. The member who stops discussion by changing the subject or interrupting is *blocking.* Becoming angry, blaming, or putting others down are considered *aggression. Seeking recognition* is observed when a member makes a special point of drawing attention to himself by expressing extreme ideas, boasting, or monopolizing the discussion. The member who introduces or supports topics related to his pet interests, beyond a point of usefulness to the group, is said to be *special-pleading.* In doing this he may pretend to speak for the entire group as if he knows what they are thinking. *Competing* is evident when members try to outdo each other or curry the leader's favor.

Withdrawal is frequently seen in groups, because everyone occasionally needs some time out. Behaviors indicating withdrawal include indifference or passivity, doodling, and whispering to others. *Dominating* is another nonfunctional behavior that is seen when a member takes over the discussion or gives directions blocking the free exchange of ideas. *Horsing around* involves disruptive behaviors, such as clowning or making fun of the situation, or joking that goes beyond the point of relieving tension and interferes with work.

Communication Pattern

It can be interesting to observe the communication pattern in a group: Who talks to whom? Who talks the most? Who talks the least? Do some of the members talk to each other but exclude certain other group members (subgroup)? Who starts and ends the group?

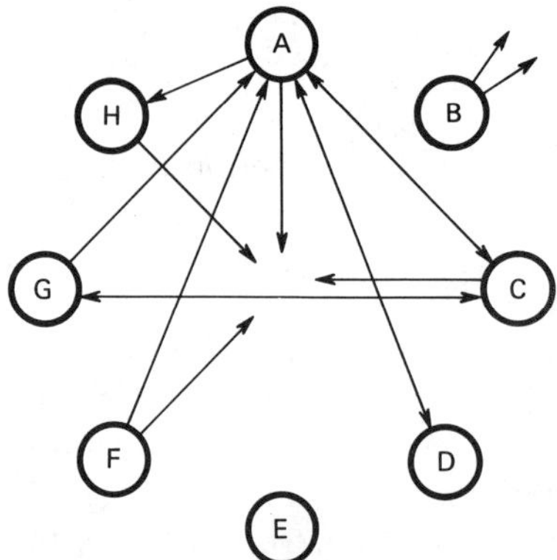

FIG. 11.1. Communication pattern.

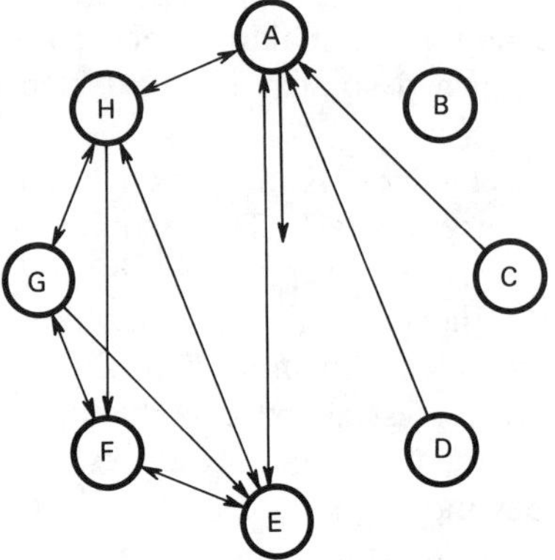

FIG. 11.2. Change in communication over time.

One method of observation is to draw a diagram representing the group members, a circle or square for each. When a transaction occurs a line is drawn between the speaker and the one to whom he speaks. If a communication is directed to the entire group, a line is drawn to the center. Figure 11.1 presents an example of a communication pattern.

On occasion there will be an individual who has talked to the group but has received no response to his communication. If he attempts enough of these interactions and gets no response from the group, he may become silent (note member B in Fig. 11.1).

It can be useful to draw communication diagrams for different periods, such as at the beginning, in the middle, and toward the end of a meeting. Another method is to draw a communication pattern each time the group moves to another major theme (this provides an objective view of the group and the process).

Figure 11.2 illustrates the change in communication over time. Who is the leader of this group? Has a subgroup formed?

HOW PEOPLE BEHAVE IN GROUPS

We have noted that an individual's prior experiences have a great influence on what he does and how he feels within a group. Some members of a group may be comfortable when expressing opinions and ideas, whereas others may be inhibited and uncomfortable about expressing their ideas. Thus a group can be a source of comfort and security, but it can also serve as a threat to some of its members. The leader, whether a therapist, a head nurse, or a teacher with a group of students, has certain responsibilities for developing a climate in which members feel free to express ideas, to grow and change. But the leader should not be the only force acting. Lieberman and associates (1973, p 428) emphasized that the leader should not harbor the conception that all change revolves around the solitary sun of the leader.

A sharing of leadership functions is more effective than an authoritarian approach. When the leader is able to share authority and other leadership functions with the members of the group, member interaction is encouraged and personal contributions are enhanced. Leadership ability and the ability to follow exist in every individual. How well these functions are performed by the group members will determine the success or failure of the group.

Leader Responsibilities

Certain responsibilities do rest with the leader. The first thing that the leader must attend to is structuring the situation. The purpose or task of the group must be identified, as well as the ground rules that are to be followed in accomplishing the task. In a therapy group this is termed the contract; it includes bits of information that every member must know. Johnson (1963) included in this contract such information as the following: (1) purpose of the group; (2) membership, especially whether others are to join later; (3) fees, if required; (4) confidentiality; (5) minutes of meetings, especially if a tape recorder is to be used; (6) length of time that the group will meet. By setting out this information and by example the leader helps the members identify what is expected of them in the group.

Group leaders should strive to foster an atmosphere of acceptance and security. The leader's attitude of nonjudgmental acceptance can do much to set the tone and build a feeling of security. A noncritical atmosphere encourages members to share more openly and to try out new behaviors. Identifying feelings, experiences, and needs that members have in common helps to build cohesion and interdependence on one another (Marram 1973). In therapy groups confidentiality is a vital factor that must be discussed. Trust is fostered if the members know that their verbalizations will be respected and will stay within the group.

Problem Behaviors in Groups

The remainder of this chapter describes some of the more common nonfunctional problem behaviors. However, certain points must be kept in mind. First, in most groups the members will be utilizing functional behaviors. Depending on the purpose of the group, the shared importance of the goals, and the stage of development, some groups may experience behavior that tends to be nonfunctional. Second, the types of interventions to be employed in dealing with nonfunctional behaviors depend greatly on the context and composition of the group. The particular interventions described here are only suggestions.

The Nontalker. Silence in any group is a frequent occurrence, especially in the beginning phase when members are reluctant to participate or are unsure of what to say. In later phases of the group's life a silence is often evidence of anger or apathy. The leader should make some judgments concerning the dynamics of the silence and intervene accordingly. For example, the leader may note that what was last said stopped everyone from talking; he then may select an intervention appropriate to follow the show-stopper. One intervention would be for the leader to comment on how the silence is perceived: "Everyone is quiet. It seems like an uncomfortable silence to me." "The group is quiet today. You all seem sad." On the other hand, the silence may be only a thoughtful interlude in which everyone is considering what has been said.

When a member's verbalizations are consistently ignored, he may respond by becoming silent. Behind that behavior is a message: "If you people won't listen to me, I just won't talk."

The nontalker may be a source of frustration to the group leader, especially if the reason for his silence is obscure. Slavson (1966) contended that there is a characterologic silence that is common to certain individuals who by nature are quiet and are not inclined to express their ideas in groups. This trait should be respected. Other members may be withholding verbalizations because they are angry, and they use silence as a means of avoiding getting involved. When a member remains quiet, the group may not immediately realize that he is angry or upset; his lack of participation can then become the focus of attention. The leader can point out that although the member is not talking he is actually controlling the process going on within the group.

People who are not comfortable in groups may feel that they have nothing to contribute, or they may place little value on their own ideas and may be reluctant to express them. If a member is fearful of the group's ridicule or is highly suspicious of the members, he will be less likely to participate. When he sees that the leader is interested in him and accepting toward him, he may start to relate to the leader and eventually to the group members.

Group members may think that the nontalker is rejecting them, and they may become angry with him for not contributing his share. It is important for the leader to acknowledge the nontalker; the leader should be supportive until it is possible for the nontalker to participate. It is not wise to put the nontalker on the spot by pointing him out; rather, a group issue can be made of his silence by asking if the members have noticed that not everyone has spoken. It must be remembered that a silent member can benefit from the group experience, even if he participates very little during the entire life of the group (Johnson 1963, Yalom 1970).

The Angry Aggressor. It is difficult to deal with an angry individual in any interaction. When anger is expressed in a group setting, it can be quite threatening, especially when the leader is the one under attack. Member-to-member expressions of hostility carry with them the threat of an altercation or disruption of the group. The members will carefully observe the leader's response to such situations. A basic understanding of anger and its derivatives in human behavior is essential, and the leader must also be aware of his own characteristic responses to anger. Techniques for dealing with anger in group therapy have been discussed by Baker and Estes (1965). Many of these techniques have application to groups other than therapy groups, and they warrant careful consideration.

It is expected that the leader of a therapy group will foster a climate of acceptance that will permit expression of feelings, including anger. The most common response to anger in everyday situations is to counter with anger. When expressions of angry feelings is encountered, but without the typical retaliation, an opportunity for new learning experiences is created. Review of an angry exchange within a group meeting also helps members explore alternative behaviors (Baker and Estes 1965).

Anger frequently is denied by individuals whose upbringing was such that angry expressions were forbidden or punished by parents or other authorities (Moore 1968). Talking about anger helps the angry person become better aware of his feelings. If necessary, synonymous terms may be used; some individuals can admit to being irritated or frustrated, but they find it difficult to admit they are angry.

Overwhelming emotions are sometimes minimized by nurses and other workers dealing with people who are disturbed. It is unproductive to say that someone is a wee bit upset when he is obviously in a towering rage. When someone is furious, the fact should be acknowledged (Baker and Estes 1965).

Rosenfeld (1969, pp 251–254) has developed specific guidelines for dealing with hostile behavior:

1. Recognize the individual's feelings.
2. Direct your responses to his concerns.

3. Accept his feelings without indicating approval or disapproval; make no value judgments.
4. Listen carefully, and refrain from arguing, giving advice, or venting personal feelings.

The Smoke-screener. Smoke-screening or intellectualization occurs in groups where there is emphasis on interaction. It is a ploy that certain people use to avoid revealing anything of significance about themselves; it is also used to avoid examination of feelings. An example of this occurred in a student group that met to discuss their feelings about their clinical experiences in psychiatry. One student spent most of the quarter talking glibly about her ego and her inferiority complex. Each time an effort was made to identify specific feelings having to do with a situation, the student would begin an explanation in terms of theory. Rather than identify a feeling, she would respond in terms of the ego and superego. The instructor and the other students finally succeeded in helping her to say what she felt, rather than what she thought or what the book said.

The Monopolizer. Who has not attended a meeting at one time or another where one of the members took over, dominated the entire time, and did not let others express their ideas? The monopolizer, like the angry aggressor, can present a major threat to the leader by taking over control of the group or by irritating and alienating group members with constant chatter or interruptions. If the leader is uncertain about how to proceed or is having difficulty in getting good group interaction going, he may allow the talkative person to fill in the gaps whenever there is a pause. Since this meets the leader's need at that moment, it may not be obvious that he is unintentionally offering encouragement to the monopolizer (Eisenberg and Abbott 1968).

Excessive talking is usually indicative of anxiety, and the person may not be aware of this behavior. The leader may intervene by asking group members to describe what is happening in the group, or the monopolizer can be asked to tell what is occurring.

One individual joined a group that had already been meeting for several months. This created tension in the group and caused her considerable anxiety. She talked continuously for the first 15 minutes; then the leader interrupted to inquire if she was aware of her behavior. The leader suggested she listen while the group members expressed their observations about the meeting. Such confrontations can help the monopolizer become aware of this behavior and the effect it has on others. Acknowledgment of the problem is the first step in reducing tension in the group.

Occasionally the monopolizing behavior is an effort to gain attention. Constant effort to be the star attraction usually results in the monopolizer becoming the object of the group's hostility; the leader should intervene and assist the group in dealing with the problem. One of the dangers of waiting for other members of the group to confront the monopolizer is that they may wait until they have exhausted their patience and then lash out in destructive anger. Close observation of nonverbal behavior within the group will reveal clues indicating that the leader should take action.

The Distractor. Like the intellectualizer and the monopolizer, the distractor is employing a defense to relieve anxiety. Whenever topics in the discussion cause him anxiety, the distractor will attempt to change the subject or stop the discussion. For example, in one group it was noticed that any time comments relating to sex were brought up, a certain member would tell a joke or start talking about pornography. After investigation of this tendency the member was able to admit that he needed understanding and acceptance before he could tolerate any meaningful discussion pertaining to sex.

Distractors should be made aware that they are interfering with progress. Group members who take over the gatekeeping functions will often point this out.

The Rescuer. "Everyone has probably met a chronic helper: over-eager to help and an initial bottomless capacity to give or do anything that is helpful" (Light 1974, p 129). Luchins (1964) called these people do-gooders. They are always ready to help someone, but they expect a favor in return. When the favor is not forthcoming they suffer disappointment and anger. In the group they will offer solutions before the problem is clearly defined. Frequently they attempt to be especially helpful to the leader; they curry the favor of authority figures by being helpful.

There was one group member who always served the other group members. She scurried to get the leaders coffee without determining whether they wanted it; if the coffee was refused she considered it a personal affront. Exploring her pattern of helpfulness enabled her to see that her service to others was based on a need to have people like her and care for her. Feedback from group members enlightened her to the fact that some people are annoyed and uncomfortable when favors are foisted on them. Few in the group were readily able to be honest about their feelings lest they offend the gift-giver.

The Saboteur. The saboteur or agent provocateur is the person whose actions tend to undermine the efforts of the group. The effect of such behavior is usually quite destructive; it may be sufficiently threatening to the integrity of the group that removal of the member must be considered.

An example of sabotage occurred in a group of five students who were assigned a group project for one of their classes. One member was angry because he wanted to be assigned to a different group. At the first meeting, when the members were trying to decide how they would approach the assignment, he disagreed with every idea. He derogated the other members; he said they were stupid for following the assigned guidelines. The group was unable to accomplish anything, and everyone left feeling angry and frustrated.

Upsetting others may be the only way some people can keep themselves comfortable. When the people around him are upset and on the defensive, the saboteur is in control. Pointing out the saboteur's characteristic pattern may suggest to him the possibility of change, and it helps the other group members understand their own distress.

The Deserter. The deserter leaves in the middle of the meeting and does not return. The dropout attends a meeting or a few meetings, then fails to come back; often he does not give an explanation to the group or to the leader. The loss of a group member usually has a detrimental effect on the group, and the feelings tend to be magnified when the circumstances of the departure are ambiguous or when the departure is the result of a stormy conflict. The remaining group members frequently feel responsible for driving the person away, and thus they feel guilty. The departure can pose a threat to the leader's feelings of adequacy, and it may arouse concern that other members might leave.

The decision whether to have someone go out to be with the deserter or to continue the meeting must be based on the circumstances. If other people are available to care for the member, such as when meetings are held in a hospital unit, the leader may opt to continue. However, if the member leaves in tears or with a threat of suicide, it may be advisable to send a group member or one of the leaders to join the person. Whichever course of action is taken, it is essential that the group explore the situation and the feelings around the incident. Sharing feelings and perceptions helps to reduce the anxiety.

The dropout also presents a problem, but it is less acute. Loss of a member poses the threat of group dissolution. Yalom (1966) researched group therapy dropouts and found that most left during the beginning phase of the group. He advised that the most effective means of preventing dropouts is to prepare the member for the group. Follow-up is indicated, and leaders should contact members who leave prematurely. Although this may not bring the individual back to the group, at least it provides the leader with information that can be helpful when exploring the loss with the remaining group members. The fact that the leader cares enough to reach out and to report back to the group reassures the members that the leader does care.

Dropouts are inevitable in groups, and they do not signify personal failure on the part of the leader. Undue concern over success and failure may prompt the group leader to pressure the member to continue, but this is contrary to the principle of voluntary participation (Yalom 1970). Supervision can help the leader sort out the feelings involved in this problem.

The Scapegoater. Often a group will single out one or two members as targets for animosity. Yalom (1970) pointed out that in a therapy group this may be a consequence of the therapist's failure to explore the anger directed at the therapist. Teachers are familiar with the tendency for a classroom of children to pick on one or two peers. In small groups (which includes the family) the members vent their anxiety and negative feelings on the scapegoat (Johnson 1963).

An example of scapegoating occurred in a committee when a new chairperson was appointed without consultation with the members. During the first meeting that she chaired, the members were angry because of their inability to reach agreement on a certain issue. One member who had arrived 15 minutes late was singled out and severely criticized for this behavior. Their anger was directed at the latecomer, but actually they were angry with the chairperson. The leader should make it known that innocent individuals have become the targets of criticism or anger.

The Seducer. Seductive behavior is a manipulative gesture with sexual overtones that is used to control others. When seductive behavior is used as the primary means of relating to others, it becomes a problem. When a group member behaves seductively with another member, this frequently is ignored at first. If the behavior continues, however, the recipient of this attention usually acts embarrassed or angry or hostile.

An example of seductive behavior occurred in an adult group. A young man often brought flowers to the women members. He would attempt to discuss sexual issues and ask for feedback from the women. Most of his comments were very suggestive, provoking nervous laughter. The leader identified this as a repeating pattern of behavior. The young man was unaware of this. The women shared the information that his attempts at "undressing them with his eyes" made them uncomfortable. He exclaimed that he thought that was what women enjoyed. He eventually changed his method of relating to the women members and established better relationships. Later in the life of the group he shared the information that seductive behavior was his way of avoiding rejection by women. If he could seduce them, he felt sure that they would like him and care about him.

The leader must be aware of the subtle interactions of the group members, because seductive behavior can start out as a covert communication pattern. Whenever the leader becomes uncomfortable with such behavior, the group should be informed of the situation. Seductive behavior is manipulative. It can be used to divert attention from the real feelings of the individual or to get something the individual wants. An honest and open approach is probably the best way to discourage seductive behavior. Beating around the bush often confuses the seducer and does not accomplish the primary goal of managing the behavior. As mentioned previously, the seducer often is unaware that he is operating in this fashion. An honest explanation of how his behavior is affecting the leader does not subjugate the seducer; rather, it gives him new awareness of his own behavior (Kelley and associates 1974). It must also be remembered that seductive behavior can be used by the leader. The reason may be the same as that of any other group member.

The Passivist. Passivity frequently results when the purpose or task of the group is nebulous or when the original purpose of the group changes. It is a common occurrence for a leader to ask for a volunteer to work on a specific task, only to have the members look at their feet as if they hadn't heard him. Even when discussion on the purpose or task does take place it is often desultory; ideas are not freely exchanged, and no one seems to be much involved.

In dealing with this passivity or apathy the leader should first assess the dynamics that are operating in the group. The following phenomena might be occurring: (1) The group's task is not well spelled out, or it is not appropriate. (2) The group is in the war stage, and members are not ready to confront the task until they work through their feelings about each other; thus, the task is taking a back seat to the real issue that is facing the group. (3) The group has lost its sense of direction; it is no longer moving toward a common goal. (4) Passive or apathetic members are in conflict over their involvement because the group is threatening and intimidating them.

After making an assessment the leader should explain to the members why he is concerned about their progress. With encouragement and support they can often renew their enthusiasm for the task and move forward. Allowing the members to unburden themselves of secret feelings will facilitate the group process and will help to accomplish the task at hand.

The Cynic. Thoresen (1972) described the cynic as the one in the group who utilizes the fighting defense. The basic premise of this individual is that the best defense is a good offense. By this means he is able to keep the attention and disenchantment of the group focused somewhere other than on himself. Thoresen (1972, p 117) stated that cynicism is "manifested by frequent challenging of the group contract and goals, skeptical questioning of genuine behavior, and attacks on stronger, threatening members." The cynic of the group may be quite comfortable challenging the group's belief that the sun rises in the east. Through his evasive maneuvers the cynic can interfere with the growth of the group and the growth of the other members.

In a group session where the members were discussing loss, one member talked about the death of her mother. She began to cry. The cynic of the group responded: "Oh this is ridiculous! I did not come here to talk about death. If this is what we are going to talk about I want to leave." The members were stunned by the insensitivity of the cynic. The leader stated, in an objective manner, "That comes across as being pretty cynical." The cynic looked at the leader and then began to cry; then she told the group that she, too, had recently lost someone. She had become overwhelmed with feelings of loss; she felt that she had to negate them by being cynical.

The most effective way for the leader to deal with the cynic is to identify for the cynic what is going on. As the previous example illustrates, the group member who uses cynical behavior is often secretly frightened. The cynic is unable to deal with his feelings; he attempts to banish them by fighting back or becoming cynical.

The Psychotic. The group member who can most easily throw a group into a tailspin is the psychotic. Group sessions conducted at inpatient psychiatric units provide many such examples. Group members on these units might have illnesses such as depression, character disorders, or psychosis. If a group member exhibits extremely bizarre behavior, the other group members as well as the leader may have difficulty in dealing with the situation.

One therapy group involved a 20-year-old man who attended a daily group session in an inpatient ward. The group consisted of about 10 members, male and female, along with the leaders. As one session started, the man began to pray. He spoke very softly. During the first half hour of the session he periodically got up and wrote religious statements on a nearby blackboard. After writing a few statements he would rejoin the group and get down on his hands and knees to resume praying. His behavior was very distracting to the group, but they did not make any comments to him. One leader decided to bring this behavior into the group's discussion. He stated: "I have noticed John acting very crazy, and no one has asked him what is going on. I'm wondering what the members think." Immediately following this statement, the man stopped his praying and began to pay attention to what was going on with the other members of the group.

When dealing with a psychotic patient in a group, the leader should consider certain factors. If a patient is unable to control his behavior and cooperate in the group, this type of therapy may not be appropriate for him. Medication adjustment or individual therapy might then be considered. The patient can be asked to join the group later, when he is able to make a contribution.

Another important factor is the psychotic patient's potential as a group member. Even though the patient may be demonstrating some psychotic behavior, he is not stupid; he can make appropriate observations about himself, about other patients, and about the group process. If the patient is acting bizarre, the leader can point this out to him. Another possibility is to help the group members express their feelings about how the psychotic patient's behavior is affecting them. The leader can help them to express their feelings rather than attack the psychotic patient. The leader should not encourage discussion of the delusional thinking of the patient; rather, a focus on reality should be emphasized.

The Interrogator. Interrogation is used to keep other members of the group on the defensive. Thoresen (1972, p 117) stated that "an individual who habitually cross-examines others in the group under the guise of 'gaining helpful information and understanding' may be fighting to keep the spotlight safely away from himself."

The interrogator may direct a barrage of questions at the other members in the early stages of the group. In some cases the members may be willing to comply with his demands; they may willingly answer all questions. In later meetings his demands may be frustrating for them; by then they may resent sharing what is going on with them if the interrogator shares little about himself.

The leader needs to help the interrogator examine his behavior so that he can see what effect it has on the group. By the time members confront the interrogator they may have reached the point where they are irritated and are reacting in anger.

There was an interrogator in a group of 8 patients in group psychotherapy, 6 of whom were court-referred. The interrogator was not court-referred. Whenever another member of the group described his situation, the interrogator asked him to justify his behavior. When the leader pointed out to the patient, in a supportive manner, that he was interrogating the other members, he was able to admit that he was not comfortable with the other members because they were ex-cons. Eventually he was able to share the fact that he was dealing largely with his fantasies and trying to keep the attention of the group diverted from himself.

The Pseudo Leader. The behavior of the pseudo leader is similar to that of the interrogator; it is an attempt by a member to hide behind a role rather than deal with his behavior and feelings. Dinkmeyer and Muro (1971) described the pseudo leader as one who uses avoidance techniques. The pseudo leader is the group member who tries to elaborate on the comments and interpretations made by the leader. He may try to present himself as a junior Freud or as the therapist's helper.

Such behavior may be threatening to the leader who has only limited experience, because his leadership role is in danger of being co-opted by the pseudo leader. Even though the pseudo leader probably desires feedback and help, he is preventing this by his effort to take over the leader's functions. He frequently fears what the group might say to him; it would be more negative than he could tolerate. The leader must help him to see that his behavior is counterproductive (Dinkmeyer and Muro 1971).

The Coalitionist. Members who want to avoid deeper involvement in the group or who fear being confronted will frequently attempt to develop alliances. This phenomenon has been called subgrouping or coalition formation.

Two members may pair up to keep the focus of the group away from themselves. A few members may subgroup to mediate or to defend a member who is under attack when conflict or confrontation occurs. There is implied an agreement between such members: "Let's keep it safe. I'll come to your aid if you come to mine" (Thoresen 1972, p 118).

Coalition formation was noted in a group of nursing graduate students. The group consisted of students from two different departments. Although the group did not sit in a particular pattern, the students in medical-surgical nursing would support and respond to each other more than to the psychiatric nursing students. The instructor noticed this trend and recorded the communication pattern. When this information was shared, the members recognized what has happening; they established a new goal to learn more about each other. The coalition formation was noted to decrease.

SUMMARY

Group processes have been presented as they relate to different types of groups. Suggestions for assessment of group development and function have been made. Behaviors that frequently present problems for the group and its leader have been described. Some examples of means for coping with these behaviors have been included.

References

Baker J, Estes N: Anger in group therapy. Am J Nurs 65:96–100, July 1965

Benne K D, Sheats P: Functional roles of group members. Journal of Social Issues 4:41, Spring 1948

Cartwright D, Zander A: Group Dynamics: Research and Theory. New York, Harper & Row, 1968

Dinkmeyer D C, Muro J J: Group Counseling: Theory and Practice. Itasca, Ill, Peacock, 1971

Eisenberg J, Abbott R D: The monopolizing patient in group therapy. Perspect Psychiatr Care 6:68, 1968

Hanson P G: What to look for in groups: An observation guide. In Pfeiffer J W, Jones J E (eds): 1972 Annual Handbook for Group Facilitators. La Jolla, University Associates, 1972

Hopkins L T: Interaction: The Democratic Process. Boston, Heath, 1961
Johnson J A Jr: Group Therapy: A Practical Approach. New York, McGraw-Hill, 1963
Jones J E: A model of group development. In Jones J E, Pfeiffer J W (eds): 1973 Annual Handbook for Group Facilitators. La Jolla, University Associates, 1973
Kelley L K, Williams R A, Eggert L L: Seductive Behavior in the Helper-Client Relationships (videotape). Seattle, Univ Washington Press, 1974
Knowles M, Knowles H: Introduction to Group Dynamics. New York, Associated Press, 1972
Lassey W R: Dimensions of leadership. In Lassey W R, Fernandez R R (eds): Leadership and Social Change. La Jolla, University Associates, 1976, pp 10–15
Lieberman M A, Yalom I D, Miles M B: Encounter Groups: First Facts. New York, Basic Books, 1973
Light N: The chronic helper in group therapy. Perspect Psychiatr Care 11:129, 1974
Luchins A S: Group Therapy: A Guide. New York, Random, 1964
Marram G D: The Group Approach in Nursing Practice. St Louis, Mosby, 1973
Mills T M: The Sociology of Small Groups. Englewood Cliffs, Prentice-Hall, 1967, p 2
Moore J A: Encountering hostility during psychotherapy sessions. Perspect Psychiatr Care 6:58–65, 1968
Rosenfeld E M: Intervening in hostile behavior through dyadic and/or group intervention. J Psychiatr Nurs 7:251–254, December 1969
Shaw M: Group Dynamics: The Psychology of Small Group Behavior. New York, McGraw-Hill, 1976
Slavson S R: The phenomenology and dynamics of silence in psychotherapy groups. Int J Group Psychother 16:397, October 1966
Thoresen P: Defense mechanisms in groups. In Pfeiffer J W, Jones J E (eds): 1972 Annual Handbook for Group Facilitators. La Jolla, University Associates, 1972
Tuckman B W: Developmental sequence in small groups. J Pers Soc Psychol 1:384–399, June 1965
Ward J T: The sounds of silence. Perspect Psychiatr Care 12:13, 1974
Yalom I D: The Theory and Practice of Group Psychotherapy. New York, Basic Books, 1970
______ A study of group therapy dropouts. Arch Gen Psychiatry 14:393–414, 1966

CHAPTER

12

ENCOUNTERING DYSFUNCTION IN THE FAMILY SYSTEM

Marilyn Peddicord Whitley
L. (Sissy) Madden

Americans have devised an ingenious method of handling family dysfunction: we have specialists who are skilled in societal interactions. These interactors are generally highly functional individuals and are considered professionals. Nurses carry this designation, and they are frequently in contact with families experiencing dysfunctional periods.

Family dysfunction is the disordered or impaired functioning of the familial system. This dysfunction may be encountered by nurses working in the community, as well as in the institutional setting. Children who have unmet physical needs or who lack skill in relating to peers and authorities often come to the attention of the school nurse. Public health nurses often see expectant mothers in poor physical health; sometimes they also discover a spouse in the home whose educational level keeps him from getting an adequate job. When a health crisis develops, such as those requiring intensive care, coronary care, or emergency room services, the hospital staff nurse usually must be concerned with the patient's entire family. The nurse employed on a medical ward encounters families dealing with long-term illness and those suffering the loss of a family member by death. The nurse in a psychiatric clinic sees families struggling with psychosis, depression, stress, drug dependence, and interpersonal conflict. The industrial nurse encounters families dealing with social pressures to acquire goods and services similar to those possessed by others in their reference group; often this effort to comply with societal norms takes a noticeable toll on the family and its members.

Both society and the family have certain expectations of the nurse who uses her skills to help a dysfunctional family. Society expects professionals to correct family dysfunction and to do it in such a way as not to disturb the societal pattern. Families expect advocacy on their behalf within the social system and assistance in restorative actions.

The specific assessment, intervention, and evaluation components of the nursing process are appropriate for use with a dysfunctional family. By using the process components the nurse is able to look closely at a family, make an assessment, help the family set goals, apply intervention techniques, and evaluate the work done toward those goals.

This chapter is designed to assist the nurse in preparing to work with dysfunctional families. The knowledge base necessary for assessment will be described. This will include definitions and characteristics of the family. It will also include a description of the equipment families need for functioning. Specific data collection techniques will be detailed. Goal setting will be discussed. The requirements necessary to effect change within the family, as well as within the nurse, will be outlined. The specific interventions of administering physical care, patient teaching, advocacy, and referral will be described. Finally, evaluation will be outlined.

KNOWLEDGE BASE

In order to be able to offer professional expertise to any family, the nurse must have a certain knowledge base. A nurse must be able to understand the family's characteristics; she must be aware of family functions and the kind of equipment necessary to carry out those functions. The nurse also needs to understand how the absence of essential components can cause dysfunction. The following sections will describe the knowledge base that is necessary before any professional can begin to make an assessment of a family.

Definition of Family

It might be said that there are as many definitions as there are families. A family partakes of the properties of a group, a support system, a communication network, a power system, an ethnic entity, and a consumer unit. Each family has both universal and particular qualities. Henry, for instance, belongs to the J. T. Wilson family on Elm Street. He also belongs to the larger family of Wilsons living on the East Coast. The Wilsons, in turn, belong to the large social system encompassing many families, as well as to the entire family of man.

The following will outline a working definition of the family unit. The term family usually designates a married couple and their children by birth or adoption who cooperatively interact for the purpose of attaining common goals. This unit forms a nucleus. It is frequently referred to as the nuclear family. Nuclear families are always two-generational, and they are time-limited. The nucleus in the American family usually endures about 20 years, at which time the members of the younger generation begin to form their own families. The adults in the nuclear family are said to come from their families of origin. The adults' families of origin are part of the extended family that encompasses the nuclear family; that is, all persons related to the two-generation nuclear family by birth, adoption, or marriage are members of the extended family. The parents in the nuclear family eventually become a family of aging, and they exist basically as members of their children's extended family. Not all Americans identify with a family constellation as just described; there are several alternatives to this definition.

Alternative Families. In order to satisfy a very important human need, those people who have no bona fide family tend to modify the standard concept to allow themselves to live in a familylike environment. While the standard family concept is two-generational, alternative families may consist of adult members of a single generation.

An alternative family may consist of two people (and sometimes their offspring) who have chosen to live together without the usual societal sanction of marriage. Such couples negotiate on various levels the rights and responsibilities included in the usual marriage contract. Another form of alternative family may include many persons who band together to live in a communal arrangement. Norms are negotiated among the members of each family grouping. The norms include privileges and responsibilities covering economic concerns, parenting, and sexual expression.

Alternatives may include adults living with substitute family members. Roommates, members of the extended family, and even pets can constitute family members for some people. Alternatives also include homosexual family units. Instances of couples of the same sex living together and interacting sexually are becoming more common and more openly recognized in American society. In many cases homosexual family arrangements will include children from previous heterosexual unions.

Single-Parent and Blended Families. Single-parent families and blended families are often included in the list of alternative families. However, since these families are frankly two-generational and include male-female contact for childbearing, they can be considered to fall between categories.

A single-parent family exists when a parent and offspring live together as a nucleus. The single-parent family is often transitory; it results from loss of one member of the parental dyad by death, divorce, or separation. One of the parents may have been included in the family only at the child's birth and early years. In any case, the lone parent must take on the parenting usually done by both mother and father. The single parent sometimes provides a substitute for the missing parent by forming a special alliance with a member of the extended family or with a dating companion. The population of single parents in America is large; it is particularly important to realize that they are often vulnerable to conditions that can cause dysfunction.

Satir (1972, p 170) defined nuclear families with missing adult members who join to form a new nucleus as blended families. Remarriage following the loss of a spouse by death or divorce is the usual precipitant for the blending of families. Blended families have many special features. They have additional sets of extended family members. They often must renegotiate previously defined family roles. In blending they may acquire members with special health problems. Sometimes blending requires changing reference groups and making adjustments in extrafamilial relationships. The blending process is often difficult for children; frequently they feel no attraction toward the new siblings or the stepparent. Numerous features of the blending process may add to conflict and lead to dysfunction of the newly formed system. Blending is a common phenomenon in American society, and it is often encountered by the nurse.

Nurses come into contact with all types of families in their professional endeavors. A clear understanding of how a person defines his family constellation is important to an understanding of a family's current dysfunction, and any dysfunction must be understood before steps can be taken to reverse it.

Family Characteristics

All families have structure. The structural framework of the family is a system of interrelated parts that form a whole. The family system includes the family members, their communication with each other, and the relationships developed; it also includes interaction with the family's environment. The family system is constantly changing. New material enters the system; other material leaves. If material can enter and leave the system easily, the family system may be characterized as an open system. Francis and Munjas (1976, p 27) stated that the degree of openness in a family is a useful indicator of a family's ability to change.

The family system functions as a whole. The movement of one part has direct effect on other parts. Information received by the system from the outside in response to its performance, as well as information exchanged within the system, affects the system. This information is called feedback. Feedback is an important concept in dealing with systems; it is the method by which one part lets another know how it is being perceived. Systems that do not permit feedback to enter or circulate are said to be closed systems. Closing the system decreases the growth possibilities and may eventually lead to dysfunction. The following clinical example illustrates a family system:

CLINICAL EXAMPLE

Mr. Roberts, an alcoholic, displayed symptoms of his illness at a neighborhood picnic. His actions angered his wife and caused her embarrassment. Their son erroneously assumed that he was to blame for his father's behavior; he tried to remember what he might have done to cause his father to drink excessively. Mr. Roberts' daughter asked him for a large advance on her allowance; she had learned that when he was drinking excessively he could be manipulated for financial gain. The neighbors informed the Roberts family that the workings of their family system were causing distress to the neighborhood. The family reacted to this internal and external feedback by not participating in subsequent social functions. They attempted to fix the blame for the damaging feedback by arguing, blaming, scapegoating, and denying. All parts of this system were affected by the father's drinking behavior. As a result, the family became more rigid and moved toward becoming a closed system.

All systems have a need to balance themselves. In open systems feedback can effect change and create a new state of balance. Closed systems block out feedback and do not allow change. The dynamics illustrated in the example of the alcoholic family demonstrate a common patterned attempt by a family system to cope with feedback. All too often the faulty coping techniques utilized by the family only serve to maintain the system in a dysfunctional state, rather than promote change. Francis and Munjas (1976, p 29) pointed out that the way a family system handles this balancing is an indicator of its stability.

In addition to structure and balance, all families have goals. All movement or change within the family system is directed toward a goal. The goal may be either natural or planned. When a family allows and encourages its young members to take on financial responsibility, it is usually planning the goal of teaching them sound financial principles prior to their separation from the family. The natural goal is the emancipation of the children. The planned goal is to provide the family's youth with knowledge and experience of the societal financial system.

Another natural goal of the family system is to maintain itself as a system. In order to achieve this, members are expected to behave in certain ways. When members fail to behave in the prescribed way, other parts of the system react with specific behaviors in an attempt to minimize the disruption and keep the family intact. Conflict and stress can occur when individual goals, family goals, and societal goals are incongruent. Inability to cope with the resulting conflict and stress can cause dysfunction.

Family Functions

A family system is task-oriented. Duvall (1971, p 149) described the natural family developmental tasks as follows: (1) physical maintenance; (2) allocation of resources; (3) division of labor; (4) socialization of family members; (5) reproduction, recruitment, and release of family members; (6) maintenance of order; (7) placement of members in the larger society; (8) maintenance of motivation and morale. American society directs its families to be self-perpetuating and to be the primary system for the transfer of social norms and values. Some of the tasks carried out by the family are family-directed; others are society-directed. Familial and societal tasks intertwine and overlap.

The manner in which the specific tasks are carried out has importance for smooth family functioning. These tasks require a certain level of mastery by family members for their successful completion. The tasks must aid, not hinder, all of the family members during their individual developmental stages.

Family Equipment

In order to accomplish their tasks, families need a certain amount of equipment. This equipment includes hardware as well as software. Hardware refers to personal possessions and the use of services granted by other social subsystems. It includes the following: (1) physical and mental health of family members; (2) ability to identify, describe, indoctrinate, and maintain family members in roles for task accomplishment; (3) access to education for economic viability. Software refers to interactional affairs; ie, interaction between the family and the greater social system. Software includes (1) the ability to gain access to and hold a desired reference group position and (2) the capacity to maintain the family system. The latter includes the use of power, communication skills, and recreation abilities. The following sections will describe this equipment and the potential for dysfunction in its absence.

Physical Health. If the proper milieu for growth and development of all family members is to be established, physical health must have high priority. Physical health is relative: If everyone in a given society is missing a few teeth, the absence of teeth is not considered to constitute ill-health. However, if only one person is without teeth, he is considered to be in poor health, and both he and his society may think it necessary to do something about his situation.

Contemporary American society has high health standards for its citizens. Billions of dollars every year are spent on the nation's physical health. There are stringent laws regarding sanitation and food handling. Dental hygiene and nutrition classes have been added to the grade school education curricula. Free lunches are provided for children from low-income families. In present-day American society the person or family unable to achieve optimum physical health is at a disadvantage. An example of a family whose male head is a quadraplegic will illustrate this point. Mr. Lopez was hurt in a logging accident, leaving him a highly dependent, multihandicapped patient. Immediately this family had the potential to become dysfunctional. The family members had to make many adjustments in order to complete their tasks together. The son just finishing high school had to reconsider his career goals in light of his perceived responsibility for the family's economic situation. Mrs. Lopez had to reassess her nonbreadwinning status. Mr. Lopez made an assessment of his entire being and his role as husband and father. With the help of a skilled nurse this family was able to meet the crisis, take in the feedback, and rebalance their system to accommodate the change (see Chapter 10). However, many family systems, when faced with such a health problem, are unable to rebalance themselves to a functional state.

There are many areas of physical health that have far-reaching implications for families. The nurse must consider dietary, congenital, and long-term illnesses as stressors. Introduction of a retarded infant into a family will add stress, temporary imbalance, and necessitate change; it will have the potential for causing dysfunction. Arthritis, heart disease, multiple sclerosis, diabetes, and a multitude of other diseases will create stress that may necessitate familial change. This stressor, physical illness, has much potential for creating dysfunctional imbalance within a family unit.

Mental Health. Mental health is also part of the equipment a family needs for successful operation. It is certainly a less obvious commodity than physical health, but it is equally important. The family struggling along with a member who is psychotic, depressed, or psychosomatic has even more difficulty coping than the family burdened by physical illness. A mother who suddenly begins to cry several times a day, who loses weight, who cannot sleep, who becomes compulsive about her housework, and who is constantly irritable in her interactions with others certainly adds stress to the family system. The schizophrenic break of a family member usually results in family imbalance and creates a dysfunctional state. This dysfunctional state may last for years if it is not corrected, and it can result in complete deterioration of the family.

The degree of mental health of a family can also be said to encompass certain factors that are usually considered in a broader category than definable mental illness. One is the factor Satir (1972) called self-worth, or the feelings and ideas one has about himself. Satir stated that people with high self-worth are characterized by integrity, honesty, responsibility, compassion, and love in their relations with others. People with low self-worth expect to be cheated, have trouble bearing responsibility, and use defense mechanisms that wall them off from others and place them in a state of loneliness and isolation.

How a family and its members feel about themselves is important. Some families try to buoy each member's self-worth. Other families work actively at keeping members in a state of low self-worth. Feelings of low self-worth may be transitory; in other cases they are a constant threat to families or their members. Functional families continually encourage their members to feel good about themselves. Lack of self-worth can strain the mental health of a family.

Roles. The members of a family must determine how they are going to accomplish their tasks together. They must decide who is going to do which task. This calls for the establishment of roles. Spiegel (1968, p 393) defined a role as a "goal-directed pattern or sequence of acts tailored by the cultural process for the transactions a person may carry out in a social group or situation." This concept of roles implies that no role is carried out in isolation; there is always a reciprocal for each role. If there is a mother there must be a child. All roles must be learned when the person first takes on the role. Roles have definite familial and societal guidelines. The American guidelines for the role of child are different from the Chinese guidelines. The Smith family's norms for the role of child will differ slightly from those of the Fulton family.

Carter (1976) stated that the roles most pertinent for families are husband, wife, lover, mother, father, son, daughter, brother, and sister. There are, of course, many subsidiary roles within this structure. Family members may occupy several roles at once.

Families have to do more than identify roles. They must decide on a method of describing the roles to each other, a method of indoctrinating members into the roles, and a method of maintaining the members within their roles. Most important, families who wish to remain functional must find methods of modifying roles to accommodate changing family needs. For instance, mothers of very young children generally feed their children. However, when the child is able to handle a spoon, the mother usually teaches him to feed himself. As the mother and child adapt to the role change, they have to communicate their intentions to each other, and both need to remain firm in their intentions. For instance, a mother cautiously gives a spoonful of applesauce to a 10-month-old child. Then the child takes the spoon; he eats a little and decorates his surroundings with the remainder. If the mother doesn't approve of this role performance, she must indicate to the child the standard necessary for proper performance. The child, in turn, must indicate his acceptance or non-acceptance of the standard. The process of indoctrination is often slow, and it usually requires negotiations by all parties. However, the alternative of continuing to feed the child herself as he continues to grow is unrealistic and could lead to dysfunction.

There is conflict over a role when the member occupying the role fails to understand the role correctly. There is also conflict if the occupant of the role is unable to learn, unwilling to accept, or unable to perform the role. There is conflict if the person occupying the role desires to change the description of the role. This is especially true if the changes differ greatly from societal and familial expectations.

Many American families are experiencing stress from role conflict at the present time. For several generations the role of mother was stereotyped in middle-class American families: Mothers bore children and resisted working outside the home while caring for those children. Mothers also did all the cooking, housekeeping, washing, ironing, and chauffeuring of children during their growing years. Besides those tasks, the role of mother often included being caretaker of the family possessions. Mothers scrubbed and polished and were responsible for the goods that the family acquired. The fulfillment of this role as described was generally liked by the society. Mothers, however, became dissatisfied.

During the past 10 years, this role dissatisfaction has caused a revolution in many American families. Many women have completely changed the description of the role of mother. The majority of women have greatly limited the number of their children. Husbands and wives in many homes are presently negotiating the chores of cooking, cleaning, and chauffeuring the children. These changes in the role of mother have far-reaching effects on all members of the family, as well as on all institutions within the American social system.

The following is a common example found in nearly every American neighborhood: Nine-year-old Richard Dobson's mother took a job outside the home when Richard entered the fourth grade. Since she was working, she was no longer able to take Richard across town to soccer practice after school. The school was no longer able to send Richard home for lunch or expect Mrs. Dobson to attend daytime school functions. Soon Mrs. Dobson found it necessary to attend night classes to improve her work skills. As a result, Mr. Dobson began to do some babysitting. This sitting reduced the time Mr. Dobson could spend working in the evenings for his company. It is easy to see how the changing of Mrs. Dobson's role of mother affected the entire family and those social institutions closely related to the Dobson family. Roles play an exceptionally important part in the maintenance of family equilibrium. Disruption of roles or unresolved conflict about roles often leads to dysfunction.

Education for Economic Viability. Education of family members is interrelated with roles. There is education for role function. This is part of the indoctrination process, and it often includes role modeling. In farm families the sons work in the fields with their fathers and learn the role of farmer by patterning themselves after the model provided by their fathers. But industrial families must go outside the family for some of the educational processes, especially as they relate to economics. Education for the role of breadwinner in an industrial society often requires extra-familial schooling. Although this is done outside of the home, it is accomplished with the financial and emotional support of the family. The same is true of education for an academic career. Parents realized a long time ago that there was a need for special skill in teaching their children to read, write, and reason in a systematic way. Individual parents began to hire skilled adults to teach their children. Eventually, many parents banded together to hire other adults to teach their children.

The school system developed out of this familial need. But in present-day American culture a dissonance has developed between families and schools. The role each has carved out and the manner in which families and schools interact with one another around these roles cause stress in many American families. Nevertheless, schools remain important to families, to family members, and to the social system at large.

Families who cannot arrange to have their members participate in the educational process or who do not have the social skills necessary to manipulate the educational system to their advantage are greatly disadvantaged in our society. Access to economic means is essential in industrial societies. Without this access a family is powerless to guide its own destiny. The social system often manages the family, whereas the family should be using the social system for the advantage of its members. The person who cannot learn an adequate breadwinner role suffers economically; he suffers in self-worth and in social status. He is forced to accept a reference group in which he may not want to participate. The individual's family may be gravely affected by this deficiency.

Impoverished groups and ethnic groups of color have long been disadvantaged in education. The education available to them has been of poor quality, and the candidate for education has had minimal adaptability to the educational situation. In industrial societies one means of relieving poverty is to provide each person an education that will enable him to obtain a reasonably remunerative job.

The Hagerty family was an example of an impoverished family economically disadvantaged because of inadequate education. Mr. Hagerty was once a functioning breadwinner, but his line of work no longer existed because of industrial change. The family lived on welfare in their grandfather's house in crowded conditions; they suffered lack of privacy and an insufficient diet. At the time the family sought help, the family members knew how they wanted their situation changed. They wanted Mr. Hagerty to get a job that paid a living wage, and they wanted to move to a house of their own. However, Mr. Hagerty was unable to make the necessary adjustments to obtain the education and retraining required for another job. His inability to reclaim the role of breadwinner resulted in a dysfunctional situation for his family.

Reference Group. It is not enough that a family have health, a division of labor held in place by roles, adequate education, and economic security; the family must also belong to a reference group. A reference group is that group of families who come into contact with each other and who find themselves in similar socioeconomic and cultural situations. Families and members of families actually have several reference groups. Some reference groups are exclusive of others. For example, the McNeal family includes no one of Italian descent. Therefore, the family has no reference to the large Italian community in the same town, even though they may have much else in common.

Reference groups give a family a sense of belonging. They also provide a standard to which the family norms can be compared. The Cooper family belongs to the reference group of schoolteachers because the male head of the family is a schoolteacher. However, the father teaches industrial arts, not English; thus the Coopers have a closer relationship to families whose fathers are industrial arts teachers. The Cooper family also enjoys backpacking. Other families who backpack have a reference group relationship with them. The Coopers belong to a Protestant church and have a special relationship with other members of that church. When the Coopers set out to acquire goods and avail themselves of society's services, they must do so in a manner similar to that of the other families in their reference group, or they will collect a societal penalty. The Coopers are not likely to buy a motorcycle to take to the mountains because a cycle would be incompatible with the backpacking reference group. Acquisition of a motorcycle would mean they would be viewed by other backpackers as different and no longer acceptable; they would have to change their reference group. Families that cannot keep up with the reference group norms, families that refuse to comply, and families that want to enter a new reference group are at risk of becoming dysfunctional.

System Maintenance. All systems must have maintenance. Every car owner knows that his automobile will stop functioning if he fails to add oil, keep the moving parts greased, use the right kind of gasoline, and treat it properly while driving. Families also have to be maintained. Maintenance requires a power structure, an effective communication system, and a certain amount of time for rest and recreation.

Families ordinarily have a hierarchical power structure. The central task for families with young children is to create a safe environment in which the children can develop. This requires a somewhat authoritarian power structure: What mother says, goes! Highly functional families work this out in different ways, but the adults hold the power. Some families have a system where mom speaks, but dad backs her up; in some families dad makes the decisions, but mom presents them to the children; in some families, when either parent speaks, the other supports. Dysfunctional families usually have trouble agreeing on who holds the power. Sometimes the children hold the power. In functional families the power system shifts somewhat as the children grow older and take more responsibility for their own functioning. In many families with older children the power structure evolves to a more democratic system in which all family members have similar input into the decisions made by the family.

The exercise of power often involves conflict. If the adults in the family do not know how to exercise the power, or if they refuse to use it or use it unwisely, the children become confused. The system begins to break down. This example illustrates the point: A student named Margaret was arrested for shoplifting. She was referred by the court for family counseling. Her family seemed to have all the equipment necessary for smooth functioning. However, Margaret said of her mother, "She won't let me be myself." Margaret's mother continued to control her 15-year-old daughter as she had done when Margaret was a 2-year-old. For example, Margaret was not allowed to choose clothes to her own liking.

In some families the adults refuse to use their power to set limits for the children. In one dysfunctional family a 16-year-old boy continually used his father's truck without parental consent. However, the adults in the family levied no penalty and made no effort to control the keys to the truck. Therefore there was chronic discord over this issue. The ineffective use of power can create stress and lead to dysfunction.

The interaction of the members in their various roles within the family is called communication. Family members are all individuals, and the roles they play are separate entities. The interaction between members while enacting their roles is the force that makes the entire system work or fail to work. Watzlawick and associates (1967) pointed out that all persons in the presence of each other communicate. The process of communication may be verbal or nonverbal. Not only must a role occupant learn how others have defined his role, he must also learn how to communicate about that definition of his role. If a mother putting her newborn to breast touches the cheek of the child that is next to the breast, the child will turn toward her ready to nurse. If she touches the opposite cheek, the child will turn away from her breast. If she touches both cheeks at the same time the child will move his head from side to side, not knowing where to nurse. Communications must be clear, say what is meant and be understood by others as the family member intends.

If a family member is unable to understand the signals communicated to him, stress will occur within the family system. If there is a family member who is retarded, deaf, blind, schizophrenic, or brain-damaged, there is considerable potential for disruption in family communication. Communication is an integral part of family life. Each member must be skilled at communicating to the others what he wants, what he needs, what he is willing to do, how he feels, and what his expectations of the other family members are. The nurse interacting with the dysfunctional family is apt to see many discrepancies between what people attempt to communicate and how others perceive that communication.

Family members' verbal messages do not always say the same thing as simultaneous nonverbal messages. Discrepancies between messages can be very confusing to the person receiving the signals. For example, a mother says, with a grimace on her face, "Here, Carol, eat this yummy liver." Many people never learn to communicate effectively. Many people are stifled in communicating what they really mean. Some people will not take responsibility for their thoughts and feelings; they continually communicate ambiguities. Family members can also play various games with communication. Some of the most common include saying they will when they won't, communicating only part of the information needed to understand clearly, passing off their thoughts and feelings as those of another family member, and overloading their own and other family members' receiving mechanisms with stimuli, thus causing anxiety. All such games lead to stress and can lead to dysfunction.

The stress on the family system caused by having to cope with all of this equipment is substantial. Families need time out from society, time out to renew their own energies. Family members also need periods of privacy and solitude. Privacy is necessary for sorting out one's thoughts and recuperating from interactions. Families also need time to enjoy each other. Some families do this over the evening meal. Others enjoy sporting or artistic activities together. All families need to close out the rest of the world for a time and enjoy being together. Laughter and lightheartedness are essential for this time together; it doesn't matter whether the family is searching for the whitest pebble on the beach, recalling an antic of one of its members, having a game of cards, or just relaxing together. A lack of rest and an absence of time for recreation cause stress and can lead to system dysfunction.

Summary. In the previous sections it has been pointed out that absence or misuse of the equipment necessary for efficient family functioning can cause dysfunction. Hardware and software play an important part in establishing and maintaining a family's equilibrium. Some families suffer multiple deficiencies in their store of wares. Other families are situationally deficient; others have only one or two deficiencies.

The nurse with a well grounded knowledge base may begin to establish a framework for behavioral action with families. Acting without thinking is risky. However, thinking without acting cannot effect change. The following sections will describe some steps that are necessary for the nurse who wishes to interact effectively with a dysfunctional family. The emphasis will be on reversing the dysfunction.

DATA COLLECTION

When working with a family, the nurse begins by asking the members what is troubling them, ie, how the family perceives the dysfunction. Sometimes people will say plainly what is bothering them: "Johnny won't stay in school." "Carol is shoplifting." "Dad is dying." "Mom is drunk all of the time." More often, families do not speak so plainly. Sometimes the things family members say are nonspecific: "We don't get along." "We fight all the time." "It's no fun to live here anymore." Nurses need to begin their assessment by listening carefully to the way family members describe their current situation. Do they identify a single person as the cause of the problem? Are they concerned about a current situation? Do they blame an outside system, or are they unable to identify the difficulty? What wares does the family indicate are missing from its equipment stores?

Family Constellation

Having heard how the family describes the current situation, the nurse begins to collect some descriptive data about the family constellation. This is easier for the family than talking about their perception of the dysfunction. Asking the family to talk about themselves usually helps to establish rapport between family members and the nurse. The family perceives the genuine interest of the nurse and begins to build a trust base at this point.

Collection of historical data must be adapted to the situation. The nurse need collect only the data that seem appropriate to the current difficulty. For instance, a public health nurse seeing a family without any food to eat should focus on the number of people in the home and their special nutritional needs rather than seek information about the family's communication patterns.

Collecting data requires the use of interviewing skills (see Chapter 2). Open-ended questions will usually elicit enough information for a brief appraisal of the family constellation. The following are examples of good beginning statements and questions:

> Tell me about the people who live in your household.
> Tell me about the other people who are important to your family.
> Who are the people who have been important to you but are no longer with your family?
> What's it like when mom's boyfriend comes over?

In situations where extended family members or adult developmental experiences appear to play a role, the nurse may want to ask such questions as these:

> What was growing up like for you?
> What kind of setting was your family raised in?
> What was it like for you when your parents were divorced?
> What was it like for you when your father was injured?

These suggested questions will give the nurse a beginning point for collecting data. She must listen carefully to the family's answers and use the more specific interviewing skills of paraphrasing, clarifying, reflecting, and summarizing to collect exact data if this is necessary in a particular area.

Health Assessment

If the health of the individual family members is not known to the nurse, she may need to make a health assessment. There are often surprises in this area. Many families have a chronically ill member or a retarded member they rarely mention. If all family members are present, the nurse may ask each member about his health, both physical and mental. If some members are absent, the nurse will have to make her assessment in part from the perceptions of other family members. The following questions are good open-ended starters:

> How does Helen's illness affect the other members of the family?
> What special things do you do for George now that he can't do everything for himself?
> When Dan began his dialysis, did it mean that the rest of you had to give up some things?
> What's it like when mom cries?
> How is it when Henry is drinking?

Questions regarding a family member's mental health must be posed tactfully. Very often the family will give the nurse some hints (openings) she can use in data collection: "Mom has her good days and her bad days." "Joanne seems different from the other girls at school." "I assume you know that Mary Ann spent 3 months last year in the state hospital." In order to increase her data base when she encounters these hints, the nurse can make a low-pressure response: "Tell me about it."

The family's self-worth is a conception about which it is difficult to gather direct information. However, it is possible to gather much information on family self-worth while the family members are telling about other aspects of their life together. Often it is best to use interviewing techniques other than open-ended questions. Paraphrasing, restating, and reflecting, as well as placing the responsibility for a feeling on a third party (or the nurse), may enable the family members to identify their feelings by a less direct and less threatening route. Here are some examples:

It sounds as if you're saying people don't treat you very well.
You say you felt rotten when you lost your job.
Other kids tell me they would feel pretty embarrassed if their dads should go to P.T.A. drunk.
I wouldn't feel very good about going to work with a black eye.

Role

In order to assess the family's ability to accomplish its tasks, questions about roles are necessary. Questioning is usually most effective if it begins open-ended; then, according to the amount and specificity of data needed, more clarifying and summarizing can be done. Here are some examples:

How are the household chores divided up?
How are the children cared for?
How does money get into your family?
How does money leave your family?
Dad earns the living; mom pays the bills. Is that right?
How do the kids get money? Do they ask mom for it?
Do they have to do something special to get it?
Does one person get more money than another?

Education for Economic Viability

Data regarding the family's access to education for economic viability may be collected by beginning with questions such as the following:

What is it like in school for members of your family?
Can you tell me about your friends at school?
Was it different for you in school last year?
What was it like for you adults when you went to school?

Is school helpful to the members of your family?
How did you learn your trade?
If you want to advance yourself in your trade, what has to be done?

Simple questions about the breadwinner's job are also important.

What kind of work do you do?
How satisfying is your job to you?
Is your job the family's only source of income?

Reference Group

Information about the family's reference group will enable the nurse to assess the family's struggle to maintain the status quo or effect change. Such data will help in identifying the family's socioeconomic status and will facilitate choices about the various support systems available. Again, open-ended questions are best for a beginning:

What kinds of people do you feel most comfortable with?
What are your friends' most valued possessions?
What things do you have that your friends wish they had?
What things do your friends have that you wish you had?
What is living in your neighborhood like for you?
How about the school the children go to? Is it right for your family?
Of all the people you know best, who would be most likely to help you out of a pinch?

Maintenance

Families who come to professionals for help gravely distressed, but who have only vague complaints, are often struggling with a systems maintenance problem. Assessment of the family power structure is extremely important. In order to plan interventions the nurse will need to know who holds the power. Some beginning questions often used are the following:

How are decisions made around your home?
Who has the last word?
How do you get that person to change his mind?
When mom tells you to do something, what happens?
When Jamie cries, what happens?

A dysfunctional family often develops a disturbed communication system. The complaints sound like this: "All we do is fight." "It's miserable to live here." The nurse can collect data by asking questions about their communication, but a more effective way is to observe the communication pattern in action. Watch how the family members describe their history together. Observe who sits next to whom. Look for coalitions and subgroups. Look to see if the members use "I" statements. An "I" statement means speaking in the first person when telling about oneself. Do the family members seem to tell only part of a story? Watch to see if one member receives, interprets, and delivers all messages to some other family member. Observe to see if the family listens when each one talks. Maybe some members are never heard. Is the family able to focus on the situation at hand, or does one member constantly interrupt and keep everyone distracted? Watch to see if the message sender is satisfied with how the receiver interprets his message. Watch to see if the message receiver gets a clear message.

Re-creation

The family's ability to withdraw from the rest of the world for a time is also important. They need that time to solve their problems and renew their energies. The nurse can ask these questions about that time:

How does your family have fun?
When some family member has a problem, how does it get worked out?
Are there any special times that are just family times, when no outsiders are allowed?
What happens when a family member is sad?

When the nurse has finished collecting data in the areas of family structure and the family's stores of hardware and software, it is then important to ask the family members to restate their problem. This time, ask them to do it in terms of what they want changed. The nurse can change her open-ended approach and become specific. This begins the process of goal negotiation and intervention.

INTERVENTION

Goal Negotiation

The nurse should begin this phase with a question for each member: "What would you like changed in your family?" The nurse must listen carefully to the first statements of change. Then she must listen even more carefully to the adjustments of those statements as other family members react.

"I don't know" statements must be reworked into specific answers. Some clinicians ask this question of family members: "If you were be be granted three wishes for the purpose of changing your family, what would you wish?" The nurse must use her interviewing skills to help the family members phrase their change statements specifically. Statements such as "I wish it would be nicer around here" must be made more specific: "I wish mom and dad would have fewer fights." "I wish mom would stop drinking." "I wish dad would get a job." These are clearly stated desires and concerns of family members, and they are sufficiently specific that they may be used by the nurse and the family as a basis for negotiating family treatment goals.

The nurse should hear from each family member. Sometimes the least likely member states the family needs most clearly. A nurse was once working with a family headed by an alcoholic male. She asked their 6-year-old child what she would like changed. The child's answer was clear: "I want dad to stop drinking, and I want him to quit hitting Patti [their baby], or I want mom to get a divorce."

The statement of desired change is the first step in the goal negotiation process. The model of goal negotiation set out by Enos and Nilsson (1975) is effective when establishing working goals for family–nurse interaction. The family members state their goals; the nurse states her goals. Then they negotiate a set of goals they are both willing to work on. The Allen family sought counseling because they wanted to decrease the number of fights between their 13-year-old twins. The nurse's goal was to improve the family's communication skills. Between the nurse and the family it was agreed that a workable goal would be to reduce conflict between the twins by teaching all of the family members to communicate more clearly with one another.

At the time the goals are negotiated, the family and nurse must also look at the ways the goals will be achieved. Enos and Nilsson (1975) suggested exploring options and barriers to achieving working goals. One option for improving family communication may be to go to a family therapist. Another option may be to sign up for a class on communication at the local church or community college. Another may be to do some well-planned reading. Sometimes a family may be able to work out the communication problem by spending a few hours with a nurse helping them clarify their messages to one another. One barrier to improving communication may be that some members of the family are not interested in the task. Perhaps some family member cannot think clearly or is schizophrenic. In one family an 18-year-old son had recently lost his hearing because of meningitis. He was opposed to family therapy, and he chose not to make the effort to understand the goals being negotiated.

Goals must be realistic for each family. They must also be attainable. It is foolhardy to agree on a goal that cannot be reached. The paraplegic person who wants to walk again may have an unattainable goal. The family who wants a dying child spared will have to negotiate and accept the goal of dealing reasonably with death. No professional can accomplish the impossible. Negotiating the goal until a workable state is reached is an extremely important step in the intervention process. To accomplish this the parties must look at all suggested goals, options, and barriers. Together they must arrive at a compromise, which is called a working goal.

When the goal has been negotiated, the family and the nurse should ask themselves how they will know when they have accomplished the goal. The Allen family might say that when the twins have only one fight a week they will have reached their goal. Turner (1974, p 28) noted that the process of evaluation is always ongoing: "Evaluation is a set of actions or a process by which it is demonstrated whether or not an objective has been achieved." It is true that one part of evaluation is the measure of achievement. However, the evaluation process also includes modification. The Allens, having succeeded in reducing the fights to one a week, may wish to set a new goal of reducing the fights to one every 2 weeks. Or possibly the original goal proved unattainable, and they wish to modify the goal and settle for a fight every other day.

Change

There are a number of requirements that must be met before change can take place within a family; they include specifics for both the nurse and the family. For the family the requirements are commitment to the goal and strength to effect change. It is useless to have a goal that dad stop smoking if he does not want to accomplish that goal. Change requires grit, unyielding courage and firmness of intent. Some families simply do not have grit. Professionals must permit such families the freedom to choose the time of their change. The nurse's door must always be left open to those who seek her help. Just because the nurse is ready for the family to change does not mean the family is ready.

Other requirements must be met by the nurse before she can facilitate a change. The obvious need for relief of physical illness requires assessment skills and the ability to deliver physical nursing care. Patient teaching skills are also important. The nurse dealing with a diabetic family member must be able to teach the proper administration of insulin. The nurse working with an aged family must be able to teach the nutritional adjustments appropriate for the aging. Dealing with a younger family requires that she be able to teach normal growth and development.

In addition to physical care and patient teaching, the nurse must learn two more important skills: referral and advocacy.

Referral

The nurse should know about the agencies in the area that offer special services to families or their members. It may be unrealistic to expect the nurse to be personally familiar with all community resources if the area is large and heavily populated. However, most large communities have a central information and referral service. Sometimes this service is available by telephone. The service will provide the name, type of services offered, and location of any agency. Resource lists of community agencies are often available through funding programs such as the United Way. Sometimes city and county health departments offer referral information. The telephone directory is also a valuable resource for locating community agencies.

Once an agency has been selected for the family, the nurse will need to give the family the following information: (1) the name of the agency, (2) the type of service provided, (3) the location, (4) the fee, and (5) the telephone number. This minimal information is mandatory in making a successful referral.

In order to become more familiar with service agencies in the community, the nurse should go out and meet the agency personnel. This allows her to refer a family directly to an individual at an agency. Referring a family directly to an individual makes the contact personal, and the family is reassured in having its own specific helper.

The nurse will want to keep current her knowledge of agencies, their personnel, and any changes made in the services offered. Feedback from the family through follow-up contact is helpful in assessing an agency. Case consultation with the other professionals at a new agency can also provide the nurse with a means of evaluating the effectiveness of the agency's interaction with the referred family. The most effective referrals are those made when the referral source, the family, and the agency all feel that a satisfactory attempt at goal attainment is being undertaken.

In some cases it is not enough to make a solid referral. The family may encounter difficulties in attempting to get assistance from the agency. Unfortunately, the larger the number of services provided, the more difficult the system seems to become for the family. Red tape, long waiting periods for appointments, and lack of personal touches are often-heard complaints when patients confront helping agencies. At this point the nurse's advocacy skills can be of advantage.

Advocacy

An advocate for a family is an intercessor, not champion of a cause. Nurses acting as advocates are likely to function as message unscramblers. The nurse is basically showing the family how to get into a system and how to make that system work for them. For example, a family finds that in order to maintain economic viability the father must apply for public assistance. The nurse advocate can inform the applicant where to apply, with whom to talk, what information to take with him, what appointment time is best, how long the process will take, and what pitfalls he might expect. In some situations the nurse might telephone the agency to clarify the family's need.

The advocate aids the family by guiding it. She does not relieve the family of the responsibility for action. Dealing with a community agency can be threatening for the family. The nurse advocate can help the family understand the workings of the agency system. However, the family must bear the responsibility for following through with the contact.

SUMMARY

This chapter has been written to assist nurses in their work with dysfunctional family systems. The knowledge base necessary for nurses to complete an assessment of a family has been presented. This basic knowledge consists of understanding the family's definition of its constellation, its functions, and its structure. The knowledge base also includes an understanding of the hardware and software necessary for operation of an American family. Hardware includes (1) physical and mental health of family members, (2) family members' uses of their roles, and (3) family access to education for economic viability. Software consists of (1) the family members' reference groups and (2) the family's capacity to maintain its own system. We have discussed how an absence of essential hardware and software can contribute to a state of dysfunction in a family.

This chapter has shown that the nursing process may be employed to assist families experiencing dysfunction. We have pointed out that the nurse is able to use her interviewing skills in the collection of data for assessment and in negotiating goals for change. The nurse can then employ the direct intervention techniques of physical care and patient teaching, or she can utilize referral and advocacy skills.

This chapter is meant to serve as an introduction to learning to interact with dysfunctional families. Nurses will find that each family is different. There is no standard formula for action. Each situation requires a slightly different application of the assessment, intervention, and evaluative process. Families often need nurses to assist them in their dysfunctional states, and nurses should continually be preparing themselves to deliver informed, sensitive nursing care.

References

Carter F M: Psychosocial Nursing Theory and Practice in Hospital and Community Mental Health. New York, Macmillan, 1976

Duvall E M: Family Development, 4th ed. Philadelphia, Lippincott, 1971

Enos M S, Nilsson B S: A Faculty Manual on Client Goals Theory. Brookings, South Dakota State University, 1975

Francis G M, Munjas B A: Manual of Social Psychologic Assessment. New York, Appleton, 1976

Satir V: Peoplemaking. Palo Alto, Science and Behavior Books, 1972

Spiegel J P: The resolution of role conflict within the family. In Bell N, Vogel E (eds): A Modern Introduction to the Family. New York, Free Press, 1968

Turner M N: Nursing process: An operational framework for nursing practice. In Hall J, Weaver B (eds): Nursing of Families in Crisis. Philadelphia, Lippincott, 1974

Watzlawick P, Beavin J, Jackson D: Pragmatics of Human Communication. New York, Norton, 1967

CHAPTER 13

FAMILY SUBSYSTEM: THE THERAPEUTIC PROCESS WITH ADOLESCENTS EXPERIENCING PSYCHOSOCIAL STRESS

Leona L. Eggert

The car is the bedroom for long but limited sex. . . .
Going to college means you're still a child. . . .
Walk down the aisle a teenager, come back a man. . . .
Beta Theta Pot. . . .
What's new, marijuana or the generation? . . .
Young people want to grow up and then get married, so they live together. . . .
Dad works harder and harder, Johnny drops out, they both want to be worth more . . . .
(Adapted from Gerzon 1969.)

And thus the whole world watches the phenomenon of youth and talks about how times have changed. The youth's criticism of the adult world is harsh: adults patch up the wounds of alienation rather than cure the causes. The adult's view of youth frequently reflects cynicism and concern; there is much comment about how times have changed for the worse. But have they really? As in G. Stanley Hall's conception of adolescence in the early 1900s, we tend to think that the problems of adolescence are recent phenomena. But look at this:

OUR YOUTH NOW LOVES LUXURY

> They have bad manners and contempt for authority. They show disrespect for their elders and love idle chatter in place of exercise. Children are now tyrants—not the servants of the household. They no longer rise when elders enter the room. They contradict their parents, chatter before company, gobble up their food and tyrannize their teachers.
> Socrates, 450 B.C.

While many of the problems encountered today by youth and by parents are different from those encountered during the time of Socrates, the fact remains that adolescence, that straddling-the-fence period of human development, has always brought great joy to some people and great concern to many others.

We prefer to think that the concern of the psychosocial nurse specialist working with children and adolescents is special—a concern that encompasses the notion of facilitating their progress toward becoming adequate adults. We are especially aware of the fact that research in psychosocial studies has demonstrated the great extent to which mental health is dependent on achieving a reasonably objective view of the self, as well as self-knowledge and self-acceptance, which is the adolescent's quest. Erikson (1956) has contributed much to our understanding of how crucial, yet how perilous, youth's search for identity can be.

Child/adolescent psychosocial nursing as a specialty is a recent addition to the human services professions. Those of us in this speciality are convinced that we have a specific usefulness that encompasses not just custodial care but therapeutic efforts and skills. We are concerned not only with those youths in turmoil but also with youth in general. We believe that there is much value in serving the needs of both, facilitating both in terms of the passage from dependence to independence, facilitating both in terms of discovering a healthy sense of self.

For many of us this interest in adolescents came about because of sudden confrontation with an adolescent encountered while working primarily with adults' psychosocial concerns. Others among us have always viewed young people as a very special group with whom we would like to work. In either case, our concerns have resulted in many of the same questions: What is normal and what is abnormal during adolescence? What causes the emotional problems of youth? What are the factors leading to the onset of certain disturbances? Answers to these questions are often sought because we need to know what constitutes a disturbance or a time of turmoil and how these disturbances can be prevented.

There are many theories about why some young people seem to be capable of smooth transit through adolescence while others are not. We have some important clues about the characteristics of adolescents who are sailing through this period of life with few problems.

In this chapter a discussion of the use of the nursing process with adolescents experiencing psychosocial stress will cover five major areas:

1. *Passage from childhood to adulthood.* It is of foremost importance that we have a thorough knowledge of what adolescence is all about before we think about how we can help. Many adults ask these questions: What are adolescents like? What can I do that will help me understand them? It is hoped that this first section will provide a perspective that will get one

over the first hurdle in working with adolescents, ie, making the alien familiar and understandable.

2. *Contemporary conflicts and sources of turmoil.* In this section we will cover some of the major situations adolescents experience, such as psychosocial stressors. Before making a nursing assessment, it helps to recall the conflict topics and the various ways teenagers handle them.
3. *Nursing assessment with adolescents.* Once we know the basic features of adolescence and the problems faced by the adolescent, we can begin making an assessment of those teenagers with whom we come in contact. This section should provide some guidelines and some tools for this task.
4. *Nursing intervention with adolescents.* After completing the task of assessment and gaining some understanding of teenagers and their experience, we can examine what guidelines there are for planning their care and intervening in their problems. There are some useful approaches for use with adolescents that differ from the approaches used with other age groups.
5. *Evaluation of therapeutic efforts.* We always want to know if our interventions have value in the lives of those we serve. This section proposes some guidelines for evaluating therapeutic efforts.

These are some of the topics that most often cause concern to those working with adolescents. No pretense of having the only answers and guidelines for each of the five topic areas is being made; what will be presented is a framework that has emerged from working with these special people called adolescents.

PASSAGE FROM CHILDHOOD TO ADULTHOOD

Many nurses and other professionals consider this topic their first concern. One problem has always been to decrease the fear or discomfort one feels in the presence of the alien, for the adolescent is an alien to most adults. In the study of adolescence it is easy to become confused because there are so many theoretical frameworks from which to consider adolescence. However, theorists do agree on some basics, even though their approaches may be different. Before considering these various approaches, we should take a look at our own current perspective.

Individual Perspective on Adolescence

How would you complete the following statements?

Adolescence is____
Adolescence encompasses the ages __________ to __________.
Teenagers are ____
They are similar to (different from) children in that________________

____

They are similar to (different from) adults in that________________

____

In order to qualify as adults, teenagers have to accomplish________________
____
Some of the greatest difficulties they are likely to encounter are____________
____.

Such a survey of ideas can stimulate us to rethink our notions about teenagers, and the accuracy of those notions will determine whether we can develop functional relationships with teenagers. In addition, the manner in which we perceive adolescents will greatly influence how we assess them and their concerns, how we select our treatment goals, and how we evaluate the therapeutic relationship. It should be interesting to compare our perspectives on adolescence with those of various theorists.

Theoretic Perspectives on Adolescence

Who Are Adolescents? Often we have heard it said that the teenager is a marginal person. Kurt Lewin (1939) described adolescents as persons straddling the fence between childhood and adulthood, free to choose whichever side of the fence serves their purposes best at the time, but not living securely on either side. This adolescent transition in life is obviously a period of change, and according to most theorists it has the potential to complicate one's life enormously. According to some theorists, people are no longer considered teenagers when they reach the age of 18 or 19 years; according to many other theorists they are still late adolescents or youths until such time as they are completely independent of their parents. Thus today many college students could be viewed as late adolescents or youths. Tosi (1974) defined adolescence as the period from 12 to 18 years of age, with youth or young adulthood encompassing the period from 18 to 30 years of age. Other writers have contended that adolescence extends to the age of 24 or 25 years, but generally it is considered the period between 12 and 20 years of age (NIMH 1973). Often adolescence is subdivided into early and late periods, early being between the ages of 12 and 16 years, late being from 16 years of age to whatever age adolescence is defined as ending.

It can be useful in gaining perspective to summarize the viewpoints of theorists from various disciplines. Such a perspective can provide further understanding of adolescents, their position in society, and the potential causes of their psychosocial stress. A summary of viewpoints from various disciplines is presented below.

Adolescence: Effect of Biologic Process. Blos (1962), a psychologist, stated that as a result of the onset of puberty the experiences of young people change in almost every aspect of their lives: emotions, interests, desires, goals, social relationships, sense of identity. These sweeping changes usually cause confusion and stress, and all this is an inevitable consequence of puberty. Blos contended that one necessary task during this developmental period is to modify former ideas about one's body in light of these many physical changes.

In an effort to sort out what they can and cannot do, find out who they are, and discover their capacities and limitations adolescents try out various roles, test limits, and see what fits. This process of testing involves rebellious, obstinate, and excessive behavior and demands; in addition to discovering their own capacities and limitations they will discover those limitations set by other people and by society. However, this whole process of finding out who they are may cause considerable discomfort: loneliness, alienation, confusion, and uncertainty. Some adolescents find these feelings so uncomfortable that they avoid making the effort to attain self-identity, and thus they remain stuck in adolescence. Confrontation with the responsibilities and expectations of adulthood can, for some adolescents, intensify their fear and confusion.

Like Blos, Anna Freud (1946) believed that the physical changes that take place at puberty complicate life enormously for young people, but they believed that all the turmoil and stress and the adolescent's emotional responses are as beneficial as they are unavoidable. They saw adolescence as a universal emotional response to a biologic process.

Adolescence: Crisis of Identity. Erikson (1956, 1959, 1964), another psychologist, emphasized the importance of cultural conditions to the adolescent experience, in addition to the universal biologic factors. To him, the search for identity is the major theme of adolescence, and it is a consequence of the way society shapes our lives. This identity crisis is especially complicated in America because of the many alternatives that our youth must choose from in patterning their adult lives: "What job, what vocation should I seek? What religion, if any? Should I marry? If so, whom? What political stance? Decisions, decisions, decisions!" In American society it is generally expected that these decisions will be made in the second decade of life. Thus the crisis of identity, finding out who one is by making all these decisions, becomes the central issue of adolescence. It is largely because of Erikson's views on the cultural factor in identity formation that adolescence has come to be considered a time of pause, of opportunity to examine alternatives and clarify values and thus establish a firm sense of self.

Margaret Mead (1950, 1952), an anthropologist, suggested that adolescence is not inherently a time of stress, turmoil, and doubts, but cultural conditions make it that. In this respect her position agrees with Erikson's. In her study of the Samoans (1950) she found that adolescence was not necessarily a difficult period in a girl's life. What determines the degree of stress is the complexity of the society, the number of choices and decisions the young person must make. These choices are relatively few in nonindustrialized societies, whereas young people in America are faced with numerous choices and a tremendous array of positions from which to choose. There are in most cases at least a dozen different ideologic viewpoints from which to choose; each group believes something different, and many of these groups have advocates ready to influence the adolescent (a parent, an aunt or uncle, a trusted friend). Other ideologies may be encountered in the books the adolescent reads. The process whereby the adolescent arrives at a clear picture of "Who Am I?" has been likened to experiencing a surrealistic film.

Adolescence: Status Phenomenon. Hollingshead (1949), a sociologist, defined adolescence in terms of behavior derived from prescribed roles in society. His view of adolescence differs a great deal from those of psychologists, physiologists, and educators. Hollingshead saw it as a matter of the adolescent's ambiguous status: adolescents are no longer children and not yet adults. There are certain roles they are expected to play, permitted to play, and forced to play, as well as roles they are prohibited from playing. He contended that the structure, content, and duration of the prescribed roles for adolescents are not determined by physiologic developments, such as puberty, but rather are determined by the society. Thus the period in the human life cycle during which the adolescent role is prescribed varies from one society to another. The important thing sociologically is the manner in which one's society treats the maturing individual.

In American society there are three major transitions that are expected to occur to persons in the second decade of life: (1) becoming physically mature; (2) shifting one's emotional ties from the family to people outside the family; (3) attaining the full status of adult. In other societies these same three shifts are expected to occur in different ways, as well as at different points in one's life cycle. Thus the important thing to remember in taking a cross-cultural view of adolescence is that we are really speaking about transitions rather than about adolescence.

Adolescence: Cognitive Awakening. Piaget (1950, 1967, 1969), as well as other educational psychologists, emphasized that adolescents are maturing in terms of cognitive and intellectual skills that give them the capacity for new levels of thinking: logical, abstract thought. These new skills provide them with greater freedom and flexibility of thought. Thus they have the intellectual capacity to solve problems and analyze and evaluate information regarding values and people.

According to Piaget, adolescents are capable of hypothetical and deductive reasoning; they understand experimental proof, and they are learning to use complex organizing systems and symbols. This increased ability to conceptualize and hypothesize enables them to understand intellectually the things they are experiencing, as well as tasks and accomplishments expected of them. It is important to remember that the late adolescent is far more capable of utilizing these intellectual skills than is the early adolescent, although both are developing and refining these skills.

Adolescence: Maturational Crisis. Theorists agree on one aspect of adolescence: it is a period characterized by change, by growth and renewal in some areas and by decay in others. Thus adolescence has the characteristics of crisis; it contains both danger and opportunity: danger of entering adulthood at an inadequate level of functioning and opportunity to enter adulthood at a high level of health and capability.

We have seen some of the various ways theorists regard adolescence: a pathway to adulthood paved by potential hazards, emotional upheavals, and many physical and mental changes; a pathway prescribed by society; a pathway with many signposts detailing tasks to accomplish, decisions to make, and possibilities to choose from. The prospect can be threatening, and adolescents justifiably experience anxiety; growth in adolescence can be characterized by chaos and confusion, both for adolescents and for those around them.

Table 13.1 contains a composite of the typical teenager. It can be valuable in synthesizing many of the terms employed, and it has value as an assessment or interaction tool for use with the adolescent.

A Helping Perspective on Adolescence

Many of the basic problems that must be understood before beginning work with adolescents have been mentioned. While the foregoing descriptions, facts, and opinions come from adolescents and from adults who are considered experts in this field, they can serve only as guidelines and approximations in the task of knowing an individual adolescent. Most important, we can never know teenagers from the perspectives of others; we must know them from their own perspectives and determine how each individual views himself. We must attempt to view them and their world from their viewpoint. This means seeking out their understandings of themselves and their opinions. It also means validating our perceptions and understanding of adolescents in conjunction with the adolescents themselves.

CONTEMPORARY CONFLICTS AND SOURCES OF TURMOIL

Once we know society's expectations of adolescents in terms of developmental tasks and role prescriptions and prohibitions, we can seek an understanding of some of the common stressors that adolescents

Table 13.1. A PICTURE OF THE TYPICAL TEENAGER*

TEENAGERS HAVE IT MADE?

Physically:

Hereditary defects appear
Anemic conditions arise
Morbidity rate increases
Permanent teeth need straightening
Disproportionate growth occurs
Sex desires rise, but can't be fulfilled

Psychologically they:

Are subject to mental disorders
Reach physical maturity without social maturity
Achieve mental capacity without required knowledge
Are developmentally out of tune with the opposite sex
Are very conscious of physique, but tend to be pimpled, skinny, fat, clumsy, flat-chested, or bare-chested.

Socially they:

Are told to act like adults, but not be adults
Are told to prepare for life, but not join in life
Are to learn to work, but not to start too soon
Are to make decisions, but be darn sure they're the right ones
Must learn to accept ideals, while watching conflicting realities
Must gear their entrance into adulthood to the social standard: eg, high school graduate, married, 18 to 24 years of age, or pregnant

The Point:

The teenage years are potentially uncertain, unstable, and full of surprises

WHAT ARE TEENAGERS SUPPOSED TO ACCOMPLISH? (QUALIFYING AS AN ADULT)

They have to:

Learn a sex role
Break the apron strings
Choose a vocation
Learn to get along with others
Develop a conscience
Achieve morality
Organize some values
Develop their intellectual skills

In other words, they must:

Gain a sense of identity and know how to answer these questions: "Who Am I? What is my role in society?"

The point:

There is real purpose in the teenage years

Table 13.1, cont.

WHAT REALLY BUGS THE TYPICAL TEENAGER?

They want to be liked by others (peers definitely, adults if possible)

Because of their first desire, to be liked, they tend toward conformity and are extremely sensitive to the opinions of others

They are interested in their bodies (girls, in fact, often rate physical attractiveness their number-one concern)

Enough money is a big problem for them

School and academic learning are a problem, but not high on the list

They are concerned about their parents, but the concern is generally directed at the teenager's welfare, not vice versa

They often wonder what lies beyond school and home (many times this is the real motivation for acquiring a college education)

The point:

Education is not first on the list of teenage priorities

WHAT DO TEENAGERS WANT?

To be liked, but they also want:

Independence, but not loss of security
Immediate satisfaction
Answers, but not leadership
Intellectual acceptance
Responsibility without restriction
Evaluation without comparison
Stability without limitations

But they are not naive enough to think they will get their way:

Maybe they don't want their way? However, they are very willing to find the limits and push them a bit

The Point:

As teenagers move toward adulthood, they set their goals high; but these are constantly tempered by societal realities

**Price J: The adolescent. In Nicholas L: The Counselor and the Group Process. Bellevue, Wash, Bellevue Public Schools Publication ASICO129/9370, 1969, pp 24–27.*

encounter as they mature and make the transition from childhood to adulthood.

Potential conflicts and sources of stress for the adolescent are listed in Table 13.2. These conflicts fall into two major categories: conflicts with self and conflicts with others (but primarily as they relate to self). Sources of conflict are not listed in the order of their importance in Table 13.2.

Depending on the extent of frustration experienced or perceived, the adolescent may be viewed as normal or abnormal. Rebellion during adolescence may be either quiet or violent. Transition through adolescence may be smooth, or the adolescent may drop out to indulge in

Table 13.2. ADOLESCENT CONFLICT TOPICS

CONFLICT	HOW TEENAGERS DESCRIBE IT
Body image conflicts	Physical changes taking place in me
Sexual conflicts	A relationship with someone of the opposite sex
Intellectual conflicts	My relationships at school
Relationship conflicts with peers and/or parents	My relationship with my friends; my relationship with my parents; what other people think of me
Role conflicts	Becoming financially independent; finding out who I am; choices I must make about my life in the next 5 years; becoming really good at something; getting a job
Ideologic conflicts	Weighing religious or philosophic values; choices I have to make about my life in the next 5 years
Continuation or exacerbation of earlier childhood conflicts	

various excesses: sex, drugs, psychotic behavior, or even suicide. Rebellion may be expressed only with parents, or it may occur as delinquent behavioral responses, antisocial responses, or sometimes psychosomatic responses. Being familiar with some of the typical responses that may be encountered with adolescents can also help in the assessment process. Recent work by Offer and his associates (1969, 1972, 1975) categorizes the responses of adolescents as (1) continuous growth, or relatively smooth sailing, (2) surgent growth, (3) tumultuous growth, or (4) abnormal growth. These forms of adaptation to adolescence will be described in terms of the conflicts experienced and the sources of turmoil encountered.

Offer and his colleagues saw the need for closer investigation of normal adolescents' behavioral responses to the transitions they must make in our society. Offer determined that the stereotype of the adolescent as a rebellious, obnoxious, emotionally unstable person is derived largely from data collected in studies of adolescents who were in therapy. Based on his original longitudinal study of 73 adolescent males (1969) and subsequent studies of thousands of normal, typical teenagers (1972, 1975), he has proposed a new theory of adolescent growth patterns and responses.

Continuous Growth

Continuous growth is the pattern of many teenagers; it is characterized by an absence of behavioral problems and by a self-assured walk. Factors contributing to the trouble-free development of those adolescents who fit this pattern include the following: trustful, affectionate, and respectful relationships with parents and the nuclear family; successful mastery of earlier childhood developmental tasks; comfortable acceptance of societal norms and expectations; ability to integrate new experiences and benefit from them. Close and comfortable relationships with peers of both sexes, a positively developed sense of intimacy during late adolescence, satisfaction with oneself, and active progress toward one's goals are also characteristic of adolescents in this group.

Surgent Growth

The pattern of surgent growth is experienced by many other young people who are also considered normal. At times their development is trouble-free, while at other times it seems to come to a standstill. Adolescents manifesting this course of development are not as self-confident as those in the continuous-growth group; less positive reinforcement from significant others has been detrimental to their self-esteem. While their family ties may be strong, these adolescents have experienced high percentages of parental deaths, severe illness in family members, and parental separations; generally there is less stability in their families than in the families of the continuous-growth group. Often the adolescents in this group will have difficulty in separating from their parents because there has been less fostering of independence and introspection. Their eventual growth through adolescence is usually as successful as that of the continuous-growth group, but it takes greater effort and energy because there are more sources of turmoil and stress.

Tumultuous Growth

Factors that characterize the development of adolescents experiencing tumultuous growth through adolescence include the following: much discord in many aspects of their lives; mistrust of most adults in their lives; disappointment in themselves and others. Common occurrences in their lives include parental conflicts characterized by poor communication patterns, wide mood swings with heightened awareness of emotional needs, early heterosexual dating patterns, and treasured peer relationships as a means of breaking away from parents. They differ from adolescents in the delinquent groups in that their parental ties are still strong and they are as successful academically and vocationally as those in the other growth groups. However, the pathway to that success is often tumultuous, and there are few trouble-free periods.

The studies of Offer and associates give us a new perspective on the clinical stereotype of adolescence as a time of inevitable turmoil and crisis. Such crises are limited to a minority of teenagers; there are other groups of adolescents who are developing and maturing by different patterns. Offer delineated three different patterns of development followed by typical teenagers, ie, those considered normal. If a teenager does not seem to fit into one of these three groups, there may be reason to suspect a maladaptive response during adolescence.

Once we know the basic facts about that period of life called adolescence, something about adolescents themselves, and something about the patterns which they may be developing, we are on our way to getting started in the helping process with a teenager. When assessment of a teenager is about to begin, questions arise: "What kinds of information would I be interested in collecting? Can I categorize this information into any meaningful framework? What tools are available to me, both within myself and outside myself, that could be used in the process of nursing assessment? For each of these tools, what theoretical framework am I drawing on for techniques and clinical judgments?"

NURSING ASSESSMENT WITH ADOLESCENTS

This section is organized around the task of assessment, the tools of assessment, and the objectives of assessment in working with adolescents. Because the process of assessment with adolescents can be difficult, especially when they are hostile and rejecting, it helps to have things sorted out: some guidelines on what information to collect, how to put it together, and how to interpret it. Table 13.3 provides an outline for nursing assessment that can be used in working with adolescents. It lists the objectives, the tools, and the theoretical framework.

Table 13.3. OUTLINE OF NURSING ASSESSMENT WITH ADOLESCENTS

OBJECTIVES (KESSLER 1966)	TOOL (SELF, TECHNIQUE, AND/OR ORGANIZER)	UNDERLYING THEORETIC/CONCEPTUAL FRAMEWORK
1. Introduce parents and the adolescent to psychosocial way of viewing the adolescent's concerns	a. Therapeutic use of self b. Organizer: Table 13.1, part 1, "Teenagers have it Made"	Eggert, Chapter 2, A Psychosocial View of Adolescents
2. Determine in what areas and to what extent the adolescent differs from others of the same age	a. Nurse's intellectual use of self	Scientific approach; Lewin's life-space interview; Fagin's marginal interview
	b. Techniques: observation, interviewing, games, interaction tools, developmental assessment tools c. Organizers: Table 13.1, part 2, "Qualifying as an Adult"; Table 13.2, Adolescent Conflict Topics	Erikson's developmental task theory; Piaget's cognitive theory; normative and maturational theories; sociologic and cultural anthropologic theories

Table 13.3, cont.

OBJECTIVES (KESSLER 1966)	TOOL (SELF, TECHNIQUE, AND/OR ORGANIZER)	UNDERLYING THEORETIC/CONCEPTUAL FRAMEWORK
3. Assess the problems or concerns and their chronicity	a. Nurse's self: interpretation of behavior and symptoms b. Techniques: interviewing, questioning regarding which problems and how long (Chapters 2 and 3); rank ordering list of concerns	Psychosocial theories regarding specific behavioral manifestations (eg, Raths et al); phenomenologic approach (Coombs and Syngg)
	c. Organizers: behavioral symptoms organizer (Tables 13.4, 13.5, and 13.6); Offer's adolescent growth patterns	Developmental theories, learning theory, valuing theory Offer's theory of developmental routes through adolescence
4. Assess areas of strength in the adolescent and the family system	a. Nurse's intellectual use of self b. Techniques: interviews; observations, strategies, etc	
	c. Organizers: Table 13.1, A Picture of Typical Teenager (What tasks have already been accomplished?); Offer's adolescent growth patterns (Which pattern seems to apply?)	Developmental theories, learning theory Offer's theory
5. Formulate some hypotheses about possible contributing factors, past and present	a. Nurse's intellectual use of self b. Techniques: problem-solving, interviewing, validating with client c. Organizer: Table 13.7, Criteria for Maladaptive Responses	Scientific approach, phenomenologic approach
6. Decide on a next step; identify and set priorities of current concerns	a. Nurse's intellectual use of self b. Technique: alternative search tool (Simon 1972)	Problem-solving approach, identifying the problem

The overall objective during nursing assessment is to identify and measure the degree of stress or vulnerability of the adolescent, as well as the behavioral responses or reactions to the stressors

Task of Assessment

According to Fagin (1972), the task of the psychosocial nurse in assessing adolescents is to gather sufficient information in four major areas: (1) relationships with significant others (parents, authority figures, and peers), (2) body image and sense of identity, (3) integrated development of various body functions, and (4) age-appropriate intellectual and behavioral functioning.

Tools of Assessment

Assessment is an active and ongoing process; many tools and strategies are employed in the process. The tools fall into three categories: (1) self, (2) techniques, and (3) organizers.

Use of Self in Assessment. The self is used both intellectually and therapeutically. For example, we as nurses use ourselves as scientists when we observe for cues and then check out our perceptions and their meanings with the adolescent. We use ourselves therapeutically by communicating clearly and concretely our warmth and concern for adolescents, our empathy with them and their experiences. By communicating our real selves, we make it possible for adolescents to get to know us and trust us.

We use ourselves a great deal in the process of establishing a relationship with the adolescent; this is a concurrent task taking place during nursing assessment, and it is one on which all else is dependent. We will examine some of the problems involved in establishing rapport with adolescents and creating a climate of trust and openness, for this is primarily where we use ourselves therapeutically during the assessment phase of the nursing process.

Establishing Rapport. How we relate to adolescents is of central concern. It is helpful to remember that the way they communicate their need for help is often through some behavioral response. This response may be antisocial; it may be directed against others, it may be directed against the self, or it may consist in movement away from others. Adolescents usually cannot clearly identify their need for professional help. Their physical and psychosocial needs are most often expressed in behavior or in word play. With younger children our efforts must be directed toward understanding their world through the language of play, whereas with adolescents our efforts are often directed toward understanding their world through their play of language and their action-oriented behavioral communication.

It is best to be honest and straightforward in communicating with adolescents. Sometimes adolescents can better accept our concern for them and our understanding of their feelings if we elaborate feelings they have only tentatively expressed. For example, we might offer a statement of empathy: "Sometimes when I have been in positions similar to the one you are in now, I have found it rather scary, sometimes confusing, maybe even a little frustrating." This leaves the door open for the adolescent to reject the analogy, to identify with the sentiment, or to elaborate the feelings. Such exchanges can also help to reassure adolescents that we are identifying with them. The human relations component in the therapeutic use of self can greatly facilitate the establishment of trust and rapport: open, constructive sharing of oneself, warm communicated respect for the adolescent, and demonstrated understanding of them and their current concerns, feelings, and experiences.

Creating a Climate of Trust. We should not ask adolescents to do something we would not do or share something we would not share. It is most helpful to adolescents if we go out on a limb first. In time, this can enable adolescents to feel secure enough to let their guard down, to have faith that we will not hurt them or take advantage of them. We must demonstrate that we are trustworthy adults; we must deliver on our promises over and over again, and we must be open and honest. This can make us predictable adults, adults to be trusted, adults with whom adolescents can be open. This atmosphere of trust and openness precludes intrusion into the life of the adolescent. Intrusion causes defensive reactions. Exposure of an adolescent's problems before they are ready to discuss it leaves them not knowing what to expect from us. They think of us in terms of challenge and attack.

There are other ways to use the self during the assessment process:

1. Staying loose. Expect to be surprised by some adolescent behaviors. Expect to be rejected. Expect changes; adolescents characteristically lack consistent behavior.
2. Be careful with words and sensitive to their nuances; the adolescent may interpret an offhand comment in a way that was not intended. This necessitates much interpretation of messages: Explain carefully; repeat if necessary; check out their impression of your words; explain exactly what is being done during the assessment, and why.
3. Remember that adolescents are frequently unsure of themselves when not on their own turf. There is a constant need to reach out and demonstrate warmth and concern, to use friendly words and behavior; without this, the first interaction with the adolescent may be the last.
4. Remember that the adolescent does not yet have the social facility of the adult. Adolescents use direct forms of communication. They point out defects bluntly; they criticize openly; they are not always gentle and sensitive in their communication with adults.
5. It is helpful to remember that the adolescent deals in powerful images and fantasies. Thus it can be enlightening to get the adolescent's perceptions of the clinical setting, the services, and the personnel.
6. The adolescent will be watching closely to see whether we as nurses align ourselves with parents, with the school, or with other adult authorities. It is ideal for us to verbalize our identification with the adolescent and negotiate communications with other adults. Helping the adolescent gain an understanding of adult positions and viewpoints usually comes later.

Use of Assessment Techniques. Assessment may involve such tools and techniques as life-space interviews, strategies, interactions, talking, drawings, and games—anything that will enable us to get to know adolescents in a comfortable, nonthreatening way. Success in the assessment process often is best achieved during an activity-oriented session, because adolescents often find it threatening to have to sit in an office and just talk. Much more can be learned while going for a Coke, taking a walk together, shooting pool in the activity center, or doing anything that is part of the adolescent's usual life experience. We can speed the process of getting to know each other by facilitating interactions in settings in which adolescents are comfortable, usually on their own turf. We must have the guts to enter the adolescent's world, not wait passively for them to come to us or be sent to us by referral. We must not assume that no-shows are necessarily resistant and not amenable to treatment. It also helps to remember that adolescents who are on the fringe, who keep adults at arm's length and send other rejection messages, often fear rejection by others; therefore, just to play it safe, they reject before they can be rejected. Often we must make the first overtures toward meeting the needs of adolescents, and we must continue to make overtures despite hostile and rejecting behavior on their part, because much of this behavior is to test our true interest and concern. Above all, a climate in which the adolescent does not feel threatened psychologically can facilitate getting started together.

Organizers Used in Assessment. The third category of tools used in nursing assessment includes organizers. Organizers that have been suggested in Table 13.3 are Price's picture of the typical teen (Table 13.1), Adolescent Conflict Topics (Table 13.2), Offer's adolescent growth patterns, the behavioral symptoms organizers of Raths and associates (Tables 13.4, 13.5, and 13.6), and Kessler's criteria for maladaptive responses (Table 13.7). Each organizer can be of value in achieving one or more of the specific objectives of nursing assessment.

An organizer that has provided a great deal of help in identifying areas of concern, areas of strength, and some hypotheses about possible contributing factors is that of Raths and associates (1966). Its three components will be referred to collectively as the behavioral symptoms organizer. It provides sets of behavioral symptoms indicating difficulty in the areas of cognitive functioning (Table 13.4), affective or emotional needs functioning (Table 13.5), and social, attitudinal or values-related functioning (Table 13.6).

It is interesting to compare the behavioral symptoms in Table 13.4 with those in Table 13.5, which are characteristic of concerns or needs related to affective functioning, ie, concerns about unmet emotional needs. These behavioral patterns that are seen in an adolescent or child suffering from

Table 13.4. CONCERNS RELATED TO COGNITIVE FUNCTIONING*

Behavioral symptoms recognizable in this area are the following:

1. *Impulsiveness in Actions.* Adolescents tend to take action without thinking, to go off half-cocked.
2. *Being Stuck.* Any situation that calls for thinking can result in their getting stuck; there is usually overdependence on adults or others for help in thinking things through.
3. *Missing the Meaning.* Not getting the point; failing to derive meaning; missing the relationship between cause and effect, between actions taken and consequences.
4. *Inflexibility of Thought.* Here the adolescent may express a need for simplicity or rigid patterns; he may evidence anxiety when faced with too many alternatives.
5. *Dogmatism.* Assertive stereotyping is the major characteristic.
6. *Fearfulness about Thinking.* Timidity and lack of confidence in expressing one's ideas; not valuing one's own opinion.
7. *Wishful Thinking.* The adolescent arrives at a conclusion first—the wish—and then, when challenged, tries to think of something to prove the point or justify the wish.

**Adapted from Raths et al: Values and Teaching, 1966. Courtesy of Charles E. Merrill Publishing Co.*

Table 13.5. CONCERNS RELATED TO UNMET EMOTIONAL NEEDS*

The set of symptoms likely to be evidenced in this area includes:

1. *Aggressiveness.* Aggressiveness may be directed at the self or at others; it may be seen in behavior such as antisocial or oppositional acts.
2. *Withdrawal or Isolation.* Withdrawal may be evidenced as physical withdrawal or emotional withdrawal—an avoidance of exploration of self, which is necessary to gain insight.
3. *Psychosomatic Illnesses or Complaints*
4. *Submissiveness.* Here there may be compliance with others in order to satisfy love and affiliation needs; relationships with others are viewed as being dependent on submissiveness.
5. *Regression.* Regression to earlier developmental behavior; there may be trust/mistrust conflicts, dependence/independence conflicts, autonomy and self-esteem conflicts, etc.

**Adapted from Raths et al: Values and Teaching, 1966. Courtesy of Charles E. Merrill Publishing Co.*

unmet emotional needs must be distinguished from those related to difficulties in thinking. It is important to consider whether the behavioral pattern is consistent and unusual, whether there are frequent occurrences and whether there is intractability of the behavior before it can be considered a maladaptive response in this category.

Table 13.6 illustrates behavioral pictures of those adolescents experiencing difficulty with role diffusion and confusion, the identity search of adolescence. These are referred to as value-related behavioral types. Because people develop in terms of cognitive, affective, and values functioning, it becomes imperative in our assessment of adolescents to employ

Table 13.6. CONCERNS RELATED TO VALUES AND ATTITUDINAL FUNCTIONING*

The set of symptoms likely to be evidenced in this area includes:

1. *Apathy.* Listlessness, lack of interest, and indifference are manifest; the adolescent goes through the motions but seems very unmotivated and uncaring.
2. *Flightiness.* There is interest in everything, but only for fleeting moments. The attention span is short, and there is a desire to do everything and perform all roles.
3. *Uncertainty.* The adolescent with this symptom seems unable to arrive at decisions on a consistent basis; there is doubt, confusion, and dependence on others in making decisions.
4. *Inconsistency.* The adolescent supports one cause today and another tomorrow; behavior is obviously inconsistent; actions and ideas are incongruent.
5. *Drifting.* Drifting is characteristic of the adolescent who seems to be without purpose in life. Nothing seems very important; there are no worries, no attempts at making changes. Not much is given, but much is expected.
6. *Conformity.* There is overconformity. Here adolescents attempt to find the norms and adhere rigidly to them. They say and do what others want of them. They have no positions and standards of their own, taking their cues from others.
7. *Dissension.* Some adolescents are persistent, nagging dissenters; they find fault with everything, irrationally dissenting and virtually thriving on contention. Their identities seem to consist only in opposition to the identities of others; they have difficulty developing identities of their own.
8. *Role-playing.* Adolescents who play roles characteristically find their identities or value bases by trying on everyone else's. They use many roles, often acting in an unreal, immature way; the roles are contrived rather than real.

**Adapted from Raths et al: Values and Teaching, 1966. Courtesy of Charles E. Merrill Publishing Co.*

data collection and organization to cover these areas. The behavioral symptoms signaling concern in each of the three areas differ, and thus they help to indicate specifically the kind of help that is needed.

The last of the organizers is presented in Table 13.7. It provides a

Table 13.7. CRITERIA FOR MALADAPTIVE RESPONSES*

Kessler's criteria (1966) for assessing maladaptive responses (and indications for referral) are as follows:

1. Age discrepancy, ie, Is behavior developmentally out of tune?
2. Frequency of occurrence of any one symptom
3. Total number of symptoms
4. Degree of social disadvantage
5. Adolescent's inner suffering
6. Intractability of behavior, ie, the efforts spent to diminish behavior are generally futile
7. General personality appraisal; relationships with family, with peers, with outside authorities are in trouble

**Adapted from Kessler: Psychopathology of Childhood, 1966. Courtesy of Prentice-Hall.*

guideline for determining if what we see and hear is normal and typical, unusual, or strongly suggestive of the need for referral.

An important point to keep in mind as we begin to arrive at conclusions based on our assessment is that our conclusions should be tentative. One look is not sufficient to see the whole picture. Accurate assessment of the adolescent's concerns and behavioral responses to those concerns requires repeated observations and reevaluation of our interpretations. When dealing with adolescents we must also check out our perceptions with them by the phenomenologic approach.

NURSING INTERVENTION WITH ADOLESCENTS

The question is not how we can cure this or that ill of youth but how can we together design a system that will enable the adolescent to take care of current specific concerns or ills and then move on with new tools for innovation, renewal, and rebirth in the future. We must think of planning and intervention with adolescents as a subtle and informal teaching–learning situation that goes both ways, the content being the self of the adolescent and the self of the therapist, the process being problem-solving. Thus the learning that occurs through therapy is transferable between parties. Using this general approach with adolescents can result in a significant learning experience for both parties. Remember that teenagers often resent the adult who works at maintaining a helping posture; they prefer not to think of themselves as dependent, as the objects of smug charity.

General Principles of Treatment

Selection of Treatment Modality. For a variety of reasons, adolescents often seem to be resistant to the therapy hour. Many authorities consider the milieu and group work approaches, which are much more like the actual life situation of the adolescent, to be more effective (Fagin 1974). Whether we use a one-to-one approach, group work, or milieu therapy, what seems to work best is to make the treatment action-oriented, just as we did with nursing assessment. This is because action communication is still highly relevant for the adolescent; verbal communication is more difficult for them than for adults.

The advantage in using group work and milieu therapy is that they capitalize on adolescent development. In group work there is the assistance of the peer group; help can be transmitted from peer to peer as well as from the adult group leader. Adolescents often are more comfortable and secure when both of these treatment modalities are used, because then they are not one-on-one with the therapist.

Creating a Climate for Change. Once a climate of trust and openness has been created in the assessment phase, a climate for change can ensue. When adolescents know that we are adults who can be counted on, that we care for them as persons, then there is reason to expect them to do their best; only then is it advisable to discuss with the adolescent the discrepancies between expressed plans and actual accomplishments. From the first encounter it is permissible to communicate expectations of change. However, it seems best to negotiate these changes. The so-called alternative search tool (Simon and associates 1972) works well in this negotiation process. Following the assessment phase, the following procedure has proved useful: (1) make a list of the concerns gathered from the discussions, (2) validate the list with the adolescent, (3) put the concerns in some sort of order, beginning with questions such as these: Which concerns do you perceive as most important? Where would you like to begin? How can we together work something out that will get you where you'd like to be? This approach helps emphasize that the concerns originated with the adolescent and that there is shared responsibility.

Communicating Expectations or Demanding Obedience. One of the worst things that can be done in working with adolescents is to make a list of rules and then demand obedience. It will not work. What seems to work best is to communicate our expectations that they will demonstrate concern for themselves and consideration for others, that they will develop mature behavior, and that we can work things out together and make responsible decisions together. This serves to prepare adolescents for making decisions based on their own values and attitudes rather than on adult-imposed rules. It is best to begin with a negotiated contract and then question behavior in terms of whether it is hurting oneself or others. Some rules are necessary, but they should be kept to an absolute minimum, perhaps two or three. These, too, can be negotiated, along with the consequences of breaking them. Rules must be enforceable, with the consequences of breaking them being known beforehand.

Our expectations of adolescent behavior are also communicated by our behavior. We must remember to use ourselves in positive ways through role modeling, we must avoid contests of will, we must avoid retaliation when we are angry, we must not seek to undermine the adolescent's self-esteem when we are frustrated. It helps to examine one's motives occasionally: "Are my expectations too great? Are they developmentally appropriate? Am I communicating faith in the adolescent's ability, and am I communicating positive encouragement? Is this rule necessary, and for whose benefit is it?"

Techniques of Therapy. Whatever techniques of therapy are chosen, they should be appropriate to the individual nurse. Effective therapists use a variety of tools and techniques taken from various theoretical frameworks. The techniques selected must be appropriate to the situation and the particular adolescent, in addition to being appropriate to the therapist. The author has found that relationship therapy is particularly suited to her therapy with adolescents. It is through the use of the relationship that growth and change occur.

These general principles do not exhaust the possibilities that may be considered in working with adolescents. However, it is hoped that they are suggestive of other principles that can be derived and that they reflect the underlying theory of a partnership in planning and in treatment.

Specific Approaches

We have looked at recognizable behavioral symptoms in three major areas: (1) cognitive functioning, (2) unmet emotional needs, and (3) values and attitudinal functioning. While many of the concerns related to thought, emotions, and values may be interrelated and may overlap, there is usually one dominant behavioral pattern with which to start.

Cognitive Functioning. Any approach planned to help resolve the adolescent's concerns about cognitive functioning should include the following steps: observing, reporting what has been observed, comparing and contrasting, asking for summarization, working together on things that require classifying and sorting. This could be accomplished by asking the adolescent to compile a list of concerns that have been identified during patient–therapist interaction and then rank them in order of importance. Planning and executing, outlining the steps to be taken in order to arrive at a certain goal, criticizing, analyzing, and looking for assumptions can also help the adolescent with problems in thinking. Games that include imagining and discovering (eg, brainstorming as if all things were possible) can facilitate the development of new alternatives. Finally, problem-solving (identifying possible solutions and experimenting with them) facilitates change and growth and provides the adolescent experience for future use. Some of the best tools to facilitate these steps are Simon's "Alternative Search Tool," "Consequence Search Tool," and "Removing Barriers to Action" (Simon and associates 1972).

Unmet Emotional Needs. Working with a so-called needs adolescent requires identifying the need (love/belonging, security, stability, dependence, independence, esteem) and then facilitating satisfaction of the need. The principle that applies is that movement toward more mature needs is not possible until less mature needs have been gratified. For example, dependence needs must be satisfied before we can expect to see movement toward independence.

It is important to remember that when adolescents evidence concerns about unmet emotional needs as well as concerns about values, it is usually necessary to deal with the unmet emotional needs first, or at least in conjunction with the values-related concerns. Meeting emotional needs takes precedence over clarifying values. Establishing such a hierarchy of concerns and needs helps us keep our perspective; sometimes it is easy to be diverted and focus on second- or third-level concerns.

Values and Attitudinal Functioning. One approach that has proven successful with adolescents is the values-clarification approach. It is particularly suited to the tasks of the adolescent in our society, and it is applicable in working with individuals and with groups of adolescents. Simon and associates (1972) have suggested strategies for this approach. Basically, the strategies are designed to help adolescents formulate a value base that can be used to guide their behavior. The theory suggests which strategies are appropriate at a given time for the individual and for the group. Processes in valuing include three major steps: choosing, prizing, and acting. The process of choosing has some substeps or contingencies that are important: choosing must occur freely. There must be a range of alternatives. Choice must be made only after considering the consequences. Prizing occurs in two steps: prizing and cherishing within oneself, and then prizing by public affirmation. The third step in the valuing process is acting; a value becomes real and permanent when we act on our prized choice repeatedly.

This valuing theory can have a great deal of relevance in our work with adolescents. If we know that the individual or the group is in the first stage of the process, then we can employ strategies appropriate to promote exploration of alternatives and free choice from these alternatives after consideration of the consequences. Often the appropriate strategies are those that permit adolescents to publicly affirm their choices. Through this process—trying a value out loud—they may find that they like the fit of that particular value, or they may find the opposite true. If the latter occurs, they move to the stage of choosing from alternatives again. Finally, strategies can be planned that facilitate acting on the values chosen.

Issues usually dealt with in values clarification with adolescents include (1) money, and how it is apportioned and treated; (2) friendship, and how one relates to important others; (3) love and sex, and how one deals with intimate relationships; (4) religion and morals, and what one has as a fundamental belief; (5) leisure, and how it is used; (6) politics and social organization, and how they affect the individual; and (7) parents and family, and how one moves toward greater independence (Raths and associates 1966, Simon and associates 1972).

A particularly valuable approach in group work with adolescents who are experiencing values concerns or attitudinally related concerns is that described in *Positive Peer Culture* (Vorrath and Brendtro 1974); many of the principles discussed here are found in this approach. It is particularly well suited to adolescents exhibiting antisocial or delinquent behaviors.

EVALUATION OF THERAPEUTIC EFFORTS

We always want to know if our efforts have made any difference. We want to evaluate our therapeutic efforts. We can measure process movement in the client: either the use of process movement scales to measure such aspects as manner of relating and problem expressions or the use of the client goal attainment scaling method. These methods reveal where adolescents were at the beginning of therapy and where they are at later times during therapy. There are also other scaling methods for evaluating client progress. Therapeutic efforts may also be evaluated with the tools presented in Table 13.8; assessment is made at regular intervals, and comments on specific events are made in the explanation column.

We cannot expect praise for our efforts from the adolescents with whom we work, nor can we expect much in the way of validation that our efforts have been successful. Many teenagers find it difficult to express appreciation and to discuss specifically what helped them. This does not mean that we should cease to try to elicit evaluation of our efforts from the adolescents with whom we work, for it is through them, their comments, their criticisms, and their helpful suggestions that we continue to increase our potential as effective helpers. Many times we do not receive feedback from the people we have worked with until years later. Thus it becomes important to set up other evaluation methods, such as having someone else observe and rate us.

WORK WITH ADOLESCENTS: AN ILLUSTRATION

Sometimes it helps to see how all these recommendations and suggestions for assessment and intervention are put into practice with adolescents. The following account is an example of a therapeutic relationship. It concerns Jeff, a young man 17 years of age, with whom the author worked.

Jeff was referred because he frequently drew illustrations on the blackboard that included skulls and crossbones, as well as other material strongly suggestive of death and suicide. During the initial sessions we got to know and trust each other, and data were collected during this assessment phase. The process and findings are given in Table 13.9. Assessment is reported in terms of Table 13.3 in order to demonstrate the tools utilized and the data gathered.

Interpretations were shared and discussed with Jeff. Goals were negotiated and clarified. Jeff wrote out what he wanted: "I want Joy as a girl-

Table 13.8. NURSE-THERAPIST CHECKLIST Measuring the Effectiveness of Help Given in Working with Adolescents

Directions: Read the questions below and rate yourself by writing in one of the numbers below according to this key: 0, not accomplished; 1, at least once or with 1 teenager; 2, at least two or three times or with 2 or 3 teenagers; 3, several times or with several teenagers.

Think through what happened today or the last time you were with an adolescent or group of adolescents. Rate yourself now and at later dates.

QUESTION	DATE: RATING	EXPLANATION
Nursing assessment		
Did you introduce both parents and the adolescent to psychosocial way of viewing adolescent concerns?		
Did you determine in what areas and to what extent the adolescent differs from others of the same age by some objective means (eg, use of tools such as Tables 13.1 and 13.2)?		
Did you assess the problems or concerns and their chronicity using the behavioral symptoms organizer, Offer's adolescent growth patterns, or some similar tool?		
Did you assess areas of strength in the adolescent and the family system by using Table 13.1 and Offer's growth patterns tools?		
Did you establish rapport and create a climate for trust and openness?		
Did you formulate some hypotheses about possible contributing factors, past and present?		
Did you make a tentative list of the adolescent's needs and concerns and verify this list with him?		
Planning interventions		
Did you decide on a next step by identifying and setting priorities of current concerns with the adolescent?		
Did you identify various methods of intervention based on the theory of cognitive, unmet emotional needs, and values-related concerns?		
Did you discuss the various methods planned with the adolescent and work from the basis of partners in planning?		
Were the methods suggested appropriate to the adolescent's identified needs or concerns?		
Nursing intervention		
Did you create a climate for change, eg, with the alternatives and consequences search tool?		
Did you communicate expectations rather than demand obedience?		

Table 13.8, cont.

QUESTION	DATE: RATING	EXPLANATION
Nursing intervention (cont.)		
Did you negotiate rules and consequences of breaking rules?		
Did you enforce the rules when necessary?		
Did you apply the principles of therapeutic use of self while maintaining relationships with both adolescent and parents?		
Did the techniques you chose to use fit both you and the adolescent?		
Did you select the appropriate treatment modality?		
Evaluation of care		
Did you develop criteria that could be used as a basis for judging outcomes of nursing interventions?		
Did you measure the effect of nursing assessment done with the adolescent and family?		
Did you assess the effect of nursing interventions employed with the adolescent during the process of treatment?		
Did you make appropriate modifications based on responses and others observations?		
Did you have someone else observe your work and rate your progress?		
Throughout the nursing process, did you gain an increased understanding of yourself as a therapist by synthesizing nursing knowledge gained from specific actions taken with the adolescent?		
		Total score

Rate yourself: Add your scores for each date. Did you progressively improve? What areas do you still need to work on? Reflect and discuss with others for more ideas on how to develop your potential in helping teenagers.

friend, but I also want to find happiness. I want to be proud of myself. I want to be liked. I want to be an individual.''

My goals were shared with him: (1) to stop suicide attempts, and eventually any ideas of suicide; (2) to learn some skills in handling personal problems, ways of getting what he wants without being left out by the kids; (3) to start working on the list entitled Qualifying as a Adult. These were to be pursued in any order he chose.

The treatment approach included involving Jeff in processes relevant to his unmet emotional needs and his concerns related to cognitive func-

Table 13.9
Process and Findings of Work with Jeff

Tool Used	Data and Nurse's Impressions
I. Objective: Determine in what areas and to what extent the adolescent differs from others of same age	
Observation, interviewing, Table 13.1, A Picture of the Typical Teenager	Small physique; otherwise normal physical development
	Comments revealed self-consciousness regarding physique (guys give him a bad time during PE)
	Above-average grades in school; vocabulary extensive, verbal skills above average (rather sophisticated communication)
Showed him the section ''Qualifying as an Adult'' and asked him to respond with his opinion of the ideas, as well as how he sees himself in relations (Table 13.1)	Three things stood out: (1) he felt left out by other kids for a long time; (2) ''My mother keeps trying to run my life and I'm tired of it''; (3) ''Someone finally treated me really nice [Joy], and because of that I really want her to be my girlfriend.''
Showed him the section ''Adolescent Conflict Topics'' and asked him to check those of concern to him and add others if necessary (Table 13.2)	Checked off body image, sexual, and relationships with peers and parents as being of concern to him
II. Objective: Assess the problems or concerns and their chronicity	
Interviewing regarding chronicity	''So far, for 1 1/2 years, she hasn't been willing to be my girlfriend—I still hope she will someday.''
	Left out by kids for a long time—''too long, and I'm tired of it—but will it change?''
Rank ordering concerns	Jeff identified relationship with Joy as no. 1 concern, relationships with peers as no. 2, relationship with parents as no. 3.
''Behavioral Symptoms Organizer''	
1. Concerns regarding cognition (Table 13.4)	Evidenced primarily:
a. Impulsivity	Suicide attempts impulsive; slashed wrists once in hallway in front of Joy to prove his point: ''If you don't change your mind, I'll kill myself.''
b. Being stuck, missing the meaning, and inflexibility of thought	Being stuck: saw only one alternative to winning Joy—threats of suicide

Table 13.9, cont.

Tool Used	Data and Nurse's Impressions
	Missing the meaning: misinterpreted Joy's natural kind, considerate behavior; despite her negative responses about being his girlfriend, he failed to get the message
	Inflexibility of thought: saw only one possibility for a girlfriend—Joy: "Joy, I'm miserable without you, so miserable that I'm just about ready to kill myself. Is there any chance you'll change your mind about being my girlfriend?" "If you don't change your mind, I'm going to kill myself."
c. Wishful thinking	"I still hope she will someday."
2. Concerns regarding unmet emotional needs (Table 13.5)	
a. Aggressiveness	Drawings were "aggressive"
	Threats of suicide and suicide attempts
b. Withdrawal and isolation	One close friend only (another very shy, quiet young man 16 years of age)
	Withdrawal from initial attempts to seek alternative to Joy
c. Psychosomatic complaints	None
d. Submissiveness	Relationship with both mother and father
e. Regression	Dependence/independence conflict with mother and many teachers
	Nurse's gut-level reaction indicated emotional and social immaturity—more appropriate for 14 or 15 years of age
3. Concerns relating to valuing (Table 13.6)	Not there yet; very few of these applied, other than "uncertainty"
III. Objective: Assess areas of strength in the adolescent and the family system	
Family interview with mother only; father not available; Offer's adolescent growth patterns	Jeff: Low self-confidence: "Nothing I do ever works out." "The kids won't change, and I'm not able to make them change."

(Continued)

Table 13.9, cont.

Tool Used	Data and Nurse's Impressions
	Wide mood swings: "Where am I as far as feelings are concerned? I've reached the end of my rope! I feel really depressed and have no more interest in life."
	Family: ties strong, mother concerned about Jeff's isolation and lack of friends; father experiencing terminal illness; stated poor communication between them (data seem to point toward tumultuous growth pattern)
A Picture of the Typical Teenager (Table 13.1)	Tasks already accomplished: strong conscience and morality; very few of the other tasks accomplished—struggling with the majority of them. Intellectual skills superior—enjoyed brain-teasers
IV. Objective: Formulate some hypotheses about possible contributing factors, past and present	
Problem solving with Jeff about possible contributing factors	Lots of "I don't know" responses at first; then, "being left out by the kids; my mother trying to run my life; my father always sick, but mostly Joy—she finally treated me different."
"Criteria for Maladaptive Responses" tool (Table 13.7) (How bad is the problem?)	
1. Age discrepancy	Suicide behavior developmentally out of tune, but a trouble sign during adolescence
	Overly strong pursuit of a girlfriend (suggestive of strong dependence needs); attempt to shift from mother to Joy?
	Lagging behind in progress on developmental tasks
2. Frequency of occurrence of any one symptom	Drawings: almost every other day now, increasing in frequency over past 4 weeks
	Suicide attempted twice—slashed wrists
	Symptoms related to cognitive functioning, five in number
	Symptoms related to unmet emotional needs: all symptoms except psychosomatic complaints

Table 13.9, cont.

Tool Used	Data and Nurse's Impressions
3. Degree of disadvantage	Very disadvantaged in terms of relationships with peers; little relationship with father
4. Adolescent's inner suffering	"I'm at the end of my rope!" Adds up to being acute in terms of suffering
5. Intractability of behavior	Efforts futile in achieving desired goals, both with Joy and with peers
6. General personality appraisal	Mother, teachers, and peers saw him as "needy" and "pathetic"
V. Objective: Decide on a next step: identify and set priorities of current concerns	
Synthesis and summary by both Jeff and nurse	Suicidal
	Strong unmet emotional needs regarding love and belonging, especially with peers
	Secondary problem in cognitive functioning related to self, but necessary to resolve in order to decrease suicidal tendencies
	Jeff's chief concern was his relationship with Joy, his desire for her as girlfriend
	Few tasks of typical teenager had been accomplished; tumultuous growth pattern

tioning. But top priority was his suicidal tendencies. The following outlines the general approaches negotiated with Jeff during the initial one-to-one therapy.

Suicide. Jeff would not break a promise. Therefore we negotiated that as long as he could promise that he would not actually commit suicide, we could proceed with his chief concern—Joy. However, if he should no longer be able to make the promise (he was to do so at the end of each session), his family would have to be involved and a referral sought. (He was currently adamant about not telling his parents about the drawings or suicide attempts.)

Joy. Joy also was seen because of the suffering Jeff's behavior was causing her. While she had no desire to hurt Jeff, she also had no desire to be his girlfriend. She was an impossible choice for Jeff: she was one of the most popular girls in the school, she was already dating someone, and she had no desire to date Jeff. She was also generally kind, considerate, and caring with those with whom she came in contact, and she had treated Jeff as she treated others. Jeff's requests and behavior were causing her great turmoil, and we worked through some approaches she could use with Jeff, as well as what her responsibilities were and were not.

To Jeff, I reported that Joy didn't seem to be responding to his methods (drawings or impulsive threats of suicide) in terms of becoming his girlfriend—he would have to work on some other methods to achieve

Table 13.10. JEFF'S ALTERNATIVES AND CONSEQUENCES SEARCH

Solution 1: Split

What I would do in this case would be to pack up all my worldly possessions and go someplace back East, likely prospects being Minneapolis, Chicago, St. Louis, or Honolulu. Of course, I would just *go* and not tell anybody except Joy.

This would solve the problem, because the problems I face here would be behind me, and the 2,000 to 2,500 miles between here and the places I mentioned aren't exactly commuting distance, so they can't easily follow me.

Advantages: Nobody would know me in a new place, and I could start all over. And my problems can't travel 2,500 miles to follow me; so from there it sounds pretty good.

Disadvantages: However, what's to stop me from thinking about the problems I have here? Especially since I think about Joy all the time. And the possibility that I might never see her again worries me. And also, there's no guarantee the same thing won't happen all over again. It did when I moved up from California. Thirdly, if I were going to do this I'd want to live alone; and that I could not afford at all. And even if I could, my parents would not allow it.

Besides, running away doesn't really solve anything.

Solution 2: Suicide

What I would do here would be, after saying goodbye to Joy and a few other people, to go off some place where I can be alone, then stab myself in the heart with a knife.

This solves the problem by ending my knowledge of any suffering I've been through. A dead person is, after all, dead.

Advantages: As I said before, I would feel no suffering: I wouldn't have my parents on my back, I wouldn't suffer seeing Joy and her boyfriend, and I wouldn't feel so generally miserable. And I would no longer be getting in everybody's way and hurting people I love.

Disadvantages: In order to end this problem, I'd have to end everything else as well. And I don't want to rush into it, because once I'm dead I can't be brought back. Since I'd be killing myself with a knife, the bloody mess might really upset people. Worse, it might cause Joy to remember me with contempt.

The really bad part is that if I do it on the spur of the moment, Ms. Eggert might lose her job. [Remember that part of the contract was that he would let me know before taking any such action, or if he felt that he could no longer guarantee he would not commit suicide.] So it would involve telling my parents. And then they'd start treating me like some kind of freak—and I would never get a chance to kill myself.

Solution 3: Finding another girlfriend

This solution was not expanded upon by Jeff at this time.

Solution 4: Making Joy change her mind

This solution was also left unexpanded by Jeff at this time.

his goal of getting a girlfriend. He agreed to explore alternatives to the problem by use of the alternative search tool. He came up with four alternatives and worked these out between two of the sessions. Table 13.10 illustrates his work.

He was making progress! His symptoms related to cognitive functioning were no longer so evident. However, he still was getting stuck—unable to work out his third and fourth alternatives. We worked on these two together, and through a very sensitive confrontation Jeff was able to see that his behavior toward Joy foreclosed any possible good relationship with her. His was a behavior pattern that would drive most girls away. Then he expressed a new problem: how to get along with girls.

Relationships with Girls. Next we explored some possible methods together, and Jeff agreed to the following: practicing some approaches with me, then practicing with some girls who would be asked in. During this process we worked with videotape to check his progress. Negative feedback from me wasn't necessary. He was very quick to voice his own dissatisfaction with himself. What was left for me to do was report the progress he was making in terms of new interpersonal skills.

Relationships with Peers. Jeff was ready to become part of a group, and he agreed to do so. Through this process his needs to belong were beginning to be satisfied.

Work continued. Jeff also needed to do some adjusting of his parental relationships, and he had his father's terminal illness to deal with. However, some of this was coming up in the group meetings; it was also encouraging that Jeff could be trusted to work out one thing at a time. He knew they were on the list.

SUMMARY

Adolescents have been objects of adult concern for many centuries. Erikson has pointed out how crucial and yet how perilous youth's search for identity can be. We must be concerned with both youth in turmoil and youth who are sailing smoothly through this stage of life, concerned that they discover a healthy sense of self during adolescence and become adequate adults. We have considered the typical teenager and have emphasized the need to know and understand the population we serve in terms of situations, tasks, and contemporary problems facing adolescents today. We have explored ways of making nursing assessments of teenagers, how they fit the typical picture and what they are currently experiencing. We have examined how we can be partners in dealing with adolescents' concerns. We have discussed other concerns: selecting appropriate treatment modalities, issues in creating a climate for change, describing our expectations rather than demanding obedience, and techniques of therapy. Specific approaches related to problems in cognitive functioning, unmet emotional needs, and confusion in values and attitudinal functioning have been discussed. We have concluded with ways of evaluating therapeutic efforts and with an example of therapy at work.

References

Blos P: On Adolescence: A Psychoanalytic Interpretation. New York, Free Press, 1962

Erikson E H: Identity and the life cycle. In: Psychological Issues, Vol 1. New York, International Universities Press, 1959

______ The problem of ego identity. J Am Psychoanal Assoc 4:1956

______ Childhood and Society, rev ed. New York, Norton, 1964

Fagin C (ed): Nursing in Child Psychiatry. St Louis, Mosby, 1972

______ (ed): Child and Adolescent Psychiatric Nursing. St Louis, Mosby, 1974, pp 135–146

Freud A: The Ego and the Mechanisms of Defense (translated by Baines). New York, International Universities Press, 1946

Gerzon M: The Whole World Is Watching. New York, Viking, 1969, p xiii

Hollingshead A: Elmtown's Youth. New York, Wiley, 1949

Kessler J: Psychopathology of Childhood. Englewood Cliffs, Prentice-Hall, 1966

Lewin K: Field theory and experiment in social psychology: Concepts and methods. Am J Sociol 44:868–897, 1939

Mead M: Coming of Age in Samoa. New York, New American Library, 1950

______ Adolescence in primitive and modern society. In Swanson G E, Newcomb T M, Hartley E L, et al (eds): Readings in Social Psychology, rev ed. New York, Henry Holt, 1952

Miller D: Adolescence. New York: Jason Aronson, 1974

National Institute of Mental Health: Facts about Adolescence. DHEW Publication (HSM) 73-9133, Washington DC, USDHEW, 1973

Offer D: The Psychological World of the Teen-Ager. New York, Basic Books, 1969

______ Offer J: Three Developmental Routes Through Normal Male Adolescence. In Feinstein S, Fiovacchini P (eds): Adolescent Psychiatry: Vol IV: Developmental and Clinical Studies. New York, Jason Aronson, 1975

______ Howard K: An empirical analysis of the Offer self-image questionnaire for adolescents. Arch Gen Psychiatry 27:000, 1972

Piaget J: The Psychology of Intelligence. London, Routledge & Kegan Paul, 1950

______ Sex Psychological Studies. New York, Random, 1967

______ Inhelder B: The Psychology of the Child. New York, Basic Books, 1969

Raths L, Harmin M, Simon S B: Values and Teaching. Columbus, Ohio, Charles E Merrill, 1966

Simon S B, Howe, L W, Kirschenbaum H: Values Clarification. New York, Hart, 1972

Tosi D J: Youth: Towards Personal Growth. Columbus, Ohio, Charles E Merrill, 1974, pp 9–10

Vorrath, Brendtro: Positive Peer Culture. 1974

CHAPTER 14

FAMILY SUBSYSTEM: WORKING WITH SCHOOL-AGE CHILDREN EXPERIENCING PSYCHOSOCIAL STRESS

Mari K. Siemon

Child psychiatry is a relatively recent addition to the human services professions. There has always been much confusion about how the treatment of children differs from the treatment of adults, and even more difficulty in articulating and demonstrating the specific role of the nurse in working with children and families under psychosocial stress.

Because of the wide variety of situations that involve child–nurse relationships, nurses have many opportunities to forestall the development of emotional illness in children. These situations involve the child who is hospitalized, the child who has contact with a nurse at school, and the child encountered by a community health nurse who is visiting a family or a new mother. Because of their training and clinical experience nurses are often called on for guidance and support.

The child psychosocial nurse is a specialist with advanced preparation in the area of secondary prevention—treating children with emotional problems. Detailing the development of the skills necessary for this kind of therapeutic effectiveness is beyond the scope and purpose of this chapter. However, in view of the small numbers of child psychosocial specialists, it is evident that there is great need for primary and secondary prevention of emotional illness by nonspecialized professional nurses and nursing students. Increased knowledge and skill in dealing with mental health in children will enable nurses in many settings to recognize psychosocial stress and act in a way to minimize it.

This chapter will provide some theoretical concepts that should be useful in general nursing practice. The concepts of psychosocial and cognitive development will be used to give an overview of normal development and to provide some understanding of the critical stresses that are related to developmental immaturity. This knowledge can be used for primary prevention in the form of anticipatory guidance for parents and teachers around such topics as problems of specific age groups and developmental characteristics. Knowledge of what the concerns of children are may also be useful in leading children's discussion groups on such topics as impending surgery, death, feelings, and sex.

This chapter will also provide some helpful hints for working with children, and it will explore specific interventions for unmet emotional needs. These concepts will be useful in the area of primary prevention, where the nurse is in a position to minimize emotional distress that results from traumatic events and stressful situations. Developmental events such as the birth of a baby or entering school bring their own stresses. There are also the stresses produced by illness, injury, or death of a parent or sibling. Trauma produced by parental discord, separation, or divorce can also affect the emotional development of the child. Such stresses may have long-lasting effects on personality development, but these effects can be minimized by skillful intervention during a critical period.

Therapeutic intervention, rather than therapy, will be emphasized. The principles of therapeutic intervention are applicable in all settings in which nurses practice. Specific diagnoses will not be dealt with, since they have little relevance in nursing intervention. Rather, specific approaches will be discussed in relation to behavioral symptoms. The underlying framework for action is based on a growth-and-development model. This takes into account cognitive, psychologic, social, and physiologic growth, as well as the child's environment. This framework is health-oriented, and the focus is on learning and growth.

The school-age child (6 to 12 years) is the subject of this chapter for some very specific reasons. Until children are 5 or 6 years old, their major social contact is with their families. In many cases the emotional problems that a child is demonstrating have already become accepted by the family as behavior that is more or less normal. Families are very adaptable; they adjust quickly to a child's behavior. Once a child's behavior becomes familiar to the parents, they tend to consider it idiosyncrasy; they excuse it: "Oh, that's just how Johnny is!" As a child enters school, more objective adults such as school nurses and teachers may become concerned about behaviors that the family has long accepted, ignored, or denied. Societal expectations enter in, and parents are faced for the first time with a new perspective on an old problem. Emotional difficulties often have their roots in the preschool or toddler years, but it is during the school-age years that children are most often referred for treatment.

A major difficulty in discussing this age group is that the school-age period cannot be viewed as a single unit. Whether viewed in terms of

Freud's psychosexual model, Sullivan's interpersonal model, Erikson's psychosocial model, or Piaget's cognitive model, this period clearly is not a single unit. Between the ages of 8 and 9 years crucial changes occur. The immature ego and intellect become more refined in their functioning. Crude interpersonal relationships and a short attention span for schoolwork are replaced by social competence and perseverance. At about the age of 9 years the child reaches a point in development where play alone is no longer satisfying. The focus of interest is on becoming an adult, and the child begins to accomplish things and deal with situations that have significance in the adult world. There is an increase in the child's ability to act and to understand. Think of the differences between first-graders and sixth-graders. What a child wants and what is found to be stressful are influenced by the level of understanding and by the enlarging sphere of social interaction. The younger child (6 to 8 years) is more family-oriented and does things for personal pleasure. The older child (9 to 12 years) begins to move toward peer gangs and is task- and goal-oriented. These differences must be considered in both assessment and intervention with school-age children.

NURSING ASSESSMENT

Objectives of Assessment

The objectives of assessment of the adolescent's psychosocial needs (Kessler 1966) have been reviewed in Chapter 13. They are essentially the same for children. Because parents and children often have misconceptions about emotional problems, the first objective is to introduce the parents and child to a psychosocial way of viewing the child's problem. Parents may perceive their child's difficulties as a reflection of their parenting skills, and they are often guilt-ridden; children may think their problems are an indirect form of punishment for some past thought or action that was "bad." It is important to explain how feelings influence behavior and to emphasize that there is no magic force influencing the child's behavior. In most cases the onset of a problem can be traced to a stressful event that was misperceived by the child because of developmental immaturity. An understanding of how children experience events will help the family see the child's responses to stress as normal and predictable. Having the emotional difficulties explained in this light can be a great relief to parents and children.

After reducing fear and guilt by showing that the child's behavior is a predictable response, the nurse can turn to the next objectives in assessment: to identify in which areas and to what extent the child differs from others of the same age, to determine how long the problem has been going on, and identify the strengths within the child and family. A child is rarely dysfunctional in all areas of his life. Emotional disturbances in a child are interwoven with normal functioning, and it is often difficult to differentiate the two.

Using these data the nurse can approach the fifth objective of assessment: to formulate some hypotheses about what past or present factors have contributed to the problem. The final step is to identify and establish the priorities of the problems that are revealed by the data. In assessment, and for purposes of planning, it is necessary to consider the areas of normal development as well as the disturbed areas within a child. If the healthy growth-producing factors are utilized, they can contribute to rapid resolution of the emotional difficulties; to neglect these factors is to consider only half of the child, and the result will be a therapeutic relationship that emphasizes deficits and problems rather than health.

Cognitive and Emotional Factors

Sorting out the information that has been gathered in the assessment and assembling it into a meaningful statement of the problem can be a confusing task. A major difficulty is determining which behaviors are normal and which are indicative of disturbance. Standard developmental characteristics and tasks of the school-age child are good criteria to use in assessing maladaptive responses. For purposes of assessing the child's emotional status, his cognitive and emotional development are of primary importance; these criteria are also valuable when planning what steps to take to relieve the child's stress. Development proceeds through a sequence of predictable stages, and the nurse's efforts to work with the child will be most effective if standard developmental tasks are taken into account and if the interventions selected are consistent with what the child needs and is able to accept.

In order to make an accurate assessment of the child's developmental functioning, it is necessary to know what behavior is typical at the child's age. This includes having an understanding of what developmental problems are characteristic of certain stages of development, so that these will not be seen as pathologic, and recognizing that the individual's process of growth is unique. Deviations from the norm are to be expected; they are not always indicative of disturbance (Fagin 1972). The therapeutic assessment must take into account both the normal developmental sequence and the child's individual patterns of development. Adequate developmental evaluation requires repeated interactions in a variety of situations to give the total picture.

When assessing the child the nurse must keep in mind that adverse events can be harmful to the child if they arouse more anxiety than he can cope with. In order to understand the impact of adverse events on the child, the nurse must know how the child perceives the world and how he experiences events at different developmental stages. Anxiety comes from different sources as the child develops. Whether a situation is stressful to the child depends on the child's developmental level and the tasks that lie ahead. In order that current anxieties may be relieved and future personality disruption may be prevented, children must have help in making sense of the world (Wolff 1973).

In working with children it is important to keep in mind that it is not the event itself, but rather the child's experience of the event, that is the crucial factor in producing trauma. Ginsberg and Opper (1969), in their interpretation of Piaget's framework on cognitive development, emphasize that the child's thinking and reasoning processes differ tremendously from those of the adult. Thus children often misinterpret their environment, and this can cause profound anxiety, especially if their misperceptions go unnoticed or are misunderstood by adults. Nurses working with children need a good understanding of cognitive and emotional development if they are to accurately assess the impact and consequences that a stressful situation may have on a child. When there has been an arrest of the child's growth because of anxiety, the nurse's knowledge of age-appropriate developmental characteristics and needs can be useful in determining appropriate interventions to facilitate resumption of the growth process.

Cognitive Development. The limitations of the child's cognitive ability greatly influences the manner in which any event is experienced. What happens to the child as a consequence of any given event will be determined by the extent to which the child can reason and perceive meanings. Despite the considerable degree of cognitive growth the school-age child has experienced, there are still numerous limitations in thinking ability at this age. These limitations are particularly significant when the nurse is assessing the child's understanding of stressful situations. By the time school age is reached, the child is moving intellectually from egocentricity toward more abstract and objective thinking (Ginsberg and Opper 1969). Eventually the child will be able to sort out events in a logical way and see causal relationships. However, development is a continuous process of growth and change, and there are no absolute times at which new abilities are incorporated. Until a child is 9 or 10 years old there are many remnants of immature thinking that cause misperceptions. The major characteristics that limit the ability of the young school-age child to interpret things accurately are egocentrism, concrete thinking, and authoritarian morality (Elkind 1970).

Egocentrism is the belief children have that events occur for their pleasure, or because they will things to happen. As a result, little logic is utilized beyond simple cause-and-effect relationships. Since this manner of thinking is not amenable to logic, magic is frequently used as an explanation for happenings. The causation of external events is focused on the self. Rituals are often employed to ward off undesirable events (Step on a crack, break your mother's back). This is the last phase in the attempt to test out causation in terms of the self before the young school-age child moves on to more rational problem-solving around the age of 9 to 12 years.

Phenomenalism is one manifestation of egocentric thinking; the child believes there is a cause-and-effect relationship between two events simply because one occurs soon after the other. An undesirable event may be linked to the child's last misbehavior, which is seen as the cause: the divorce of the child's parents may be thought to be the result of the fact that the child spilled milk at dinner 2 days earlier. Another remnant of preoperational thought that often lingers is animism. Young children believe that everything happens on purpose, and they often give inanimate objects human characteristics. Piaget postulated that for a child there is no such thing as a chance or natural event (Elkind 1970). Thus, on tripping over a chair, the child may believe that the chair is carrying out punishment for something the child has done. This may also be combined with magical thinking, in which thoughts are considered to be as powerful as deeds. Children believe that what they think about will come true. A child can become very frightened after wishing that a baby sister were dead, or after wishing that Daddy would break his leg so he couldn't go away on a trip.

Concrete thinking confuses issues even further for the child. During the school-age stage of concrete operations, children are just learning how to decipher symbols in speech. They are also becoming acquainted with the multiple meanings of words. Until children are 10 or 12 years old, words continue to be taken literally. The phrase "Bad boy!" may be taken literally and personally; the child may not understand that it is meant to apply only to the current situation. If he is given the message often enough, the child will begin to behave badly because he believes he is inherently bad. Adult speech is often symbolic, and children get confused notions of the world when they hear adult symbolism: "He's in bed with a bug." "He's burning up!" "There's a fork in the road." "Daddy is tied up at the office." Taking words literally can lead to magical thinking, and even everyday events can be stressful to children if they misinterpret the language being used to describe those events.

The morality of young children is authoritarian. Rules are seen as absolute and unchangeable. A young school-age child experiences guilt directly proportional to the amount of damage done. The child does not take into account considerations of intentions; the same amount of guilt is felt whether a lamp is broken accidentally or intentionally. An integral part of authoritarian morality is the concept of imminent justice: crime incurs punishment; falling down after stealing from the cookie jar is seen as punishment. Guilt and fear can be overwhelming in the child's world; there morality is strict, and crime soon brings punishment. From the child's perspective, divorce, illness, and death may be seen as fitting punishments for misbehavior, rather than as adult problems and decisions or as natural happenings.

Emotional Development. Erikson drew attention to the links between childhood experiences and adult personality. His developmental approach considers the stages of growth in terms of particular problems in relationships with others that are of concern at different ages. Each stage has its own problems and sources of anxiety as children move toward independence. The resolution of problems depends on the life experiences the child has.

According to Erikson (1963), school-age children have already completed three stages in personality development: they have acquired a basic sense of trust in themselves and others, they have achieved a sense of autonomy as individuals, and they have developed a sense of initiative for exploring their world. Children in this stage have accomplished the basic skills of walking, talking, and toilet training; they are busy consolidating the gains they have made. The challenge that faces the child at this point is the development of a sense of industry and competence. The problems the child may encounter will involve developing feelings of inadequacy and inferiority should success experiences prove elusive and social encouragement too weak.

The school-age child is curious and eager to explore and master new experiences. The major theme is to do things better than before. The child is further establishing a sense of identity. A conception of the future becomes a consideration, and having a conscience becomes an important varible. Children begin to think ahead to the consequences of their actions and feel a sense of guilt. Guilt combined with faulty logic can cause considerable emotional distress.

In summary, Erikson's theory of personality development and Piaget's theory of cognitive development provide a foundation for determining the emotional status of the school-age child (Kessler 1966). Development proceeds in sequential stages, and each stage uses tools acquired in the previous stage. Stress can cause a child to regress to an earlier stage if his resources are not adequate to deal with his situation. Understanding how children perceive and interact with the world is crucial for identifying possible stressors caused by developmental immaturity. This is the first step in working effectively with children and families.

Critical Developmental Stressors. The emotional and cognitive developmental factors that characterize school-age children also make them vulnerable to stress and anxiety. Because of the developmental factors that are operating, there are some things that can create problems for school-age children but usually not for children at older and younger developmental stages. Loss and separation experiences such as death and divorce often lead to emotional distress in this age group. Because they are still egocentric and still relate all events to themselves, children may perceive parental separation as personal rejection, and they may also believe that they have caused the separation. A loss may also be perceived as punishment for being naughty. As misconception builds on misconception, the child can be overwhelmed by guilt, grief, and anxiety.

Similar thought processes and misintepretation of information contribute to suicide in children. The most prominent symptom in children who kill themselves is anxiety precipitated by parental rejection (either real or imagined). Lukianowicz (1968) stated that, for children, suicide is not related to despair and a desire to terminate an intolerable situation; rather, it is related to an immature way of processing information. A history will often reveal a recent loss. Even as the child is coming to grips with the concept of causality, the irreversibility and finality of death are misunderstood. If the loss by death of a loved one is seen by the child as a rejection, the child may attempt to rejoin or "visit" the lost loved one. The methods used are usually classified as accidental deaths. Drowning, shooting, hanging, and darting in front of a car can result from magical thinking and misperceptions.

Another area of concern for school-age children is in being different in any way from their peers. It is in the school-age group that comparisons of abilities, physical appearances, and families first take place. Competence and participation in group activities are of primary importance. Handicapped and learning-impaired children become painfully aware of differences in ability, and this can easily lead to feelings of inadequacy and low self-esteem.

Summary. It is important to keep developmental characteristics in mind when assessing children, as well as situations that may cause problems because of the child's developmental immaturity. The child will probably not be able to verbalize these concerns. Knowing such things in advance will enable the nurse to make some predictions as to what the concern may be and to initiate some secondary prevention to decrease the traumatic effects.

Framework for Assessment

Once the assessment data have been sorted into adaptive and maladaptive behaviors, a closer look must be taken at the areas of functioning that are impaired. A framework for determining the specific area in which the child is having difficulty has been presented in Chapter 13.

Symptoms may indicate a problem in the area of cognitive functioning, affective functioning, or social, attitudinal, or values-related functioning. Categorizing symptoms into these broad categories will be helpful in planning specific interventions (Raths and associates 1966).

This chapter will focus on the area of affective functioning, since this is one of the most troublesome areas for children. Confusion in values can occur only when there is more mature cognitive development than is seen in the school-age child. As has been discussed, problems in thinking can certainly contribute to increased stress in children; however, interventions in the cognitive area are difficult with children, because correcting the deficit usually requires development and maturation. Thus clinical assessment of which area is causing problems for the child will usually reveal unmet emotional needs in the affective area of functioning.

Problems in Affective Functioning. Behavioral symptoms indicative of problems in the affective area may include consistent and unusual manifestations of one of the following: aggressiveness, withdrawal, psychosomatic illness, submissiveness, or regression.

Aggressiveness. An aggressive child is belligerent; he is often in fights. He may be the one who steals, sets fires, or displays extreme cruelty to animals. Aggression can also be directed inward, producing such manifestations as head-banging and accident-proneness.

Withdrawal and Isolation. The withdrawn child does not participate in activities with peers; she has no friends and is extremely quiet. She is the loner.

Psychosomatic Illness. For children, psychosomatic illness can mean chronic headaches and stomachaches with no physiologic basis, although it can also include asthma, eczema, and colitis.

Submissiveness and Passivity. Submissive children always give in, don't stand up for themselves, and don't complain about pain. They wait for someone to tell them what to do and do not initiate action on their own. Physically handicapped children often fit this category.

Regression. The regressed child may manifest all behavior that is characteristic of an earlier stage of development, including soiling, wetting, whining, thumb-sucking, and clinging.

If the child's behavioral symptoms seem to fit into the area of affective functioning, there is a further kind of organization that can be carried out before formulating a care plan. It is possible to formulate hypotheses about past and present contributing factors by identifying which specific emotional need has not been adequately met.

Emotional Developmental Tasks. The emotional needs of the child are related to developmental tasks. Tasks are simply learning experiences that must be accomplished during a particular period of growth in order to prepare a child for the next period. The task of childhood as a whole is to prepare an individual to function productively and independently. Each stage of development contributes a necessary step to the overall process.

If everything goes according to schedule, the child will master one period of growth and acquire all the necessary skills before moving on to the next. If the necessary experiences are not provided, there will be gaps in the child's learning. The child may move on to the next phase of development, but with incomplete knowledge.

Thus it is possible that a school-age child may be in one stage, and also struggling to master a task of an earlier stage. Development can also be uneven. A child may be age-appropriate in some areas (eg, physical appearance, relationships with adults, body movements) but be immature in other areas (eg, emotional reactions, relationships with peers). Nursing intervention with the emotionally disturbed child must be based on the idea that if some of the child's basic needs can be met, tension will be reduced and development can proceed on a normal course, preventing personality disruption in the future. There are only four emotional needs that could possibly be unresolved issues for a school-age child: trust, autonomy, initiative, and industry (Erikson 1963).

Developing trust is a task of infancy; it consists essentially in gaining a sense of predictability and security about the world. The particular relationship experience that is crucial is that of dependence. An infant's first dependent relationship will set the stage for relationships in the future in which the child must be dependent on another person (Wolff 1973). Inadequate experiences will result in feelings of pessimism and mistrust. The child with such a background can certainly move on developmentally, but the remaining mistrust will affect how the child relates to other people. A nurse may encounter a 7-year-old child who is age-appropriate in many areas but who is behaving in a way indicative of unmet trust needs. This can happen in two ways: A child can crave dependence and be clinging, whining, and extremely fearful of new situations, with a lot of thumb-sucking or nail-biting. An opposite reaction to the same need is the child who resists all forms of dependence, particularly illness. The child in this case will refuse to go to bed, will not admit to being ill, will fight being held or cuddled, will act aloof, and will have difficulty establishing a relationship with the adult who is providing care. Such children are reticent about sharing thoughts and fears, and they have a cautious, superficial manner of relating. A nursing history may reveal events that were contrary to the life experiences needed to develop object constancy. Events that could be contributing factors to problems with trust are frequent separations from parent, emotional or physical battering and abuse, and a variety of caretakers while an infant (foster home, orphanage, group home, lengthy hospitalizations).

A school-age child may also manifest delay in the development of autonomy. This is actually a task of the toddler period. The crucial experience is a cooperative relationship with a person who is more powerful. Having determined that the world is a safe and predictable place, the child needs to feel an ability to exercise control over some areas of life and develop confidence in the capacity to please others (Fagin 1973). Since the overall purpose of the childhood period is to acquire the ability to be independent, the child needs help in moving from the complete dependence of infancy to the emancipation that adolescence brings. Adults can assist this transition by allowing children to make decisions on their own about areas they really can control. Letting children dress themselves and wear what they choose is a safe place to start (color combinations are not nearly as crucial to children as they are to adults). Another way to give children a feeling of confidence is to give them choices between things that are acceptable to adults (peanut butter sandwich or bologna sandwich for lunch). Negative experiences during this period will result in feelings of shame and doubt. Without a healthy resolution of this phase, the child may give up the notion of having a cooperative relationship and become excessively compliant. An alternative reaction would be continued struggle for control, which could result in behavioral symptoms that would tend to give the child a sense of power over others. If adequate skills are not developed in this earliest social training period, children craving power resort to aggression: taking toys away from younger children, arguing about anything an adult suggests, being irrationally obstinate, refusing to eat, soiling and wetting (the ultimate control, because no one can make them stop), or "forgetting" to take the prescribed insulin ("No one can tell me what to do!"). Without an opportunity to develop a healthy and appropriate sense of power, the child may overcompensate and become obstinate and manipulative. Factors revealed by the child's history may provide clues that autonomy is an unmet need: parents who have rigid rules of what is right and wrong; punishment for assertiveness or disagreement by the child; parental discouragement of trying any new skills; physical handicaps. Handicapped children are a special concern in this area. Children with crippling diseases (cerebral palsy, spina bifida, arthritis) may have difficulty moving about on their own; generally they must rely on an adult to move them, feed them, or dress them. Without careful management such children can easily become very passive. If the child doesn't have the ability to control things physically, control may be gained by crying, by tantrums, or by refusal to participate in therapeutic regimens. If nurses can develop the habit of looking at difficult patients as being emotionally needy, some real benefit can accrue for both child and nurse.

Developing a sense of initiative is the psychosocial task of the preschooler. The aspects of relationship development that are important in this stage are experiences of life in a family group. The struggle is between being curious and comfortable with experimenting and being anxious, inhibited, and withdrawn (Wolff 1973). The continued physical development of this period gives children new motor skills that facilitate exploration and the development of initiative. At the same time, these new abilities can lead to situations that leave children feeling guilty and fearful that they have gone too far in exploration (eg, getting lost at the store, breaking a lamp). The development of initiative starts with a firm sense of the self as separate; it progresses through these stages: awareness of being able to do things without adults, mastering physical skills of independence, and setting goals (but not necessarily finishing the initiated task). Children who have not developed an adequate sense of initiative will be afraid to try new things; they will decline when asked to perform a task, they will ask for adult help frequently, and they will wait to begin a task until told to do so. A history may reveal overly solicitous and anxious parents, an environment that lacks the stimulation to evoke curiosity, or immobilization during a critical period (body cast, rheumatic fever, physical handicaps). A special concern here are children with sensory deprivations such as blindness or deafness. Because they miss essential cues from the environment, they may find it frightening to try new experiences. There is a very realistic fear of being hurt, and they need sensitive management to complete this stage of development.

School-age children are in the process of developing a sense of industry. This is the time when experiences of working in groups are crucial and when attitudes toward work are developed. The tasks of the school-age child involve moving outside of the family toward peer relationships, seeing oneself as an individual in relation to others, developing skills that will win recognition and aid in the movement toward independence, and moving intellectually from egocentric, inductive reasoning to deductive reasoning (Fagin 1972). If experiences are unsuccessful or if they provoke too much anxiety, the child may grow up with feelings of inferiority about the ability to work and relate to peers. This will affect motivation for schoolwork or therapeutic regimens, as well as the ability to cooperate with other children.

The emotional problems children experience during this time are centered around the developmental tasks of the period. The means of coping with difficulties are by use of the skills available to the child to accomplish the developmental tasks. For the school-age child, competition, compromise, and cooperation are the behaviors that help in mastering the intricacies of social relationships (Fagin 1972). No matter how inadequately these skills may have been learned, it is through them that the child attempts to cope with problems. The child who is having difficulty developing a sense of industry may react by avoiding any type of competitive behavior, even to the point of shunning any social interaction with peers. This can even extend to the ability to learn. The child's learning may be inhibited because of fear of competition, which may be followed by failure in school and development of psychosomatic illnesses to avoid going to school or playing with other children. Such children may also demonstrate their feelings of inferiority by apologizing profusely for accidents or failures; they often have a standard preface for their work: "It's not very good." At the other extreme, the child may react to difficulties in developing a sense of adequacy by being fiercely competitive in all areas. These are the children who always have to win, who have to have the first choice, who find it impossible to compromise and who always need to be the best in sports or grades. There are many home and school situations that foster feelings of inferiority rather than industry. An interview may reveal causative factors: parental emphasis on attaining perfection; comparison of the child with siblings; lack of appreciation for individual differences and areas of strength. The message the child receives is discouraging: "Don't do a thing if you can't do it well." The message should be encouraging: "It's OK to try. Some things you'll be better at than others."

Summary. Assessment information can be classified in three major areas: the cognitive system, the values or attitudinal system, and the affective system. The majority of behavioral symptoms exhibited by school-age children will fall under the affective system. This broad classification can be further broken down to identify which specific unmet emotional need is causing difficulties: trust, autonomy, initiative, or industry. Because the symptoms differ for each need, the behaviors the child exhibits will signal the kind of help that is needed. Specific interventions for unmet emotional needs will be discussed later.

Emotional difficulties experienced by school-age children are expressed in characteristic ways. The behavioral expression is influenced by the skills available to the child to accomplish the developmental tasks of the period. In addition to identifying the emotional difficulties the child is experiencing in regard to the developmental tasks of the school-age period, repeated observations will help the nurse to determine the degree to which a child uses behaviors of an earlier developmental stage to express needs and achieve satisfaction (eg, thumb-sucking, whining).

Use of behaviors from earlier developmental periods is particularly noticeable in school-age children, because they are clearly so immature (eg, wetting, thumb-sucking). Unsatisfied needs from an earlier period can be a considerable problem, because the behaviors being manifested prevent the child from accomplishing the tasks of the school-age period.

In the school-age period children should be moving out of the family and exploring and experimenting with the environment in order to learn about themselves and others. If the child is struggling to master an earlier developmental task, the turmoil will have an effect on self-esteem and on the manner of relating to others. The symptoms that are characteristic of unmet needs result from anger, fear, and frustation; they generally go hand in hand with difficulty in peer relationships, disturbed family relationships, and poor academic functioning.

Tools of Assessment

Observation. Assessment is an ongoing process. There are many tools a nurse can use to obtain information and organize it. Observation is an excellent means of assessing the child's emotional status. Children lack the verbal expressive ability of adults; they are naturally action-oriented. Observation will yield a wealth of information about how children regard themselves and their world. It is essential to remember that a single observation is not sufficient for nursing diagnosis and intervention. Only after observing a child in a variety of activities and situations can an accurate assessment of behavior patterns be made.

When observing a child, it is useful to keep some general considerations in mind:

1. What are the developmental tasks and needs of a child in this age group?
2. What areas could present concerns because of the child's developmental stage?
3. What type of play is most typically seen at this stage and why is it useful?
4. What are the characteristics of a good environment for a child this age (eg, safety factors, toys, stimulation)?

With these broad areas as a basis for sorting adaptive and maladaptive behavior, the nurse can begin looking at much more specific categories in order to get an impression of how the child is functioning in crucial areas. Carbonera (1961) has done a good job of identifying the major areas that should be observed.

Physical appearance is an important consideration. How the child looks and dresses, along with an estimate of general health, will give a good idea of the general care received. For younger children, physical appearance will indicate parental concern; for older children who can groom themselves, grooming is a gauge of self-esteem. Children who do not feel good about themselves will generally disregard even the basics of grooming.

Body movement and use of the body will indicate the degree to which the child feels comfortable with the body. The nurse should determine whether movement is quick or slow, clumsy or assured, and whether development of the large and small muscles is uniform or uneven. Another important area to consider is how much of what a child is feeling is expressed by the body. Children who feel good about themselves and the world will be spontaneous and will move spontaneously.

Observing facial expressions is a good way to determine whether the child reflects what is felt minute by minute, or only when something is felt intensely. A constant deadpan expression may indicate real denial of feelings or abnormal reluctance to show feelings.

Speech can give clues to cognitive development; it is also an indicator of moods. Consider how much of what the child is feeling is expressed through the tone of voice; note the nature of the speech pattern under stress. Is speech an important way of communicating, or does the child communicate better in other ways?

A child's emotional reactions can be a good measure of trust in other people; emotions can reveal how safe the child considers the immediate environment. How and when the child exhibits happiness, sadness, anger, or any other emotion is a factor in assessing the child's awareness of feelings. Another aspect to consider is control over feelings. Is there too little, too much, or a healthy balance?

How and when the child seeks out relationships with other children is a factor in social development. Does the child wait for others to initiate contact? What is the interaction like? Is there sharing, fearfulness, bossiness, or inhibition? Is the picture one of immaturity, advanced maturity, or age-appropriateness?

Relationships with adults comprise a crucial area, especially in determining a child's level of trust. Note how easily the child goes to an adult, how often, whether there is a need for physical closeness, and whether the child is different than others of the same age. Are adults used for comfort, and does the child accept limits?

The final area to consider in an assessment of the child involves the play activities used. Play is more than just fun. It is also an essential part of social and emotional development and a means for enhancing self-concept. Through play, children test out ways of interacting; they form schemata of identity: "Who am I?" "How do I relate to others?" "How do others relate to me?" Both the content and the structure of play parallel cognitive and psychosocial development and reflect emerging intellectual functioning, the changing view of the self, and increasing social awareness. There is gradual movement from random motion and play centered around the self to play with objects and play near other children; eventually there is cooperative play with others. A good way to begin an observation is to determine whether the child is more involved in solitary play or group play; one should also consider the kinds of toys that are being used. It should be determined whether play is primarily for social pleasure, sensory pleasure, or expression of feelings, as well as what activities are the most pleasing or frustrating. The expression of fantasy is a crucial consideration: Are there major themes? Is it aggressive? What roles does the child take? Observing play activities is an excellent way of gathering information about the sense of initiative. The nurse should notice whether a child tries new things, is curious about people and toys, and exhibits any special skills.

Interviewing Methods. When an interview with a child is used as part of nursing assessment, it is important to keep in mind some basic characteristics of children. First, children are action-oriented. A sit-down conversation is not a natural situation. Information can be elicited more easily while drawing or playing a game, rather than in a straight face-to-face encounter. Second, children see size as power. It is usually helpful in establishing rapport to keep to the child's eye level. This may mean sitting on the floor or on pillows rather than on chairs.

The third factor to keep in mind has to do with the differences between working with children and working with adults. Children rarely seek help for illness or distress on their own; it is the adult who notices problems and seeks help. Children are passive recipients of the process, and they are often confused about what is happening to them. With cognitive immaturity playing a part, younger children will see illness as an indication that they have been bad and are being punished; older children will resent being different from their peers or being restricted in their movement toward competence. Since denial is a primary defense mechanism, even with older children, problems will tend to be ignored. This means that in the initial interview the child may be fearful, hostile, rebellious, guilty, and confused (Erikson 1963). Beginning a relationship under such conditions can be very discouraging unless the nurse is prepared for such possibilities. An added dimension is that children do not verbalize problems and fears as adults do. Expression will be by motor activity or will be phrased in a kind of code: "All those other kids are crybaby sissies!" The real meaning must be interpolated: "Is it OK not to be brave all the time?" It is at such times that observation skills are useful for getting the whole picture.

Another difference in working with children is the tendency they have toward growth and health. Even though they may exhibit symptoms of an earlier, unresolved developmental stage, children are still in the process of maturing. Unlike adults who may be stuck in an unfinished developmental stage, children are still growing and moving through developmental periods. Cognitive and psychosocial maturation alone will correct many emotional difficulties. It is this power of the ego that Erikson (1963, p. 83) had in mind when he said that children fall apart, but unlike Humpty Dumpty they grow back together again.

During an initial interaction, children need the same information that adults need to ease anxieties and fears. Keep in mind that children have a different perception of illness and treatment. Knowing that they use denial when anxious or threatened, and that they often keep silent or try to hide their most troublesome concerns, the nurse must anticipate anxieties and respond to them even if they are unexpressed. A good place to start is to explore any fantasies the child may have regarding why he was brought in for treatment. Ask the child to share the information given by the parents about coming to the hospital or clinic.

Armed with an idea of how the child is experiencing a situation, the nurse can then correct misperceptions. The child should know in nonthreatening terms what the nurse knows. Major areas to touch on are what the concern is, who is concerned (parents, teachers), and why people are working with the child. The final task is to explain the therapeutic value of treatment. Even though it may not be stated, children will wonder "What's in it for me?" They need to know in general terms that treatment will make them feel better, be happier, walk better, or have more friends.

This process of sharing information provides a good opportunity to assess the child's mental status. This important aspect of assessment has been greatly facilitated by the work of Goodman and Sours (1967), who developed a child mental status examination that provides a procedure for doing a comprehensive psychosocial assessment.

Summary

Assessing the psychosocial development of a child and identifying emotional difficulties is a considerable task. The first step in doing this is recognizing age-typical behavior; the nurse must know what developmental problems are characteristic of certain periods and what situations are likely to be stressful. Another thing to keep in mind is that each individual develops in a unique way, and deviation from the norm does not necessarily mean disturbance. While children have considerable individuality, they are also influenced by significant people in their lives and events in their environment. Examination of a child's behavioral symptoms, as well as past and present factors influencing that behavior, will allow determination of which emotional needs are causing the child problems. Two tools of assessment that nurses are well prepared to use are observation and interviewing. It should be kept in mind that an assessment must be flexible, so that it can be changed as more information is added or initial impressions are seen in a different light.

NURSING INTERVENTION: CARRYING OUT THE CARE PLAN

General Considerations

Peplau (1963) identified two types of counseling in nursing practice. One type is immediate situational counseling, as in explaining surgery to a child. The second is developmental counseling. Here the task is to encourage latent capacities and enhance healthy development. It is developmental intervention that will be the focus here. This is certainly an area for which nurses are qualified, and it is an area where they are important because of their contacts with children and families.

Before the nurse enters into a helping relationship with a child, it is important that she clearly understand the purpose of nursing intervention. Fagin (1972, p. 7) has identified three general purposes:

1. To assist the child with new learning in regard to himself and his world;
2. To assist the child and family with relearning of roles and relationships and with expectations;
3. To assist in restoring those aspects of living that show deprivation.

When dealing with children, it is easy to be caught in the trap of wanting to save them from harm. As a result, many nurse-child contacts continue past the point of resolving the problem because the nurse thinks that she needs to help the child "just until this new situation is past." Waiting for the child to stabilize and cease experiencing confusing events will take until adulthood. It is not realistic to think that the nurse can always save the child from hurt, nor would it be beneficial to do so. Such thinking does not recognize the child's strength, adaptability, and capacity for problem-solving. The task of intervention is to help a child over a developmental hump on which the child is temporarily stuck. From that point the normal process of development can take over; the child can do very nicely alone, at least until another hump is encountered. This allows a child the experiential learning so crucial for development.

In addition to defining the purpose of intervention, the nurse should consider the medium for intervention. Verbal techniques are useful, and they should be part of an interaction; however, because of the limited expressive ability of children, activity is a necessary component for problem-solving. A helping relationship can be seen as an educational process. If Elkind's (1970) interpretation of Piaget's work is used as a framework, it is clear that, in order to learn, children need to manipulate things and physically act on their environment to incorporate concepts. Also, children are most interested and learn best when an experience is novel enough to involve them in an activity. Lastly, children will learn only what they are developmentally ready to learn. These ideas about how children learn illustrate the importance of activity in planning nursing interventions with children. What children do is often more significant than what they hear, and the type of experiences provided will influence what is learned.

For example, in the case of impending surgery, explaining the procedure is not all that is needed to make the child feel less anxious about the unknown. An opportunity to handle a syringe, explore the recovery room, and bandage a doll in the way the child will be bandaged will be a great help. Even older children need these tactile experiences, as well as a chance to draw what they know about body parts and how they function.

Tools of Intervention

Play Techniques. Play as a medium of expression is one of a number of tools available to the nurse in the treatment process. Children play out their feelings in much the same way as adults talk them out. By using play materials symbolically and giving them personalized meanings, children can project their feelings and attitudes through the play medium (Erikson 1950).

Play activities are an integral part of a helping relationship, not a separate process. An accepting and empathic attitude on the part of the nurse enhances the effectiveness of play for the child. It is important to realize, however, that not all play is therapeutic. Some play is simply an age-appropriate expression, with no real relevance to a child's concerns. This kind of play is not useful in the treatment process, nor is play that is overstimulating or that produces overwhelming guilt or anxiety (Burns 1970). It is the nurse's responsibility to control the situation so that play is therapeutic. This can be done by removing certain toys, redirecting play, stopping a play activity, or setting out certain toys that will provide therapeutic expression. Each child must be seen as an individual who uses play in a unique way toward a unique end. What is useful to one child may be inappropriate for another. The use of play in a nurse–child relationship should be kept within the context of individual goals and needs.

Play is most useful in helping a child to discharge anger and anxiety (Burns 1970). This occurs in four stages. At first, feelings will be diffuse and pervasive, with no real focus. At this point the child may pound clay or throw beanbags. An older child may refer to everything as stupid and walk around hitting the wall or furniture. A general feeling comes through, but it is not clearly connected to a person or situation.

Gradually, anger and anxiety will be directed at an object. This is usually the family, siblings, or the nurse. Feelings are not so generalized, and a child will start to show feelings when a certain person is present.

As further expression of feelings is encouraged, anger remains specific, and some positive feelings begin to emerge. The child begins to feel the ambivalence of both loving and being angry with someone. In this stage the child may ignore or be angry with the nurse when she visits; the child may cry and cling, or protest when the nurse leaves: "Don't leave yet!"

Finally, positive and negative feelings become distinct and focused. Emotions are consistent with the reality that motivates them. The child will be able to have positive interactions with the nurse, but may get angry when it is time for an injection or unpleasant treatment.

Burns (1970) has identified seven ways in which play may be used with children to accomplish the process of discharging feelings. Ventilation is a play technique that encourages a child to pour out feelings that have been unexpressed. Tension is relieved, and energy can be focused on problem-solving. Such play is facilitated by the use of a punching clown, beanbags, a dart gun, clay and almost any large muscle activity. Ventilation is useful after a painful procedure or a traumatic event.

Play can also be used as a means of binding anxiety and calming a child who is immobilized by a threatening subject or a frightening situation. Giving a child something to do during a break in treatment or while talking can pave the way for proceeding with the business at hand (physical therapy, explaining surgery, talking of death). Here, play is really a secondary activity to help a child maintain control and avoid panic. Children sometimes express themselves better while playing with clay, shooting darts, or doodling.

Working through is an important function of play. The child is helped to play out conscious and unconscious conflicts to arrive at a resolution. This can mean allowing the child to play out having surgery or going to a funeral, until some degree of comfort with the information is reached. Toys that promote this kind of play are puppets, dolls, dollhouses, and blocks.

Play used for communication is a good way of identifying problems. Dramatic play is useful here to help the child reveal concerns about a divorce or a handicap, for example, through repeated themes in play. Through the choice of play materials, the child gives many clues about the level of awareness of problems and the amount of directness that can be tolerated. Pretending to shoot at inanimate objects or animals shows less ability to deal with feelings than playing with human figures. Anger directed at toy soldiers rather than at dolls representing mother, father, or baby shows that the child cannot focus anger yet. Responding with direct statements of what the child may be feeling, or taking a role in a fantasy, can facilitate expression of concerns.

If a child must reexperience elements of an earlier developmental stage before completing a more mature level, play can be used for regression. The entire personality need not regress if this can be expressed in a safe environment. Regression in play frequently occurs with younger children after the birth of a sibling, or if a child is under the prolonged stress of a chronic illness. Regressed behavior or play can be comforting because it is familiar. Clay, a baby bottle, and finger paints are useful toys.

For older children who are having difficulty with acquiring a sense of industry, play can be used for the development of the necessary skills. Inability to perform the tasks and skills of the peer group can be damaging to the self-esteem of the child. Kinds of play that can be used include educational games to increase mathematics skills, shooting baskets, building models, or learning how to play cards. This type of play can be useful for children who have lost the use of their limbs and who need to be exercising them; it is also good for developing age-appropriate skills.

Another way in which play can be used is in modification of a life style. When the child's basic approach to tasks is self-defeating, play can be used to modify the approach. The style of playing is usually representative of approaches to other situations. This may include such things as building a model wrong because of refusal to follow directions, and cheating at checkers. Such approaches will set the child up to fail at school tasks and in peer relationships. Pointing out the consequences of actions and helping the child to try alternative styles can help change self-defeating patterns.

Communication Techniques. Besides play, there is a variety of activities that allow the nurse to communicate with the distressed child. There are many books available for children on understanding feelings, death, divorce, sibling rivalry, and problems at school (see Bibliography at end of chapter). It is sometimes useful to read a book with a child and either talk generally about the characters in the story or talk about how the story directly relates to a child's situation. Children like books and stories, and this is a natural medium for relating to them.

Another technique is to cut pictures out of magazines and paste them on cards. A child may either tell a story about a picture, which will probably be a projection of the child's own feelings, or talk in general about the emotions expressed in the picture.

In cases where children have come from very confused and chaotic backgrounds, it is often useful to help the child write a life history. The nurse can help to fill in confusing gaps and put events in proper perspective. This is a concrete and entertaining way of dealing with emotion-laden material. This can be adapted to writing a story about impending surgery to find out what the child knows or fears.

Specific Approaches for Unmet Emotional Needs

In order to plan appropriate nursing intervention for the school-age child, the nurse needs to assess the child's cognitive development and identify specific needs the child is expressing, using the structure suggested by Raths and associates (1966). Keeping in mind what the primary conflict of each developmental stage is, activities can be planned to provide opportunities to complete developmental tasks.

Tables 14.1, 14.2, and 14.3 give some examples of specific approaches. The tables are not meant to be exhaustive, but rather a reference place from which to begin. Specific interventions can be planned in terms of the structure of the contact or nurse–child relationship, the kind of toys that will be useful, and the kinds of activities that will provide appropriate developmental experiences. Consideration should be given to how these three components can be used together in a helping relationship to assist the child complete developmental tasks and continue moving toward independence. A crucial consideration is to determine what is of interest for the individual child. For older children the structure may be more important than the toys or activities.

Only the three tasks of development prior to the school-age period are discussed. Since the development of a sense of industry is a normal task of the school-age child, the task may be in various stages of completion until about the age of 12 years. Problems in this area will be of a more acutely situational nature. A child who has not mastered tasks of an earlier stage is a more immediate concern, since these difficulties are more chronic. Failure to complete earlier developmental tasks can interfere with or arrest progressive personality development and impair the child's capacities for accurate perception of the world, impulse control, learning, and establishing satisfying relationships with others.

CONCLUSION

This chapter has described a framework for nursing assessment and intervention to be used in working with school-age children under psychosocial stress. Behavioral symptoms of a child can be indicative of problems in the cognitive area, problems in the affective area, or problems in the value or attitudinal area. Each area has a distinct set of

Table 14.1. EXAMPLES OF SPECIFIC APPROACHES FOR UNMET TRUST NEEDS

STRUCTURE	TOYS	ACTIVITIES
Retain sameness with respect to time and place for meeting, or have same nurse each shift.	Allow the child to bring familiar objects from home for transition in adjusting to a new situation: blanket, toy, comics, clothing, pictures	Send a card during vacation to help maintain the relationship during physical absence
Be consistent in limit-setting so that a child knows what to expect and can feel secure	Make it clear the child is accepted: "Whatever toy you choose is OK."	Games of predictability: hide and seek, catch, peek-a-boo (this can be done with a child 6–8 years by ducking into a doorway and surprising the child while walking down a hallway)
Display appropriate affect with expression of feelings, so that messages are clear and consistent		
Follow through on promises made		
Physical comfort is important; consider things that will enhance the comfort of the child, such as sitting on a chair, on the floor, or on pillows; going to the park; having a snack		
Offer help if it is needed: "Would you like me to hold that for you?"		
The closer a relationship becomes, the more the child will check out the caring by testing limits or refusing to talk, to see if you'll stay close anyway		

Table 14.2. EXAMPLES OF SPECIFIC APPROACHES FOR UNMET AUTONOMY NEEDS

STRUCTURE	TOYS	ACTIVITIES
Allow the child to have choice of time and day to meet (between alternatives acceptable to the nurse)	Have many toys available that the child can choose from	Give alternative list of activities the child can choose from
Don't make decisions a power struggle ("I'm bigger than you."); when deciding which exercises to do first or what game to play, flip a coin or draw straws	Use toys that allow for control: guns (6–9), marbles (6–12), billiards (9–12), puppets (6–9), darts (9–12), pounding a pegboard (6), beanbags (6–9), "Bozo" punch clown (6–8)	Use activities that allow a child to push things around: games where objects get pushed around so people don't have to be (checkers, chess, 9–12); knocking down a block tower (6–7); pushing dolls around (6–9)
Give the child a chance to say no without retaliation		Use games that involve being in control or gaining territory: Monopoly (9–12), Captain, May I? (6–9), king of the mountain (6–9), tug-of-war (6–9)
Respect decisions the child makes		Encourage the child to claim territory and assert rights by making signs for the room or bed: STAY OUT, DO NOT DISTURB, JOE'S ROOM
Give verbal reinforcement and praise for something done by the child		Allow for modeling by the child without getting into a power struggle: When a meeting is over, say, "I'm going now." The child is free to go on his own.
Let children finish projects on their own, no matter how long it takes		Side-by-side activities allow a child to follow without the adult demanding that the child do something; this is good for teaching. Let the child know: "I'm going to add this much water to my paint mix." He will follow.
Allow many choices: not if something will be done, but when (Now or 5 minutes from now?), or how (This dressing first, or that one?), or what (Your cereal first or your juice?)		Keeping a secret diary is a way of having some territory that no one else knows about
Allow the child to do as much for himself as possible; this requires patience and freedom to move at a child's pace, not adherence to a rigid schedule		

Table 14.3. EXAMPLES OF SPECIFIC APPROACHES FOR UNMET INITIATIVE NEEDS

STRUCTURE	TOYS	ACTIVITIES
Give the child permission to explore: "It can be whatever you want it to be."	Use toys that can be taken apart and put together in a new way: paper dolls (6–9), Tinkertoys (6–8), Lincoln Logs (6–9), Erector set (9–11), blocks (6–8), clay (6–9), Mr. Potato Head (6–8)	Encourage activities that evoke curiosity and risk: treasure hunt (6–8), find the hidden toy (6–8), dramatics (6–12), guessing games (Twenty Questions) (9–12), charades (9–12)
Offer encouragement to try things in a new way: "Let's try to do things in a different way today!"	Use toys that can change shape and form and be manipulated: paints (6–12); finger paint (6–9); scissors, paper, and paste (6–12); soap bubbles (6); building a model (9–12)	Recognize that speech is a tool for exploration, not a commitment to action. Encourage fantasy exploration. Act out different endings for stories. Encourage talking through: "What if I do this? What will happen?" Focus on the emotion, not the absolute content.
Structure new experiences in stages so that they are not so threatening		Encourage exploring the environment and making collections of rocks or leaves or making a scrapbook
Express interest in a task, without intruding on it and defining it: "Looks like you're having fun with that!" Not: "That looks like a new belt for your Grandpa!"		
It isn't fair to ask the child what he is producing. He doesn't know what he will end up with. Imposing such boundaries discourages experimentation.		
If there is a struggle about trying things out, find ways in which trying is safe at first: have puppets or dolls act out; fantasize with a story character		
When the child asks for an answer to a question, indicate where to look up the information, but let the child find the answer		

symptoms associated with it, and each requires different interventions. Many school-age children under psychosocial stress exhibit symptoms related to problems in the affective area. Behavioral symptoms are the result of some unmet emotional need during the process of development. The broad problem area of affective functioning can be further broken down to identify which specific emotional need is a problem: trust, autonomy, initiative, or industry. Tools of assessment that are readily available to the nurse are observation and interviewing.

Once an assessment has been made of the areas that are of concern for the child, a treatment plan can be formulated. The basic theory underlying the therapeutic intervention described in this chapter is the growth and development model. The focus is on learning and growth experiences, not on pathology. There are really two types of intervention. The first is designed to alleviate immediate situational stresses. The task is to supply some information through puppets or stories to enhance cognitive understanding of a situation. A more complicated intervention involves developmental needs. Here the aim is to develop and encourage latent abilities in the child to promote healthier, more productive living outside of the nursing situation. The task of this type of intervention is to supply experiences needed to complete some unfinished developmental learning. A crucial consideration for both types of intervention is to determine at what level the child is functioning. Providing experiences that the child is not developmentally ready for, regardless of chronologic age, will be frustrating for the child as well as the nurse.

This chapter has made no attempt to cover the full range of approaches and methods available in working with children. Instead, the purpose has been to map out a problem-solving process that can be used by any nurse with any child in any situation. Helping a child with emotional problems is within the capabilities of nursing students and graduate nurses if specific problem areas can be identified.

Nurses in health and hospital centers, schools, and any setting serving children and families constitute a valuable and virtually untapped resource in the field of child mental health. Nurses are uniquely suited for primary and secondary prevention with disturbed children and families because of the wide variety of possiblities for nurse–child contact in hospitals, in schools, and in the community. It is hoped that the expanding role of nursing to include emotional support in the role of counselor will open up more opportunities for nurses with varying backgrounds to participate in all phases of child psychosocial nursing. This chapter has been aimed at increasing knowledge of emotional development and providing a framework for assessment and intervention with children under psychosocial stress to aid in the process of expanding nursing roles.

References

Burns B: The use of play techniques in the treatment of children. Child Welfare 49:37–41, January 1970.

Carbonera N T: Techniques for Observing Normal Child Behavior. Pittsburgh, Univ Pittsburgh Press, 1961, pp 21–25

Elkind D: Children and Adolescents: Interpretive Essays on Jean Paiget. London, Oxford Univ Press, 1970, pp 7–25, 50–71

Erikson E H: Conference on the problems of infancy and childhood: Growth and crises. In Senn M J E (ed): Symposium on the Healthy Personality. New York, Josiah Macy Jr Foundation, 1950, pp 17–91

——— Childhood and Society. New York, Norton, 1963, pp 209–222, 247–255

Fagin C M: Nursing in Child Psychiatry. St Louis, Mosby, 1972, pp 1–12, 28–45

Ginsburg H, Opper S: Piaget's Theory of Intellectual Development: An Introduction. Englewood Cliffs, Prentice-Hall, 1969, pp 270–285

Goodman J D, Sours J: The Child Mental Status Exam. New York, Basic Books, 1967

Kessler J W: Psychopathology of Childhood. Englewood Cliffs, Prentice-Hall, 1966, pp 68–83

Lukianowicz, N: Attempted suicide in children. Acta Psychiatr Scand 44:415–435, 1968

Maier H: Three Theories of Child Development. New York, Harper & Row, 1969, pp 13–79

Peplau H E: Counseling in nursing practice. In Harms E, Schreiber P (eds): Handbook of Counseling Techniques. New York, Macmillan, 1963

Raths L, Harmin M, Simon S B: Values and Teaching. Columbus, Ohio, Charles E Merrill, 1966

Wolff S: Children Under Stress. Harmondsworth, England, Penguin, 1973, pp 17–64

Bibliography

UNDERSTANDING CHILDREN

Aries P, Blishen E, Hostler P, Jacobson D, Laski M, MacInnes C, et al.: The World of Children. New York, Hamlin Publishing Group, 1966

Chapman A H: Games Children Play. New York, Berkley Medallion Books, 1971

Child Study Association of America (ed): Insights: A Selection of Creative Literature about Children. New York, Jason Aronson, 1973

Dileo J: Children's Drawings as Diagnostic Aids. New York, Brunner/Mazel, 1973

______ Young Children and Their Drawings. New York, Brunner/Mazel, 1969

Lewis R: Miracles: Poems by Children. New York, Simon & Schuster, 1966

______ Journeys: Prose by Children. New York, Simon & Schuster, 1969

DEALING WITH DEATH

Buck P: The Big Wave. New York, Scholastic Book Services, 1947

A little boy comes to grips with losing his family in a tidal wave in Japan. 8–14 years

Coburn J B: Annie and the Sand Dobies. New York, Seabury Press, 1964

An 8-year-old boy narrates his struggles to understand the death of his dog and baby sister. 8–14 years

Fassler J: My Grandpa Died Today. New York, Behavior Publications, 1971
A child comes to see the death of his grandfather in a new light. 6–9 years
Haig-Brown R: Return to the River. New York, Crown, 1946
A rather long but sensitively written book on the life of a Chinook salmon; shows death as a natural process and part of the life cycle. 9–14 years
Miles M: Annie and the Old One. Boston, Little, Brown, 1971
A little Navajo girl does everything in her power to stop her grandmother's death, until her grandmother explains that death is natural and time can't be held back. 4–8 years
St Exupery A: The Little Prince. New York, Harcourt, Brace, World, 1943
A lovely classic about what we have of others in our memories even after they are gone. 9–adult
Sawyer R: The Year of Jubillo. New York, Dell, 1940
A story of a girl who loses her father and learns to deal with her pain and loneliness. 9–12 years
Stein S: About Dying. New York, Walker, 1974
A well-done book for young children, beautifully illustrated with photographs; a good book for education and preparation. 4–8 years
Steinbeck J: The Red Pony. New York, Doubleday, 1966
Originally published in 1937, this is a classic about the death of a pony who is a boy's best friend and what the boy learns about life. 9–14 years
Viorst J: The Tenth Good Thing about Barney. New York, Atheneum ,1973
A sensitive story of a cat who dies and how a little boy comes to understand death as part of a natural cycle for all living things. 6–9 years
White E B: Charlotte's Web. New York, Dell, 1972
A classic about the death of a spider; all her friends learn special things about grief and memories. 5–10 years

DEALING WITH SIBLING RIVALRY

Arnstein H: Billy and Our New Baby. New York, Behavioral Publications, 1973
A lovely book about how Billy learns that there are special things about being a big boy and that there is enough love to go around for him and a new baby. 6–8 years

DEALING WITH DIVORCE

Gardner R: The Boys and Girls Book about Divorce. New York, Prentice-Hall, 1971
An informed and honest book that deals directly with feelings children have and what they can do about them. 6–14 years
Zolotow C: A Father Like That. New York, Harper & Row, 1971
A little boy who has never known his father fantasizes about the kind he would like and makes a decision about the kind of father he will be. 6–9 years

DEALING WITH SEXUAL ADJUSTMENT

de Schweinitz K: Growing Up. New York, Macmillan, 1963
A nice book for younger children, with many photographs of animals and their babies, as well as people. 6–8 years
Pomeroy W: Boys and Sex. New York, Dell, 1968
______ Girls and Sex. New York, Dell, 1969
Well-written and well-illustrated books on puberty, sexual urges, physical development, and feelings. 10–14 years

Widerberg S: The Kids Own XYZ of Love and Sex. New York, Stein and Day, 1971

Nicely done story of a little girl talking to her mother and father; simple and adequate explanations for all the questions of children. 6–9 years

DEALING WITH COGNITIVE HANDICAPS

Fassler J: One Little Girl. New York, Behavioral Publications, 1968

Well-done story about a retarded child and her frustrations in making friends. 6–8 years

Gardner R: The Family Book about Minimal Brain Dysfunction. New York, Jason Aronson, 1973

This book is in two parts: one has explanations for parents, and one is to be read to children to explain reasons and feelings. 6–12 years

Gold P: Please Don't Say Hello. New York, Behavioral Publications, 1975

Story of an autistic boy. This would be a good book to be read to siblings. 6–8 years

Klein, G: The Blue Rose. New York, Lawrence Hill, 1975

Lovely book about a retarded girl and feelings and how Jennie is special in her own way; illustrated with photographs. 6–8 years

COPING SKILLS AND PROBLEM-SOLVING

Berger T: I Have Feelings. New York, Behavioral Publications, 1972

Illustrated with photographs of children in different feeling states. A good way to teach a child about feelings and open a discussion. 6–9 years

DeMille R: Put Your Mother on the Ceiling. New York, Viking, 1955

A book of children's imaginative games. A very useful tool for developing listening skills, for use as a stimulus to imagination, and for dealing with the concerns of the child. 6–12 years

Fassler J: The Boy with a Problem. New York, Behavioral Publications, 1971

A good book to use in initiating talk about children's concerns. A story about a little boy who can't eat or sleep because of anxiety and how it helps him to talk. 6–8 years

Freed A: T.A. for Tots. Sacremento, Jalmar Press, 1973

A nicely illustrated book to aid in teaching about relationships and ways of relating to get needs met. 6–8 years

Garcia E, Pellegrini N: Homer the Homely Hound Dog. New York, Institute for Rational Living, 1974

Homer felt sorry for himself because others didn't like him until he found out what he could do to make friends. 6–8 years

Gardner R: Fairy Tales for Today's Children. Englewood Cliffs, Prentice-Hall, 1974

An alternative to some of the traditional fairy tales. The new versions make use of psychologically sound problem-solving: the ugly duckling does not become a swan, but learns to deal with loneliness and make friends. 6–12 years

Gardner F: Stories about the Real World. Englewood Cliffs, Prentice-Hall, 1972

A book that presents real-life school, family, and peer problems with real-life solutions that inspire discussion and action. 6–12 years

Sobel K: Stories from Inside/Out. New York, Bantam Books, 1974

A number of short stories on real-life situations for children, such as cheating, taking dares, and running away. The stories are open-ended, so that the reader can end them. 6–10 years

Stein S: A Hospital Story. New York, Walker, 1974
Illustrated with photographs of a hospital, this is a good book for exploring fears and concerns. 6–8 years

Williams M: The Velveteen Rabbit. New York, Doubleday, no year given.
A lovely story about being real, and how much feelings hurt sometimes. 6–8 years

Wittels H, Greisman J: Things I Hate. New York, Behavioral Publications, 1973
Nicely done book about a little boy and all the things he hates, but still has to do. A good book for ventilation of feelings. 6–8 years

CHAPTER

15

SOCIAL NETWORKS

P. M. MacElveen

An individual manages his concerns involving health and illness within the context of his life style, and this means dealing with other people. These others may include family members, neighbors, friends, employers, fellow workers, teachers, and classmates. Additional people may be ordered in groups, clubs, or organizations of which the individual is a member. These people, with their connections to the individual and to each other, constitute the individual's social network.

Being connected with or linked to others is an important aspect of the human experience that is particularly important for achieving and maintaining a high level of individual function and life satisfaction. The individual's self-image, his sense of belonging, the meaningfulness of his existence, and his sources of love, approval, reward, and support are most frequently derived through primary group interactions with others (Cooley 1955). Throughout history one of man's most severe punishments has been to isolate a person from his social network: physically by imprisonment, solitary confinement, or exile; socially by ostracism.

The sharing of attitudes, values, and norms with others generates cohesion among people. This traditional sense of connectedness and belonging is the antithesis of the alienation so common among today's young people. Bronfenbrenner (1974) associated alienation with the increasing social disorganization in American society that is reflected in our high rates of violent crimes, infant mortality, runaway mothers, and divorce, as well as in the new form of custody fight: who gets stuck with the children. The young person, not being well integrated into society, feels "uninterested, disconnected, and perhaps even hostile to the people and activities in his environment" (Bronfenbrenner 1974, p 53). Alienation is also reflected in our rising rates of youthful runaways, school dropouts, and destructive acts against the self and others. It is not surprising that some young people are seeking alternative ways of establishing a connectedness in communal living arrangements and commitments to fundamentalist religious groups.

In preindustrial societies people frequently lived out their lives in one place, maintaining a fairly stable social network. The important primary group relationships, defined as being face to face, affective rather than instrumental, and permanent, were available to most people (Cooley 1955). Simmel (1957) was one of the first to question whether primary group relationships could endure in the modern industrial society characterized by mobility. Propinquity, or the nearness of people to each other, is one determinant of the possibilities of interaction and the establishment and maintenance of relationships.

Frequent change of residence is disruptive to networks, and it changes people's relationships. The urban industrial demands for occupational mobility and the opportunities for social mobility strain kinship and nonkinship bonds by increasing the geographic and social distance between the individual and those in his social network. Workers move to where their labor is needed. Education and expanding job opportunities allow children access to occupations other than those of their fathers; these new occupations are often associated with different life styles and social classes. Thus the farmer's child can become a lawyer or a dentist and live in the affluent section of a large city.

Litwak and Szelenyi (1969) pointed out that primary groups are not being replaced by industrial bureaucratic organizations; rather, primary groups are enduring, but with some modifications. In today's society telephones are considered to be household necessities, and new forms of transportation make travel so easy that geographic distance is no longer a significant barrier; both of these developments contribute to integration and cohesion of networks. Societal norms support upward mobility, change, and incorporation of newcomers in work and neighborhood environments. Thus it has become easier to leave nonkinship networks in one place and enter new networks in another place. Kinship networks have increasing potential for surviving over great distances with the help of modern communication and transportation systems.

It is important to note that a social network does not exist as a concrete reality. Social network is an abstraction or symbol used to organize our thinking about a set of relationships among an individual and others with whom he interacts. The social network is not a social whole, and it is not enclosed by a common boundary (Bott 1957, p 276).

This chapter will be limited to a consideration of the supportive nature of the social network. Many daily needs are met within the context of the network, and in times of illness or other trouble special resources may be mobilized from relatives, friends, and neighbors. The social network will be examined in order to assess productive and counterproductive aspects of a person's social environment and to determine nursing actions to assist the person toward optimal function and life satisfaction.

NETWORK STRUCTURE

Kinship and Nonkinship Networks

The kinship network includes the nuclear family and the extended family, or those who are related biologically and legally. The nonkinship, or friendship, network includes neighbors (people living near each other who have frequent face-to-face contact) and friends (persons freely chosen for affectional reasons, common interests, and shared value systems). Often friends are similar in age, sex, and stage in the family life cycle. Kinship and friendship networks are not mutually exclusive; a friend may also be a relative who lives next door.

Other persons may be included in the social network who are not in a primary group relationship. These are persons with whom there is face-to-face contact and with whom special interests and activities are shared. Such persons might be members of clubs, organizations, teams, community task forces, or other groups. Lopata (1973) called these people associates, implying a connection of a secondary rather than primary order. The focus of their interaction is on the shared interest or activity. In these relationships there are not likely to be the strong affectional bonds, sense of obligation, or exchanges of goods, services, and emotional resources that are common among relatives, friends, and neighbors.

Connections may also be made with people in agencies designed to deliver special services associated with legal, health, financial, housing, or other needs. Sources of help preferred by many individuals and families in times of stress are primary groups (relatives, neighbors, and friends) rather than professionals, agencies, or institutions. Often the latter are never used, even when their services would be quite appropriate. Assistance from known persons seems more acceptable than asking for help from strangers (Croog and associates 1972, Sussman 1953).

Size

Whether a network has many or few members is influenced by several other considerations. The kinds of relationships available, the strength of the ties, and the geographic nearness of members are important determinants of the value of the network in satisfying the individual's needs. Very small networks have limitations; resources may become exhausted if demands are prolonged or extensive. However, that a network has many members is no guarantee that resources will be available or forthcoming.

Connectedness

Connectedness relates to the numbers of people in a network knowing each other. A network where almost everyone knows everyone else is highly connected. Bott (1957) termed this a close-knit network. A network where few members know each other is described as a loose-knit network. Kinship networks are likely to be close-knit, as most relatives usually know one another. If friends are drawn from a variety of places, such as from work, school, and leisure activities, many of them may not know each other.

Social networks of primary group relationships can be illustrated by considering an individual (or family) surrounded by a circle of points, each of which represents a person in the individual's kinship, friendship, or neighborhood groups. A line drawn between the individual and one of the points indicates a link or connection between them. Lines between points in the network indicate which persons are linked to each other either by kinship or by social relationship. In Fig. 15.1, an individual designated X is connected to eight other persons, few of whom are connected to each other, except indirectly through X. In Fig. 15.2, individual Y has eight people in his network who are directly connected to each other as well as indirectly connected through Y.

The network in Fig. 15.1 is more loose-knit than the network in Fig. 15.2, which is more close-knit. Bott (1957) found that the greater the degree of connectedness in any couple's social network the greater the degree to which domestic tasks were defined as male or female responsibilities. She also found that in the close-knit networks people kept in touch with one another, gave help when needed, shared norms and values, and exerted pressure on the couple to conform to the norms. Persons in the network also provided the husband and wife with numerous sources of emotional satisfaction, thus lessening the emotional demands between them. Couples with loose-knit networks had less access to external help, support, or sources or emotional satisfaction. They were also less subject to social control or pressure to conform to a set of norms. These couples depended more on each other and tended to share more family tasks, with less concern about sex-role stereotypes.

NETWORK PROCESSES

Basic elements of network processes are entrance and exit, construction, maintenance, and repair. While this list is not exhaustive, these particular processes are important in the nurse's work with clients and families.

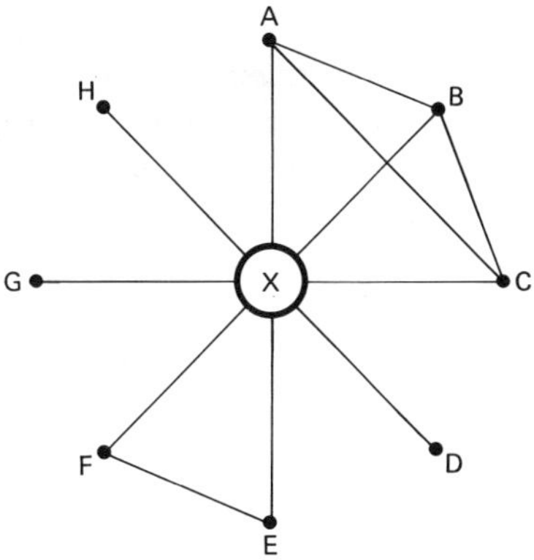

FIG. 15.1. X's network, loose-knit.

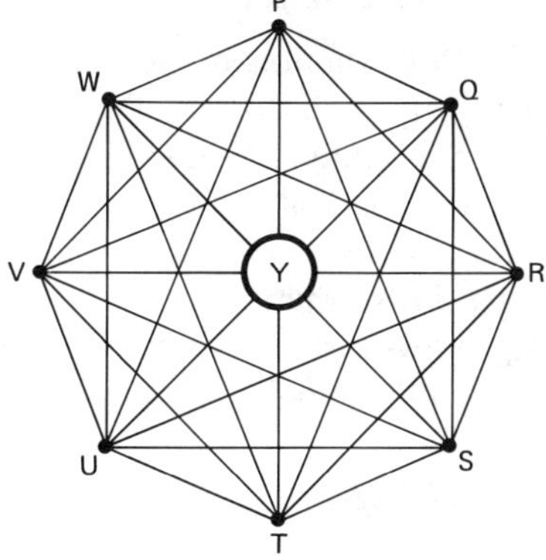

FIG. 15.2. Y's network, close-knit.

Entrance and Exit

Entrance into kinship networks occurs by birth, adoption, and marriage. Kinship bonds are relatively permanent (eg, parent–child or sibling ties); however, marriage bonds can be dissolved by divorce. Outside the kinship network, entrance and acceptance into groups where a person may be present on a regular basis is determined by group norms as well as by the person's network skills. Such groups may be composed of people at work, in the neighborhood, at school, at church, or in other local groups. Entrance into such groups is often facilitated by orientation programs and welcoming committees, by norms that favor accepting newcomers, and by norms that long-term residents are friendly to newcomers. The communications media and compulsory education have contributed to a common language and a shared culture that also facilitate the rapid incorporation of newcomers. Entrance into such groups provides opportunities for making friends and adding to the friendship network.

Exiting from networks is facilitated by the same processes that assist one's entrance into networks; like entrance movement, exit movement is often expected and orderly. Leaving for marriage, school, advancement, or better job opportunities is accepted behavior. Terminating relationships in a satisfying manner is very important and requires skill. Losses of relationships and support systems frequently make individuals and families vulnerable until such time as they become familiar with new surroundings and begin to establish a new network. A move to a new city can be especially difficult for women who stay home caring for the home and young children. They may have less opportunity and less energy to invest in making new friends than their husbands, who may meet many people in their work away from home.

Construction

Construction of new networks requires an investment of time and energy, as well as taking certain risks, especially if one is alone in the task. Searching for individuals and groups who share goals, interests, or values is difficult in a strange community. For example, people who are unsure of their self-value and their skills in communicating and getting along with others in the past are often handicapped in building friendship networks. These people may need help in mobilizing the necessary social skills and finding opportunities to meet others.

Maintenance

Maintenance of the kinship network is enhanced by face-to-face contact, reciprocity and sharing of family occasions, and other activities. Because of its structural basis, the kinship network is more resistent to neglect and abuse than the friendship network, which is based on mutual affection. A major responsibility for maintaining the kinship bonds is usually part of the female role in the family. Women most frequently take care of correspondence, initiate phone calls, and set up visiting patterns (Reiss 1962, Mirande 1969). They collect and disseminate news from other relatives and keep people up to date on family events occurring in the network. Where distance intervenes, communication is important; it lends substance to the structural bonds of the kinship network.

Maintenance of friendships requires that the relationship remain mutually rewarding. Since these relationships are based mainly on affection, a decrease in affection easily leads to dissolution of the link. Frequency of face-to-face contact is likely to intensify the bond (Homans 1950). Maintenance of long-distance friendships is difficult without communication of a nature that is satisfying to both persons. An important factor in the continuation of relationships is the content of the contacts, eg, social interaction, shared recreation, participation in family celebrations and rituals, and exhanges of goods, services, and emotional support.

Repair

Bonds between the individual and members of the network may be damaged by behavior that threatens the safety of the individual or the network members, by withdrawal (which may be interpreted as rejection of the other persons), or by unusual behavior (which is unacceptable). People usually will have been having problems in their interactions with family members, friends, neighbors, employers, and fellow workers for long periods before seeking help or before hospitalization is necessary. Repair of these relationships requires the reopening of communication and reestablishment of the bonds. Failure to repair the network may be counterproductive, as sources of support and help may be lost to the individual at a time of vulnerability and heightened need for network support. If help from the network remains unavailable, other alternatives must be sought.

Network bonds may also be jeopardized by absences from the network. Situations where young adults are establishing their own lives away from home or where people move to other cities because of new jobs or promotions do not constitute network absences. Network absences are those periods of time when the individual is physically separated from the network and, although communication may be maintained by letters or telephone calls, face-to-face interactions are limited. These are absences such as imprisonment, lengthy hospitalizations, military service away from the family, being at sea half the year in the case of fishermen and merchant seamen, and other extended travel periods required by one's occupation. These departures and returns are events that can be stressful, especially for family members. Where absences are predictably intermittent, as with some occupations, mutually satisfying patterns of communication and interaction need to be established. These patterns may be different from what they would be under other conditions.

A major change in one relationship, such as occurs in divorce, results in adjustment of other relationships, for example, those with the former in-laws and mutual friends. Some relationships may be lost; others may need redefinition.

NETWORK FUNCTIONS

Within the network different relationships can exist and a variety of needs can be met. Relationships are the source of many satisfactions. It is unlikely that any one relationship can provide all the satisfactions and meet all needs. Weiss (1969, pp 38–40) proposed that certain relationships meet specific needs that are essential to well-being. He defined five categories of relational functions:

Intimacy. Intimacy provides for effective emotional integration: a safe, warm closeness where one can be expressive. Intimacy ameliorates loneliness and is usually found in close relationships with a spouse, friend, sibling, or parent. Sexual involvement is often, but not always, associated with emotional intimacy.

Social Integration. Social integration is provided by persons sharing similar situations or working toward similar goals. Interaction frequently involves the give and take of experiences, information, ideas, and favors. Lack of social integration produces a sense of social isolation and may be associated with feelings of boredom. This function is usually found in relationships with friends and colleagues.

Nurturing Behavior. Opportunity for nurturing behavior is provided by relationships where the person cares for and is responsible for a child. Frustration of this function can result in a sense that one's life is unfulfilled and empty of purpose.

Reassurance. Reassurance of worth is provided when one's competent behavior in a role is recognized and validated. The competence may be in occupational or family roles and may be attested to by colleagues, family members, and friends. Absence of this recognition results in reduced self-esteem.

Assistance. Assistance is provided through help and resources from family, friends, and neighbors. Only close relatives can be expected to provide extensive or long-term help. Absence of any relationship to provide assistance results in a sense of anxiety and vulnerability.

Weiss found that for some people a relationship providing guidance was important. This kind of support was found in relationships with mental health professionals, clergy, and others.

NETWORK STYLES

The dominant pattern of behavior with members of the social network may be referred to as the person's network style. Four network styles were identified in two studies of home dialysis patients (MacElveen 1971, MacElveen and Smith-DiJulio 1976) that are described briefly below: kinship, friendship, associate, and restricted styles. Criteria for determining network style were the following:

1. Contact: the frequency of face-to-face visiting
2. Reciprocity: how often goods, services, and emotional support were exchanged
3. Holidays: the sharing of significant family occasions, events, and vacations

No patients were found who had pure styles that excluded all other interactions.

Kinship Network Style

Persons and families with kinship network styles spend much time with relatives engaging in many kinds of interactions and activities. The frequency of contact is high; there is considerable exchange of goods, services, support, and information and help in solving problems and making decisions. Sussman and Burchinal (1962) and Sharp and Axelrod (1956) found that in kinship networks large amounts of help and support flow from parents to young married couples; later, in another phase of the family life cycle, help and support flow from middle-aged couples to aging parents. These patterns of assistance occur across social classes and do not seem to be influenced by education or financial status. Important family occasions, celebrations, and vacations are shared with relatives.

Friendship Network Style

The friendship style is very similar to the kinship network style, except that friends and neighbors rather than relatives are the important members of the network. The frequency of contact is high, as is reciprocity and sharing of important occasions, celebrations, and vacations. The friendship network is used by some people as a substitute for a kinship network when relatives live far away. However, other people maintain strong friendship networks though relatives are readily available; for them, kinship connections simply are not preferred.

Associate Network Style

Another style of network behavior, which we term associate, is characterized by fairly large numbers of people. Contact may be regular, but it is not necessarily of high frequency; a very important factor is that reciprocity is limited. The associates in the network are often members of recreational, social, or occupational groups. These relationships survive as long as the mutual interest brings the persons together. Associates are usually not included in important family occasions, celebrations, or vacations. While associates may be resources for approval and rewards related to the mutual interest, these relationships are not likely to involve sharing of problems or troubles, and therefore mutual assistance patterns are not likely to develop. The network with large numbers of people is not necessarily a valuable resource for help.

Restricted Network Style

Some people have networks that are restricted in size, reciprocity, and sharing. At the extreme in this group would be the hermit who seeks to live independently and alone, not seeming to need or value interaction with others. Society is hardly overrun with hermits. However, we do observe many isolated persons who are strongly bonded with no one or bonded only tenuously with a few people, who themselves are often isolated. Visiting is infrequent; these are often lonely people who are vulnerable in times of trouble because they lack resources for help and support. Some persons and some nuclear families value their independence, believing that they are responsible for solving their own problems or that they do not have the right to ask for help from others. These people may give little help or support to others. They tend to restrict sharing of important family occasions and vacations to the nuclear family. While this style functions well for many people, prolonged or multiple crises may quickly exhaust their limited personal resources.

NETWORKS AS RESOURCES FOR SUPPORT

Caplan (1974) defined the social support system as a group of people who provide feedback to the individual about himself, who validate his expectations about behaviors from others, and who help in communicating more effectively with the external world. The support system may be utilized frequently in the course of daily life, but it is particularly significant in times of illness and trouble. At these times three basic elements are necessary in the support system: (1) significant others who assist the individual to use personal strengths to cope successfully with emotional problems; (2) people to assist with daily living tasks that cannot be accomplished alone, and (3) persons who have access to specific kinds of resources the individual needs, such as financial help, information, and material goods to ease the difficulties being experienced (Caplan 1974, pp 4–7).

Individuals and families are subject to times of difficulties and problems when external help is useful and sometimes necessary for survival. Acute illnesses, accidents, and deaths are major events likely to evoke helpful responses in most networks. Other crises result from job loss, trouble with the police, financial problems, failure to achieve expected occupational or educational goals, unwanted pregnancies, divorce, or other disruptions of the family system.

Help comes from the kinship network not only in times of stress but also at holidays, birthdays, anniversaries, and family life cycle events such as weddings, births, graduations, and deaths. These occasions may be used to disguise material support in the form of gifts, loans, transfer of property, or other material aids.

The findings of Litwak and Szelenyi (1969), from a study of primary group structures and their functions, suggested that neighbors are called on for help with urgent, short-term problems that need immediate response, especially in the form of services such as lending a tool, babysitting, or providing a ride to the hospital emergency room. Relatives give more substantial help with larger or long-term problems, providing assistance similar to that provided by neighbors if the relatives are nearby. If they are at a distance, relatives may still provide material goods, emotional support, and financial aid. Friends help with middle-range problems and are consistently seen as helpful and emotionally supportive in a wide range of situations.

Croog and associates (1972) investigated the sources of help received by males experiencing first myocardial infarctions. These cardiac patients utilized help from numerous sources: relatives, friends, and neighbors. Services from nonrelatives were seen to be equal to those received from relatives, if not better. Except for physician and hospital services, minimal contact was made with professionals or agencies, although many problems might have been appropriate for those resources. Instead, needs were met by the primary groups. Patients identifying help from any one primary group source also reported helpfulness from other primary group sources. In addition, there was a significant correlation between patterns of frequent visiting before illness and patterns of help and assistance during illness. The investigators suggested that the underlying phenomenon may be the level of social integration. Well-integrated persons have favorable relationships that are characterized by "solidarity, including mutual visiting and emotional and material support" (Croog and associates 1972, p 39).

An important aspect of social networks is that in the linking of the individual with the others in the network, role relationships are observed. Being born into a family establishes the first set of connections and, concomitantly, the first set of roles: eg, daughter/sister/granddaughter or son/brother/grandson. Later other roles may be added: friend, student, employee, spouse. Each role requires interaction with persons in reciprocal roles: daughter–parent, sister–sibling, granddaughter–grandparent, friend–friend, student–teacher, employee–employer, wife–husband. In addition, other persons may be in the same roles and sharing similar experiences, such as other students or employees. The set of roles in large measure structures where and when a person will be and what activity is likely to be occurring. Individuals who have very limited networks, either because they do not have many roles or because they are not connected with many people, may have little structure to their lives, and they often have difficulty getting through the long days. Patients discharged from mental hospitals who do not have a family and who are unemployed may live alone, having little or no significant interaction with anyone. It is difficult for them to see any sense or meaning in their lives if they have no place to go and no one waiting for them. The elderly widow whose life once revolved around her husband may also suffer from role deprivation. More numerous roles provide increased opportunities for seeing the self as worthwhile; there is more feedback from role reciprocals who validate role performance as competent.

Special kinds of information, experience, support, or other resources are sometimes not available in the network for particular kinds of problems, and this can cause considerable discomfort to the persons involved. In this respect, the emergence of self-help groups is a notable phenomenon. These groups usually arise when society has failed to provide a structured means to deal with a specific problem or need. When a number of people with the same difficulty come to know each other and find that there are no means available to meet their needs, they may form a special group. Help is often obtained by sharing experiences, and sometimes professional and community resources are mobilized for the group's own purposes. Self-help groups have developed in response to problems with particular diseases and treatments, drug abuse, obesity, widowhood, single-parenthood, child abuse, and even dying. These groups meet regularly, providing acceptance, understanding, education, and mutual assistance. They link the individual to responsive others at a time when his social network is an inadequate resource for special needs and help is not available through profesional, institutional, or agency sources.

A promising application of social network theory has been developed by Speck and Attneave (1971): use of social network intervention as a therapeutic modality that is preferred in specific cases to individual, family, and group therapy. The social network members are assembled; for an average middle-class family the group may include 40 persons who meet in the client's home with the network team for a series of usually six to eight meetings. These tribal-type meetings mobilize the energies of a large number of participants; they provide opportunities for the healing of torn bonds. The shared problem-solving and the experience of unity in this cooperative endeavor are described by the authors as being an "antidote to the aura of depersonalized loneliness characteristic of post industrial society" (Speck and Attneave 1971, p 331).

Network intervention is based on faith in human beings and on the rewards of watching them mobilize their potential to deal with their problems. This is an alternative approach to the therapist's use of knowledge (or magic) and self to help the client. The primary goal in network intervention is to enable people to cope with their problems and to share their coping abilities. In these large groups of 40 or more people who care enough to commit themselves to a series of meetings, a network effect occurs. In the process of trying to solve the original problem, the intense interactions, exchanges, and collaborations ramify throughout the entire group. Over a period of weeks the effects of the process are reflected in changes in such areas as relationships, personal goals, and attitudes. Network intervention is an unusual way of helping, and it requires a special team; its effectiveness has not been evaluated.

NURSING ASSESSMENT

As the nurse assists the client to formulate goals in response to an identified problem, it may become clear that solutions or strategies may be limited if they depend entirely on the client's own physical and psychologic strengths and resources. Exploration of alternative approaches to the client's goals would include an assessment of resources available through the client's relationships with other people. The nurse would want to know the following facts:

1. Nature of the available network regarding:
   a. Kinship and nonkinship members
   b. Members nearby and at a distance
   c. Connectedness (loose- or close-knit)
2. The client's dominant network style:
   a. Kinship
   b. Friendship
   c. Associate
   d. Restricted
3. The client's relationships that fulfill the following needs:
   a. Intimacy
   b. Social integration
   c. Opportunities for nurturing behavior
   d. Reassurance of worth
   e. Assistance
4. The network potential to assist with current client goals:
   a. Strengths, resources, supports
   b. Client's history of use of the network in previous times of trouble

Assessment of resources is made within the context of specific needs related to the client's current situation and goals. These needs may involve goods, services, emotional support, or relationships. Helpful responses to the needs may be one-time events (such as assistance finding a job) or short-term responses (such as transportation to physiotherapy sessions following surgery). Help continuing for extended periods of time may be necessary for the family and child with physical or mental developmental disabilities. Intensive help may be needed by the family with a terminally ill member prior to the person's death and during the grieving period that follows.

Assessing how the client meets general needs for achieving maximum function and life satisfaction is closely related to network style: some people depend mainly on themselves, others are interdependent with relatives and nonrelatives. Network behaviors may also be influenced by the client's developmental stage and the particular tasks involved. During adolescence, for example, the young person struggling with independence and dependence is likely to be spending larger amounts of time and energy with peers (in the friendship network) than with family (in the kinship network). The adolescent may seek support from peers for such things as acceptance, borrowing money, and solving problems, rather than asking for such help from parents.

Let us look briefly at two people who are 20 years old and who have high school educations and similar socioeconomic backgrounds. Their social networks, however, are quite different.

CLINICAL EXAMPLE I

Ann has been moving around working at ski resorts for the past 2 years and has been in this city for only a few months. Her family lives in another state, and she has not seen them or talked to them for about 6 months. She writes occasionally and tries to remember to send cards on holidays and birthdays. Her friends from high school are now far away, working and going to school. Ann has a small apartment and is collecting unemployment. The neighbors she knows both work, but they are often around evenings and weekends. She had been working as a cook's helper, but was laid off recently. She also has clerical skills, but she has been unable to find a job.

CLINICAL EXAMPLE II

Eve and her new husband Tom live in the city where she was raised. Her husband's family moved there 3 years ago. Eve works as a checker at a local supermarket; Tom works for an insurance company. She sees her church friends when she attends services and maintains contact with several high school friends. The couple sometimes spend social evenings with friends from Tom's office. They also participate on numerous occasions with both families. Tom's parents have a small trailer, which Eve and Tom have been helping to fix up. They plan to borrow it for vacation use later in the summer.

Figures 15.3 and 15.4 illustrate the primary relationships in each network. Interviews with Ann and Eve also revealed some data about the patterns of interactions and exchanges that were occurring and some of the direct connections between persons in the networks. Information about all the connections in their networks was gathered over more than one interview, but it is presented here in total for convenience of discussion.

Suppose Ann and Eve met with similar misfortunes, perhaps a fractured hip sustained in an auto accident. How might their experiences be similar or different during emergency hospitalization for surgery and the postoperative and rehabilitative phases? How might the sudden death of a parent be experienced within the respective networks? How would Ann and Eve cope with an arrest requiring bail and a trial? What might happen after discharge from a brief hospitalization for having made a suicide attempt?

It is easy to recognize in Eve's network the greater potential for many kinds of support available from a number of different sources, all nearby, that might be mobilized to assist her and Tom during any of the above situations.

Ann's family is distant; neighbors are gone workdays, and her high school friends are not nearby or available. One option that Ann might consider in such a situation is returning to her parents' home until she is well enough to take care of herself. Another would be for a family mem-

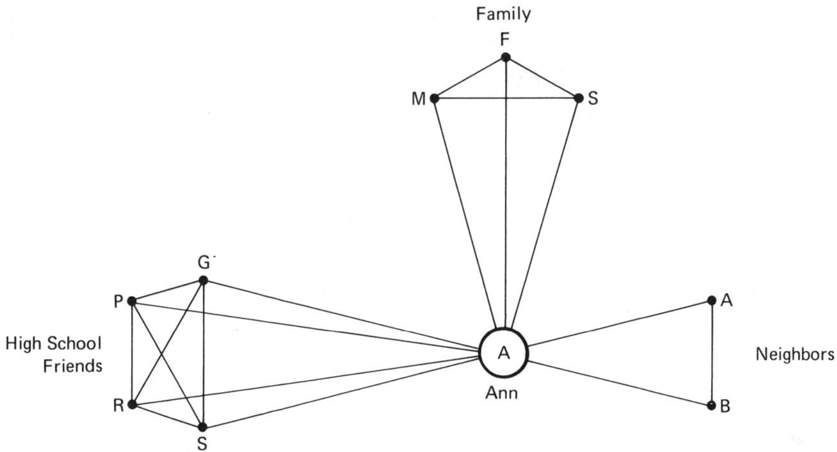

FIG. 15.3. Ann's network.

ber to come to be with her. Financial aid, emotional support, help with problem-solving, and other aids might be forthcoming from her distant network in response to her time of trouble. If family help were unavailable, Ann might seek help through existing local agencies, self-help groups, and outpatient services. The transition period between institutional care and being able to manage life independently can present serious problems for the person with a limited social network and limited financial resources. Attempting to cope entirely alone with any of the troubles described above might be overwhelming for someone in Ann's position.

Together the nurse and the client should identify what needs to be done and how best to do it. The nurse should respect the client's priorities and preferred style of means to meet needs. She should assist the client in planning and implementing the chosen course of action. These nursing activities of helping to identify special needs and the available options and their consequences enable the client to make informed decisions, to have an investment in them, and to maintain some determination over what is happening.

Awareness of developmental tasks is clearly important in using the networks of both of these women. Ann, for example, might be working on establishing her independence from her family and working toward identifying herself as a competent adult. The nurse will want to know how Ann feels about turning to her parents for help. It may or may not be all right with her to be in a dependent position in relation to her parents at a time of special difficulty. She may need to solve her problem independently.

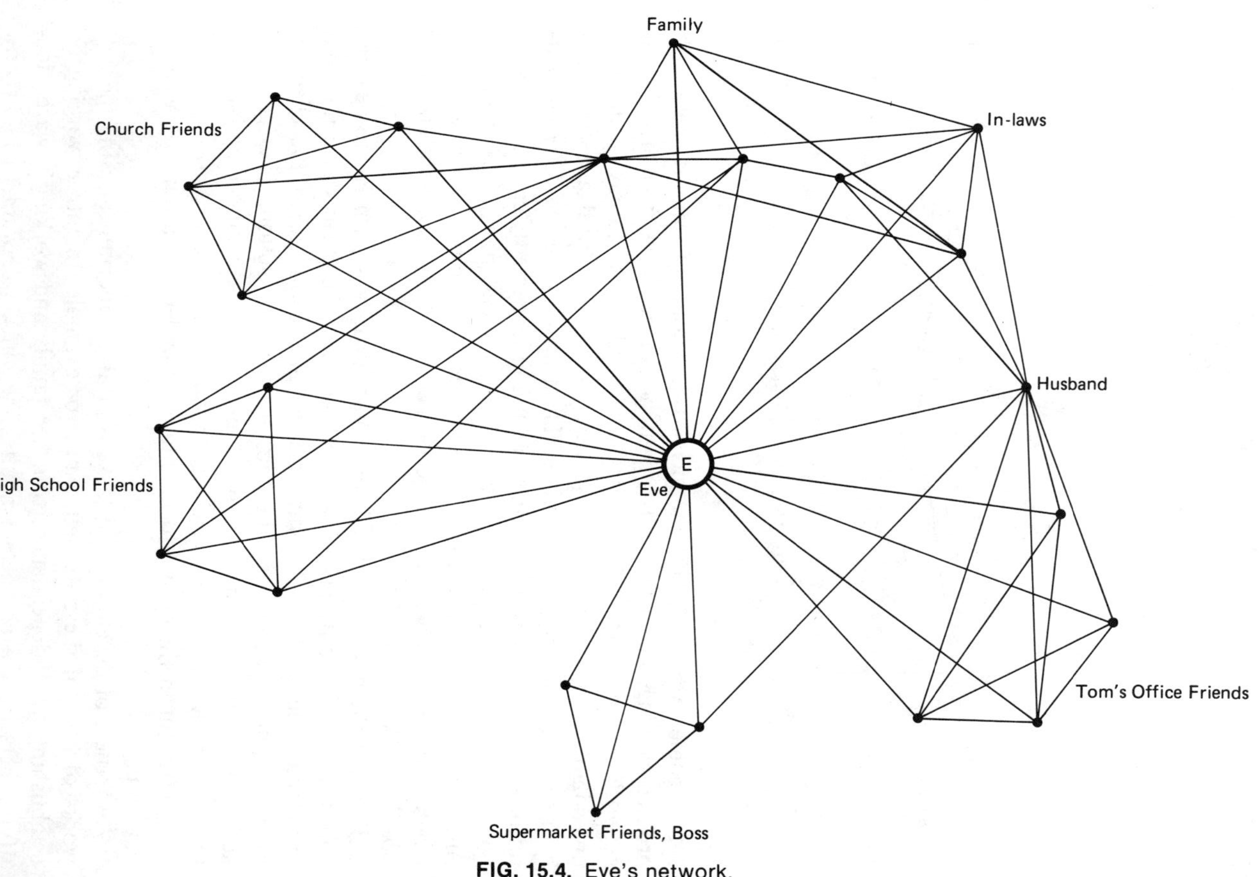

FIG. 15.4. Eve's network.

Eve, also, may still be emancipating herself from parents, and she has a new husband besides. It may be significant to Tom whether she turns to him or to her parents in a time of great need. The young couple who have been married only a short time are likely to be still adjusting to their new life and building their relationship, while each of them is also striving toward adulthood. Can Eve have confidence in Tom and trust his abilities to meet her needs or to help mobilize other resources to meet her needs? How does Tom define the situation, and where is he in his own emancipation from parents? Is he likely to be threatened or overwhelmed by the magnitude of Eve's needs and his perceived ability to meet them? Sensitive assessment in this situation, appreciating the interplay between developmental tasks, network relationships, and the need for help, is a challenge. Long-term and short-term client outcomes could differ considerably depending on the plan of action chosen. Ideally, the nurse could assist Ann and Eve to use this difficult time to grow in awareness of themselves, to recognize their own strengths and weaknesses, to gain satisfactions in their relationships with significant others in their networks, and to enhance their problem-solving skills for future use.

In our society much value is attached to achievement of independence, while dependence is associated with weakness, inferiority, incompetence, and subordination. Dependence, by definition, implies a relationship to another person. Independence means freedom from the influence and control of others, self-sufficiency and self-determination. For some people, independence excludes the right to sometimes feel weak, weary, or lonely, or to want to be taken care of for awhile. Making it through life alone is a difficult task; yet little emphasis is placed on interdependence as a societal value. Interdependence in the network implies mutual accepting and understanding, giving and receiving, helping and being helped, sharing happy times and bad times.

NURSING INTERVENTION

Interventions based on assessment of the client's network are aimed at mobilizing resources to meet special needs during times of illness or other problems and assisting with skills needed for maintaining mutually rewarding relationships within the network. The sense of being connected and belonging, of sharing norms and values with others, contributes to the general well-being of the individual and of society.

Transportation to the clinic, a babysitter, someone to stay with the client for a while, help in finding a job or housing, financial assistance, information and support, or whatever the client or family needs may well be available from members of the network. Being able to tap those resources involves making needs known and being able to accept offered help; the nurse can assist the client with these processes. If assistance cannot be elicited from the social network, the client can be referred to agencies in the community and can be connected in that way to some resources.

The kind of emotional support that may be needed in working through the death of a parent may be available from family, neighbors, or friends. Self-help groups for people dealing with losses are emerging in many communities. For some clients, community mental health services may be appropriate. The nurse, with the client, determines how best to meet the needs.

For the client who is threatening suicide, staying with a friend or neighbor overnight rather than being alone may be more comfortable until other interventions are implemented. Several significant others from the social network can be mobilized around a client who needs frequent supportive contacts initiated by others for a brief period.

The person discharged from an inpatient psychiatric unit may have to negotiate reentrance into the family and other parts of the network if the absence has been lengthy or if the exit was associated with conflict or negative interactions. The client may need some new verbal and nonverbal behaviors to rearrange previous interaction patterns in order to promote more positive relationships. Interaction skills necessary for rewarding relationships can be generated and practiced with the nurse and with other clients. Role-playing, assertiveness training, and small group interaction are ways in which such skills might be acquired. There are many opportunities provided in the nurse–client relationship for trying out new ways of interacting in a safe environment. These behaviors can then be tried with others. It is not likely that the nurse can effect radical change in the network styles of individuals during times of prolonged trouble, especially those who pride themselves on independence and who avoid incurring obligations to others. During periods of crisis, however, clients may be assisted in trying alternative problem-solving behaviors; this can include legitimizing the acceptance of help in times of need and the establishment of a few network links that include reciprocity. Where clients refuse to consider accepting help from their social network, the nurse should support the client in exploring alternative strategies or community agency assistance.

Besides those who are resistant to accepting help, there are other individuals and families who may be at high risk because of network deficiencies. Many elderly people have outlived their relatives and friends, or they may have no people who care about them nearby. They may suffer from relationship deficits and experience loneliness, boredom, isolation, low self-esteem, and vulnerability. Physical mobility and financial problems limit their abilities to move toward others. Single-parent families, where one parent carries the load of both parents, may have little or no means of meeting personal needs for intimacy and respite, and there may be minimal time and energy for network development and maintenance. Connecting older people with such families in a foster grandparent program has made many older people feel wanted and needed; it has assisted the single parent by providing time for more activities, and it has enabled children to receive attention from a caring adult other than the parent. Nuclear families with both parents working may also have little time and energy to invest in network activities. Working women may have little time for the responsibilities of network communication and maintenance. Individuals and families who have problems of extended duration or a series of crises may exhaust the abilities of their networks to respond. The nurse's knowledge of community resources is particularly significant in working with these high-risk groups.

SUMMARY

Networks composed of primary relationships (relatives, friends, and neighbors) are important sources of support essential to well-being. Networks differ in terms of size, membership, connectedness, patterns of contact, sharing of significant occasions, and reciprocity. Knowledge of clients' networks and their styles of interacting in their networks is valuable as the nurse works with clients toward promoting and maintaining maximum opportunity for maintenance of health and efficient problem-solving in times of crisis.

References

Bott E: Family and Social Network. London, Tavistock, 1957

Bronfenbrenner U: The origins of alienation. Sci Am 231:2, 1974

Caplan G: Support Systems and Community Mental Health. New York, Behavioral Publications, 1974

Cooley C H: Primary groups. In Hare P, Borgatta E F, Bales R F (eds): Small Groups. New York, Alfred Knopf, 1955

Croog S H, Lipson A, Levine S: Help patterns in severe illness: The roles of kin network, non-family resources, and institutions. J Marriage Family 34:32–41, February 1972

Homans G C: The Human Group. New York, Harcourt Brace, 1950

Litwak E, Szelenyi I: Primary group structures and their functions: Kin, neighbors, friends. Am Sociol Rev 34:365, 1969

Lopata H Z: Widowhood in an American City. Cambridge, Schenkman, 1973

MacElveen P M: Exploration of the cooperative triad in the investigation of home dialysis patient outcomes. Unpublished doctoral dissertation, University of Colorado, 1971

———, Smith-DiJulio K: Network behaviors in a long term illness situation. Seattle, University of Washington, unpublished paper, 1976

Mirande A M: The isolated nuclear family hypothesis. In Edwards J N (ed): The Family and Change. New York, Alfred Knopf, 1969

Reiss P J: The extended kinship system: Correlates of and attitudes on frequency of interaction. J Marriage Family 24:333–339, November 1962

Simmel G: The metropolis and mental life. In Hatt P K, Reiss A J Jr (eds): Cities and Society: The Revised Reader in Urban Sociology. New York, Free Press of Glenco, 1957

Speck R V, Attneave C L: Social networks intervention. In Haley J (ed): Changing Families. New York, Grune & Stratton, 1971

Sussman, M B: The help patterns for the middle class family. Am Sociol Rev 18: 22–28, 1953

———, Burchinal L: Kin family network: Unheralded structure in current conceptualizations of family functioning. J Marriage Family 24:231–240, August 1962 August 1962

Weiss R S: The fund of sociability. Trans-Action 6:36, July–August 1969

APPENDIX A

GLOSSARY OF PSYCHOSOCIAL TERMS

This review of terms is presented to assist the nurse in becoming familiar with some of the terms that are frequently used in the psychiatric mental health setting but that are not often found in formal glossaries. Many of these terms are used in everyday speech, but they take on special meanings when used in this area of nursing. In addition, many of the terms are used to define or explain one another, and some are used interchangeably.

Although standard psychiatric glossaries and dictionaries were consulted in compiling this list, no specific definitions of these terms could be found. Many verbs that originated with psychoanalysis are now being used outside the analytic framework, and here they take on less specific meanings and are used by mental health professionals of various disciplines to mean various things. The definitions were compiled from the author's understanding of the terms, and in presenting the explanations no source of validation is claimed aside from collegial consensus.

Most texts and learning materials that nurses use define their terms in relation to the symptomatology and psychopathology of patients. Only a few help the nurse clarify the details of what she and the patient do together or how nurses communicate with one another about what they are doing with the patient and how the patient is responding. This is certainly not an exhaustive effort; however, individual instructors and nurses can begin with this outline and then redefine terms as they are used in their own settings and frameworks.

AT ONE LEVEL
AT SOME LEVEL These phrases are used to denote levels of unconscious, preconscious, and conscious processes that influence behavior. For example, a patient may say adamantly that he does not want to participate in any group activities, and

This glossary was developed by Dianne C. Longo.

yet he manages to get to his group on a regular basis. One might say that at some level the group must have meaning for him because he attends.

ACTING ON
TO ACT ON

These terms refer to putting feelings, thoughts, or fantasies into action or behavior. Impulsive people are people who act on their thoughts, feelings, or fantasies immediately, without any (or very little) intervening consideration of the consequences. Frequently people believe that if they think about or fantasize about something, then that's actually what they want and what they should do. This is not necessarily true. One does not have to act on fantasy or feeling if one chooses not to. However, the closer that fantasy and thoughts come to being put into action, the more likely it is that they will eventually be acted on. The more detailed the plan and the more concrete the planning, the more likely it is that thoughts and feelings will be put into behavior. For example, suicidal fantasies (ideation) become more dangerous as the plan becomes more specific and the means that are selected become more dangerous and more readily available. In a positive vein, the same pattern holds true: the more specific the plan and the more readily available the means, the more likely it is that the problem can be solved. Patients with problems but with no plans for solving them have little to act on. Thus one measure of a patient's progress in problem-solving is the amount of energy and interest that is put into the planning phase.

ACTIVE ROLE

Students and nurses often hear the phrase "be more active with the patient." This means that the nurse initiates interaction with the patient and continues in an intiative stance. For example, she consistently seeks the patient out, rather than waiting to see if the patient will approach her; she follows through on discussions; she makes appropriate suggestions, rather than waiting for the patient to bring up a list of ideas; she initiates the topic of conversation, rather than letting the patient structure the conversation. An active role is best demonstrated by crisis intervention: in the context of an ongoing relationship the nurse may call the patient on the telephone without being asked by the patient to do so. The nurse is also responsible for bringing up suicidal or homicidal ideations for discussion, rather than waiting for the patient to spontaneously share this information. Obviously, whether to take an active or a passive role (or a combination of the two) depends on the patient, the situation, and the goals of the relationship.

ANTICIPATORY
GUIDANCE

If people know what to expect, they can be better prepared to deal effectively with a situation. In this sense anticipatory guidance can be used to prepare a patient for a concrete procedure (eg, ECT) or to prepare a patient for a difficult interpersonal encounter. Examples of anticipatory guidance include the following: role-playing with a patient about the possibilities for handling an impending encounter with another person; making a list of things to remember so that the patient will not forget to cover specific details during an anxiety-provoking discussion.

BASELINE Baseline can be used either as an adjective or as a noun. It means the customary pattern of behavior, feelings, and reactions of an individual without interference from extraneous or extenuating circumstances (eg, extreme stress, large doses of medication).

CONCRETE To make something concrete is to make an idea or a concept understandable in a less abstract way. Students usually ask for specific examples of principles, something they can understand in down-to-earth terms, something they can act on, something solid. A concrete answer is whatever will answer these questions: "What do you mean exactly?" "Give me a specific example." "How do I translate this idea into behavior?" This term also refers to cognitive abilities in general. The phrase "he's really concrete" usually means "he cannot abstract or use ideas freely," either because of organic impairment of intelligence (eg, mental retardation) or emotional impairment (eg, schizophrenia).

DEAL WITH See HANDLE.

EXPLORE
EXPLORATION These terms refer to an important aspect of the communication process with a patient. To explore usually means to discuss significant issues in detail. Exploration is usually carried out from a variety of perspectives over a period of time. Frequently the same theme is explored over and over again in the nurse–patient relationship as the level of the relationship changes and the patient's level of self-knowledge increases. Exploration is best approached with the idea that there are no absolute rules about what is true or untrue, good or bad, changeable or unchangeable. The discussion is one in which many possibilities may arise. The nurse should approach the patient without prejudging the patient's response, and she should not hold the patient to a commitment because of what was said during the exploratory phase in problem-solving. Exploration is simply an attempt to investigate uncharted territory.

HANDLE This term is used interchangeably with the term deal with, or sometimes the term integrate. Essentially what transpires when one handles something (eg, a confrontative response) is that feedback is accepted and considered by the patient without the patient becoming extremely anxious or panic-stricken or resorting to seriously dysfunctional patterns in order to maintain equilibrium. If the patient automatically denies what is said, if he forgets, represses, or cannot integrate a response, fact, or event into his conscious experience of the world at the time, it is said that he cannot handle the material.

HURTING

People who hurt, who may be described as hurting, are experiencing emotional pain. The term is not used in the colloquial sense meaning lacking.

LOSSES
LOSS

These terms do not refer exclusively to death; they are usually used to refer to loss that occurs through changes in a patient's life style (loss of a role), family (child leaving home), or physical health (new diagnosis of a medical disease). Williams and Holmes (Chapter 4) list the common changes that imply losses. For example, getting married imples loss of single status, with all the positive and negative ramifications of that change in status. Being pregnant implies temporary loss of one's customary physical appearance, wardrobe, and eating habits. Becoming a parent implies loss of the nonparent state. Once one becomes a mother or a father the old experience of being a nonparent is lost forever. Losing an arm and losing a job are losses that are easier to recognize because they are more concrete.

LIMIT SETTING

Setting limits with patients is very important, but it is sometimes difficult to do. In setting limits, the nurse is telling the patient something specific: "You can go this far over here, this far over there, but you cannot go past this point or you will suffer certain repercussions." All of us have limits set for us: classes are only so long; we only have a limited time to prepare for an examination or a deadline. Likewise, patients need limits set for them when they cannot set limits for themselves. Nurses can and do limit how much time and attention patients receive, as well as number of staff working with an individual patient when this is appropriate. Setting limits also implies rules and regulations. For example, inpatients are given definite limits: "If you drink alcohol on the unit you will be discharged. Those are the rules." "If you go out on pass you must return by 11:00 P.M., or you will not be issued a pass in the future." Patients who push limits abuse the privileges that accompany their rules and regulations: the patient who drinks alcohol in the lobby and comes to the inpatient unit drunk; the patient who returns night after night from a pass exactly 2 minutes past 11:00 P.M. Sometimes these patients push limits within the nurse–patient agreements; an example would be trying to lengthen the time for an interaction past the point initially agreed on.

MATERIAL

This term is used synonymously with thematic content, or content of an interaction. Therapists refer to this content as material (eg, sexual material, conscious material, unconscious material).

MOBILIZE

To mobilize a patient usually means to get him moving: walking, talking, eating, sleeping, working, thinking, behaving. This term is best illustrated by the nurse working with the severely depressed person who is immobilized and can be described as having psychomotor retardation. The patient is withdrawn; he is slowed down to the point of not being able to walk, talk, eat, sleep, work, think, and behave.

PROBLEM SOLVING

Everyone could probably use some assistance in problem solving. When the nurse problem solves with the patient, she does not solve the patient's problem or tell him what to do, but she does take him through the problem solving process. The nurse should recognize that her task is to provide an atmosphere in which the patient can solve a problem, or she may structure their interaction so as to increase the likelihood that the patient can arrive at a solution. In order to do this the nurse must be familiar with the problem solving process and know how to employ the process with the patient.

RESOLVE

In order to grow and develop as individuals, all people must adjust to major changes in their lives. A certain amount of emotional work is required in order to integrate new experiences into our perspectives of ourselves and our life goals. The most concrete example is the need to resolve the death of a loved one. It is known that people resolve grief in stages, usually within a certain period of time; in order to arrive comfortably at the substitution phase, it is important to have worked through the previous stages successfully. If this does not occur, then it is said that someone has not resolved his grief or that someone is exhibiting symptoms that are indicative of an unresolved grief reaction. Resolution of any loss (or conflict) takes time; it does not occur in one or two interactions with a patient. The amount of time involved depends on many factors; multiple losses take longer to resolve than isolated changes; persons with poor ego functioning usually take longer than healthier individuals to resolve changes. Resolution is the end result of what is usually considered a working-through process. To resolve an event, change, or incident usually means to come to terms with the reality of a change in a way that does not block future growth. That is, further development must not be blocked by strong unresolved feelings concerning past events that negatively influence present and future coping behaviors. Many people are not aware of the amounts of emotional energy and time that are involved in resolving a life change or a conflict about an important issue. People are often surprised when they discover that past losses, changes, or conflicts are still very much with them. With exploration of present crises they may come in touch with feelings of sadness, grief, anger, or guilt over past events. Frequently in the process of working through a present crisis, many past feelings can be resolved.

SANCTION

It is often necessary to sanction a patient's expression of feelings. Sanction in this sense means to allow or to positively reinforce the patient's expression of feelings. Sanctioning expression of feelings is in some ways mental health teaching. Traditionally, patient teaching has been kept within the realm of concrete medical facts. Examples are numerous: how insulin works, how to recognize the seven warning signs of cancer. In mental health nursing a certain amount of teaching is also necessary. This is accomplished not only by verbal instruction but also by allowing patients to experience a different kind of relationship in which nurses give patients permission, or sanction, for verbal expressions of feelings and thoughts by listening and accepting any feelings the patients may wish to express. Sometimes nurses strengthen this sanctioning with comments to the patient: "It's normal, it's OK, it's not harmful to be angry with someone." "Most people feel helpless in this situation. Is this true for you, too?" Verbalizing the implied frequently has the effect of sanctioning thoughts and feelings that people sometimes consider bad or evil. The nurse who calmly accepts statements such as "I hate my children," "I'm so angry with my mother I sometimes think about hurting her," or "I feel so guilty I ever got married" is allowing the patient to understand that any and all feelings are an essential part of being human and that having negative feelings does not imply that someone is inhuman. Although some feelings need not and should not be acted on, everyone has a right to his feelings.

STAFF SPLITTING

Staff splitting occurs when a patient successfully manipulates the staff into taking sides for or against the patient. That is, the staff members do not agree on the patient's intentions, concerns, degree of honesty, etc. One side believes the patient and sympathizes with his position; the other side is hostile to the patient and does not believe the patient is honestly sharing his concerns and problems. This happens when the patient tells one nurse one thing and then tells another nurse an entirely different thing. The two nurses meet, and conflict ensues, each nurse believing she has the true picture of the patient's position. Patients who indulge in staff splitting frequently try to engage the nurse in a special relationship: "Promise me you won't tell anyone if I tell you this." "Miss Jones, you are the only person who really understands me." Staff splitting must be guarded against; it can be destructive not only to the patient (who is not receiving consistent care) but also to the staff, who may become unnecessarily angry, fearful, and suspicious of one another. Inpatients particularly must always be told that although information is confidential it must be shared with those people who are also involved in their care. Staff splitting also points out the need for open communication between staff members about consistency in patient planning.

STRUCTURE

This term is used in many ways. As a noun it refers to an environment that is organized in a clear and unambiguous fashion (eg, a structured inpatient setting or milieu). Similarly, an experience can be structured or unstructured (eg, a lecture with a beginning, a middle, and an end, versus a seminar where ideas are discussed in a more random fashion). The verb to structure means to provide concrete organization for an activity or an interaction (eg, the nurse–patient interaction where the nurse structures the conversation so that the patient rather than the nurse is the focus of the conversation). Most of us need a certain amount of structure. We impose that structure on our environment from within when we set our own timetable and our own deadline and meet our objectives without any external source of control. Others rely more heavily on external structure: directions from others on how to focus their time, when to do what and for how long. Likewise, patients need varying degrees of structure. Patients who are highly anxious or very disorganized in their thinking need and respond best to concrete, simple structure in the form of verbal directions (eg, "Do this now. Do that at 5:00 P.M.") or written guidelines ("This is your schedule for the morning: at 8:00 A.M. take a shower and dress; at 9:00 A.M. attend a group meeting; at 10:00 A.M. meet with your nurse; at 11:00 A.M. go to crafts; at 12:00 have lunch."). When their anxiety lessens, when they become more organized in their thinking, or when new learning

SUPPORT

This term generally refers to time and attention. It does not refer to agreeing with the patient about an issue or taking the patient's side in a dispute with another staff member or a family member. The following are examples of support in the nurse–patient relationship: being available to the patient under a clear, consistent agreement; spending time with the patient; accompanying a patient to a stressful event; working with the patient on a difficult task.

occurs, the focus for control can again come from within. At this point it is usually said that the patient can handle a less structured approach.

TERMINATE
TERMINATION

To terminate means to end a relationship in a systematic fashion. Termination refers to the final phase of the nurse–patient relationship. To terminate with a patient does not refer just to saying goodbye, or even to the final meeting with a patient. It refers to the entire phase, which has a number of elements. During termination the nurse is responsible for structuring this phase in order to fully explore with the patient a number of significant issues: (1) progress of the relationship, (2) the patient's progress, (3) the patient's feelings about termination in general, (4) the patient's reaction to terminating this specific relationship. The termination process is very significant, and the more comprehensively this phase is approached the less likely it is that the patient will leave the relationship with unresolved feelings about it.

VENTILATE
VENTILATION

Ventilation refers to a free, uninterrupted flow of thoughts and feelings. It's what we all do when we "just talk." In providing an atmosphere for ventilation the nurse accepts whatever feelings are expressed, concentrates on listening, and provides a nonjudgmental setting. This is not the time to problem-solve with the patient. People who need to ventilate usually need to express their feeling first and respond logically afterward; this sequence usually happens of its own accord. After a patient has ventilated significant material, he usually has released enough tension so that problem-solving is more efficient and is internally structured. Ventilation allows a better perspective on a problem; after ventilating, one can decide on a course of action: what to act on, what not to act on. Whether action is taken or not, ventilation is a legitimate activity in itself and should be sanctioned with the patient.

WORK
WORK THROUGH
WORKING THROUGH

Nurses often make statements about work: "That's a lot of work for that patient." "The patient is really working hard." Work, in this sense, usually refers to the expenditure of emotional energy on a problem; the most common example would be expression of thoughts and feelings. Emotional work may not result in a concrete end point, but it is expenditure of energy nonetheless. Working through is likewise the process of becoming aware of uncomfortable feelings, risking self-disclosure, resolving a loss, problem-solving, exploring painful topics, or attempting to learn new ways of relating to others.

APPENDIX B

*SCHEDULE OF RECENT EXPERIENCE (SRE)**

Thomas H. Holmes
Richard H. Rahe

This questionnaire consists of two sections, a personal history section and a recent experience section. Each item of the questionnaire is to be answered on the answer sheets according to the instructions. Read each item and the choice of answers carefully, judge the answer as it applies to you, and mark it on the answer sheet.

SECTION I: PERSONAL HISTORY

This part of the questionnaire deals with information about your personal background. Most questions can be answered by placing a check-mark (√) in that bracket which best describes your situation. Each of these questions has only *one* answer that is appropriate. Other questions in this section require that you write your answer in the given space.

Example: What is your religious preference?

( ) Protestant
(√) Catholic
( ) Jewish
( ) Other
( ) None

This means your religious preference is Catholic.

 Further information about the cost and use of the Schedule of Recent Experience (SRE) can be obtained from Thomas H. Holmes, M.D., Department of Psychiatry and Behavioral Sciences RP-10, University of Washington, Seattle, Wash. 98195.

Please mark your answers on this sheet.

1. What is your sex?

   ( ) Male
   ( ) Female

2. What is your age in years?

   ( ) Under 21
   ( ) 21–30
   ( ) 31–45
   ( ) 46–65
   ( ) Over 65

3. What is your occupation?

   ____

4. What is your racial background?

   ( ) White
   ( ) Black
   ( ) Native American
   ( ) Chicano
   ( ) Asian
   ( ) Other

5. What is your religious preference?

   ( ) Protestant
   ( ) Catholic
   ( ) Jewish
   ( ) Other
   ( ) None

6. What is your present marital status?

   ( ) Married
   ( ) Divorced
   ( ) Separated
   ( ) Widowed
   ( ) Never married

7. How many times have you been married?

   ( ) 0
   ( ) 1
   ( ) 2
   ( ) 3
   ( ) 4+

8. How many times have you been divorced?

( ) 0
( ) 1
( ) 2
( ) 3
( ) 4+

9. How many times have you lost a spouse by death?

( ) 0
( ) 1
( ) 2
( ) 3
( ) 4

10. What is the highest level of education you have obtained?

( ) Grade school
( ) High school
( ) Technical school
( ) College
( ) Graduate degree

11. Approximately how long have you been at your present residence?

( ) 1 year
( ) 2 years
( ) 3 years
( ) 10 years
( ) 10+ years

12. How many times have you moved in the last 5 years?

____

13. In what country were you born?

____

14. In what area of the U.S. has most of your life been spent?

( ) East
( ) South
( ) Southwest
( ) Midwest
( ) Rocky Mountain
( ) Alaska
( ) Pacific Coast
( ) Hawaii
( ) Other
( ) Not applicable

15. What is the population of your birthplace?

( ) Rural
( ) 5000–
( ) 5000+
( ) 50,000–
( ) 50,000+

16. Where is your father's place of birth?

____

17. Where is your mother's place of birth?

____

18. How many brothers do your have?

____

19. How many sisters do you have?

____

20. What is your birth order in the family?

( ) Oldest
( ) Youngest
( ) Middle
( ) Only child

21. What was your age when your mother died?

( ) Mother living
( ) 0–5 years
( ) 6–10 years
( ) 11–15 years
( ) 16–20 years
( ) 20+ years

22. What was your age when your father died?

( ) Father living
( ) 0–5 years
( ) 6–10 years
( ) 11–15 years
( ) 16–20 years
( ) 20+ years

SECTION II: RECENT EXPERIENCE

Part A (Items 1 through 12)

This section of the questionnaire is different from the first part in three ways. First, the questions have to do with whether an event did or did not happen *and* when. Second, the answers to these questions are to be marked on a separate answer sheet. Third, the answer sheet has been separated into the following four time periods.

0 to 6 mo   6 mo to 1 yr   1 to 2 yrs ago   2 to 3 yrs ago

For each numbered question in the booklet:

1. Think back on the item event and decide if it happened to you and when it happened.
2. If the event in question did happen in any of the time periods, mark the answer by circling the "yes" in the appropriate time period. Y means Yes.
3. If the event in question did not happen in any of the time periods, mark the answer by circling the "no" in the appropriate time period. N means No.

When in doubt of the event happening, then circle the "yes." If you are not certain of the time period, do not worry; just try to be as close as possible. There must be a circle each time period.
Example:

Item No. 1: Mark under the appropriate time periods when there has been either a lot more or a lot less trouble with the boss.

0 to 6 mo	6 mo to 1 yr	1 to 2 yrs ago	2 to 3 yrs ago
(Y) N	Y (N)	(Y) N	Y (N)

This means that you have had either a lot more or a lot less trouble with the boss in the past six months and also 1 to 2 years ago. You had neither a lot more nor a lot less trouble with the boss 6 months to 1 year ago and 2 to 3 years ago.

Item Number

1. Mark under the appropriate time periods when there has been either a lot more or a lot less trouble with the boss.
2. Mark under the appropriate time periods when there was a major change in sleeping habits (sleeping a lot more or a lot less, or change in part of day when asleep).

3. Mark under the appropriate time periods when there was a major change in eating habits (a lot more or a lot less food intake, or very different meal hours or surroundings).
4. Mark under the appropriate time periods when there was a revision in your personal habits (dress, manner, associations, etc.).
5. Mark under the appropriate time periods when there was a major change in your usual type and/or amount of recreation.
6. Mark under the appropriate time periods when there was a major change in your social activities (e.g., clubs, dancing, movies, visiting, etc.).
7. Mark under the appropriate time periods when there was a major change in church activities (e.g., a lot more or a lot less than usual).
8. Mark under the appropriate time periods when there was a major change in number of family get-togethers (e.g., a lot more or a lot less than usual).
9. Mark under the appropriate time periods when you had a major change in financial state (e.g., a lot worse off or a lot better off than usual).
10. Mark under the appropriate time periods when you had in-law troubles.
11. Mark under the appropriate time periods when you had a major change in the number of arguments with spouse (e.g., either a lot more or a lot less than usual regarding child-rearing, personal habits, etc.).
12. Mark under the appropriate time periods when you had sexual difficulties.

Part B (Items 13 through 42)

This part of Section II is similar to Part A, except that the question now asks you to indicate the *number of times* an item event happened in each of the appropriate time periods.

Each of the time period columns is numbered 0, 1, 2, 3, 4+. These numbers represent the number of times the event happened. The last number, 4+, means the event happened to you four or more times. If the event did not happen, circle the 0. There needs to be a circle in each time period.

Example:

Item No. 19: Mark the number of times in each appropriate time period that you have had a change in residence.

0 to 6 mo	6 mo to 1 yr	1 to 2 yrs ago	2 to 3 yrs ago
0①2 3 4+	⓪1 2 3 4+	0 1②3 4+	⓪1 2 3 4+

This means that you changed residence once in the past six months and twice 1 to 2 years ago. You did not change residence 6 months to 1 year ago or 2 to 3 years ago.

Item Number

13. Mark the number of times in each appropriate time period that you experienced major personal injury or illness.
14. Mark the number of times in each appropriate time period that you have lost a close family member (other than spouse) by death.
15. Mark the number of times in each appropriate time period that you have experienced the death of spouse.
16. Mark the number of times in each appropriate time period that you have experienced the death of a close friend.
17. Mark the number of times in each appropriate time period that you have gained a new family member (e.g., through birth, adoption, oldster moving in, etc.).
18. Mark the number of times in each appropriate time period that there has been a major change in the health or behavior of a family member.
19. Mark the number of times in each appropriate time period that you had a change in residence.
20. Mark the number of times in each appropriate time period that you have experienced detention in jail or other institution.
21. Mark the number of times in each appropriate time period that you have been found guilty of minor violations of the law (e.g., traffic tickets, jaywalking, disturbing the peace, etc.).
22. Mark the number of times in each appropriate time period that you have undergone a major business readjustment (e.g., merger, reorganization, bankruptcy, etc.).
23. Mark the number of times in each appropriate time period that you married.
24. Mark the number of times in each appropriate time period that you divorced.
25. Mark the number of times in each appropriate time period that you had marital separation from your mate.
26. Mark the number of times in each appropriate time period that you had an outstanding personal achievement.
27. Mark the number of times in each appropriate time period that you had a son or daughter leave home (e.g., marriage, attending college, etc.).
28. Mark the number of times in each appropriate time period that you have experienced retirement from work.
29. Mark the number of times in each appropriate time period that there was a major change in working hours or conditions.
30. Mark the number of times in each appropriate time period that you had a major change in responsibilities at work (e.g., promotion, demotion, lateral transfer).

31. Mark the number of times in each appropriate time period that you have been fired from work.
32. Mark the number of times in each appropriate time period that there was a major change in living conditions (building a new home, remodeling, deterioration of home or neighborhood).
33. Mark the number of times in each appropriate time period that your wife began or ceased working outside the home.
34. Mark the number of times in each appropriate time period that you took a mortgage greater than $10,000 (e.g., purchasing a home, business, etc.).
35. Mark the number of times in each appropriate time period that you took a mortgage or loan less than $10,000 (e.g., purchasing a car, TV, freezer, etc.).
36. Mark the number of times in each appropriate time period that you experienced a foreclosure on a mortgage or loan.
37. Mark the number of time in each appropriate time period that you have taken a vacation.
38. Mark the number of times in each appropriate time period that you have changed to a new school.
39. Mark the number of times in each appropriate time period that you have changed to a different line of work.
40. Mark the number of times in each appropriate time period that you have begun or ceased formal schooling.
41. Mark the number of times in each appropriate time period that you had a marital reconciliation with your mate.
42. Mark the number of times in each appropriate time period that you had a pregnancy.

SECTION II: ANSWER SHEET

Part A

	0 to 6 mo	6 mo to 1 yr	1 to 2 yrs ago	2 to 3 yrs ago
1.	Y N	Y N	Y N	Y N
2.	Y N	Y N	Y N	Y N
3.	Y N	Y N	Y N	Y N
4.	Y N	Y N	Y N	Y N
5.	Y N	Y N	Y N	Y N
6.	Y N	Y N	Y N	Y N
7.	Y N	Y N	Y N	Y N

8.	Y N	Y N	Y N	Y N
9.	Y N	Y N	Y N	Y N
10.	Y N	Y N	Y N	Y N
11.	Y N	Y N	Y N	Y N
12.	Y N	Y N	Y N	Y N

Part B

	0 to 6 mo	6 mo to 1 yr	1 to 2 yrs ago	2 to 3 yrs ago
13.	0 1 2 3 4+	0 1 2 3 4+	0 1 2 3 4+	0 1 2 3 4+
14.	0 1 2 3 4+	0 1 2 3 4+	0 1 2 3 4+	0 1 2 3 4+
15.	0 1 2 3 4+	0 1 2 3 4+	0 1 2 3 4+	0 1 2 3 4+
16.	0 1 2 3 4+	0 1 2 3 4+	0 1 2 3 4+	0 1 2 3 4+
17.	0 1 2 3 4+	0 1 2 3 4+	0 1 2 3 4+	0 1 2 3 4+
18.	0 1 2 3 4+	0 1 2 3 4+	0 1 2 3 4+	0 1 2 3 4+
19.	0 1 2 3 4+	0 1 2 3 4+	0 1 2 3 4+	0 1 2 3 4+
20.	0 1 2 3 4+	0 1 2 3 4+	0 1 2 3 4+	0 1 2 3 4+
21.	0 1 2 3 4+	0 1 2 3 4+	0 1 2 3 4+	0 1 2 3 4+
22.	0 1 2 3 4+	0 1 2 3 4+	0 1 2 3 4+	0 1 2 3 4+
23.	0 1 2 3 4+	0 1 2 3 4+	0 1 2 3 4+	0 1 2 3 4+
24.	0 1 2 3 4+	0 1 2 3 4+	0 1 2 3 4+	0 1 2 3 4+
25.	0 1 2 3 4+	0 1 2 3 4+	0 1 2 3 4+	0 1 2 3 4+
26.	0 1 2 3 4+	0 1 2 3 4+	0 1 2 3 4+	0 1 2 3 4+
27.	0 1 2 3 4+	0 1 2 3 4+	0 1 2 3 4+	0 1 2 3 4+
28.	0 1 2 3 4+	0 1 2 3 4+	0 1 2 3 4+	0 1 2 3 4+
29.	0 1 2 3 4+	0 1 2 3 4+	0 1 2 3 4+	0 1 2 3 4+
30.	0 1 2 3 4+	0 1 2 3 4+	0 1 2 3 4+	0 1 2 3 4+
31.	0 1 2 3 4+	0 1 2 3 4+	0 1 2 3 4+	0 1 2 3 4+
32.	0 1 2 3 4+	0 1 2 3 4+	0 1 2 3 4+	0 1 2 3 4+
33.	0 1 2 3 4+	0 1 2 3 4+	0 1 2 3 4+	0 1 2 3 4+
34.	0 1 2 3 4+	0 1 2 3 4+	0 1 2 3 4+	0 1 2 3 4+
35.	0 1 2 3 4+	0 1 2 3 4+	0 1 2 3 4+	0 1 2 3 4+
36.	0 1 2 3 4+	0 1 2 3 4+	0 1 2 3 4+	0 1 2 3 4+

37.	0 1 2 3 4+	0 1 2 3 4+	0 1 2 3 4+	0 1 2 3 4+
38.	0 1 2 3 4+	0 1 2 3 4+	0 1 2 3 4+	0 1 2 3 4+
39.	0 1 2 3 4+	0 1 2 3 4+	0 1 2 3 4+	0 1 2 3 4+
40.	0 1 2 3 4+	0 1 2 3 4+	0 1 2 3 4+	0 1 2 3 4+
41.	0 1 2 3 4+	0 1 2 3 4+	0 1 2 3 4+	0 1 2 3 4+
42.	0 1 2 3 4+	0 1 2 3 4+	0 1 2 3 4+	0 1 2 3 4+

APPENDIX C

AMERICAN NURSES' ASSOCIATION STANDARDS OF PSYCHIATRIC AND MENTAL HEALTH NURSING PRACTICE

Psychiatric Nursing is a specialized area of nursing practice employing theories of human behavior as its scientific aspect and purposeful use of self as its art. It is directed toward both preventive and corrective impacts upon mental illness and is concerned with the promotion of optimal mental health for society, the community and those individuals and families who live within it. The dependent area of Psychiatric Nursing Practice is implementation of physicians' orders. The independent areas are assessment of nursing needs and development and implementation of nursing care plans, including initiation, development and termination of therapeutic relationships between nurses and patients. Psychiatric Nursing is practiced largely in collaboration and coordination with those in a variety of other disciplines who are working concomitantly with the patient. Thus, a high degree of interdependence with colleagues from other professions is inherent.

The Practice of Psychiatric Nursing is characterized by those aspects of clinical nursing care that involve interpersonal relationships with individuals and groups as well as a variety of other activities. These activities include: providing a therapeutic milieu, concerned largely with the sociopsychologic aspects of patients' environments; working with patients concerning the here-and-now living problems they confront; accepting and using the surrogate parent role; teaching with specific reference to emotional health as evidenced by various behavioral patterns; assuming the role of social agent concerned with improvement and promotion of recreational, occupational and social competence; providing leadership and clinical assistance to other nursing personnel. Joint planning or cooperative and collaborative efforts with other professionals are an essential part of providing nursing service. Most psychiatric settings employ an interdisciplinary team approach which requires highly coordinated and frequently interdependent planning.

Direct nursing care functions may involve individual psychotherapy, group psychotherapy, family therapy and sociotherapy. Psychiatric Nurses engaged in these therapies may employ a variety of approaches, particularly in the rapidly emerging area of sociotherapy and community mental health. With the national trend toward community mental health, Psychiatric Nurses are more and more involved in providing services aimed toward prevention of mental illness and reinforcement of healthy adaptations in addition to corrective and rehabilitative services.

The indirect nursing care roles of the Psychiatric Nurse are those of administrator with emphasis on leadership functions; clinical supervisor with emphasis on leadership functions as well as clinical teaching; director of staff development and training in a clinical facility; consultant or resource person; and researcher. In some of these indirect care roles, nurses will also be involved in providing some direct nursing care services to improve their own clinical skills and to serve as role models. All of these roles require coordinative and collaborative efforts with other disciplines.

The purpose of Standards of Psychiatric Nursing Practice is to fulfill the profession's obligation to provide and improve this practice. The Standards focus on practice. They provide a means for determining the quality of nursing which a client receives regardless of whether such services are provided solely by a professional nurse or by professional nurse and nonprofessional assistants.

The Standards are stated according to a systematic approach to nursing practice: the assessment of the client's status, the plan of nursing actions, the implementation of the plan, and the evaluation. These specific divisions are not intended to imply that practice consists of a series of discrete steps, taken in strict sequence, beginning with assessment and ending with evaluation. The processes described are used concurrently and recurrently. Assessment, for example, frequently continues during implementation; similarly, evaluation dictates reassessment and replanning.

These Standards of Psychiatric Nursing Practice apply to nursing practice in any setting. Nursing practice in all settings must possess the characteristics identified by these Standards if patients are to receive a high quality of nursing care. Each Standard is followed by a rationale and assessment factors. Assessment factors are to be used in determining achievement of the Standard.

STANDARD I

Data are collected through pertinent clinical observations based on knowledge of the arts and sciences, with particular emphasis upon psychosocial and biophysical sciences.

Rationale. Clinical observation is a prerequisite to realistic assessment of a client's needs and for the formulation of appropriate intervention. Observations can be facilitated through knowledge derived from a broad general education. In addition, scholarship acquired in the study of psychosocial and biophysical sciences fosters acuity of perception and alerts the nurse to psychologic, cultural, social and other relevant clinical data.

Assessment Factors

1. Data collecting activities involve observation, analysis and interpretation of behavior patterns of clients which indicate a need for growth promoting relationships.
2. Data collecting activities involve identification of significant areas in which clinical data are needed.
3. Data collecting activities involve utilization of knowledge derived from appropriate sources to gain a comprehensive grasp of the client's experience.
4. Data collecting activities involve inferences drawn from observations which contribute to a formulation of therapeutic intervention.
5. Data collecting activities involve inferences and treatment observations which are shared and validated with appropriate others.

STANDARD II

Clients are involved in the assessment, planning, implementation and evaluation of their nursing care program to the fullest extent of their capabilities.

Rationale. To a very large degree, the therapeutic process is a learning process. The same principle that applies to learning also applies to therapy; that is, the learner or client must be an active participant in the process. The ability to participate in such a process will vary from person to person and, at times, even within the same person. The word "therapy" is used here in its broadest sense; that is, any behavior or planned activity that promotes growth and well-being. Thus, "nursing care program" and "nursing therapy" are interchangeably used, although it is recognized that many other forms of therapy exist.

Assessment Factors

1. Clients' capabilities to participate at any given time are assessed, always keeping in mind the ultimate goals mutually determined by the client and nurse.
2. Plans for achieving and re-examining the goals are developed with the client, making whatever readjustments are necessary to progress toward them.

3. Problems are identified in collaboration with the client to determine needs and to set goals.
4. Progress of clients toward mutual goal achievement is assessed.

STANDARD III

The problem-solving approach is utilized in developing nursing care plans.

Rationale. A nursing diagnosis is based on pertinent theories of human behavior. It is used to plan therapeutic intervention taking into consideration the characteristics and capacities of the individual and his environment in order to maximize the treatment program for the client.

Assessment Factors

1. The individual's reaction to the environment is observed and assessed.
2. Themes and patterns of the behavior are observed and assessed.
3. Nursing care plans are used as a guide to nursing intervention.
4. Nursing care plans are interpreted to professional and nonprofessional persons giving care.
5. Observations and reports of others are incorporated in the nursing care plans.
6. Nursing care plans are designed, implemented and reviewed systematically by the nursing staff.

STANDARD IV

Individuals, families and community groups are assisted to achieve satisfying and productive patterns of living through health teaching.

Rationale. Health teaching is an essential part of a nurse's role in work with those who have mental health problems. Every interaction can be utilized as a teaching-learning situation. Formal and informal teaching methods can be used in working with individuals, families, the community and other personnel. Emphasis is on understanding mental health problems as well as on developing ways of coping with them.

Assessment Factors

1. The needs of individual, family and community groups for health teaching are identified and appropriate techniques are used in meeting these needs.
2. The principles of learning and teaching are employed.
3. The basic principles of physical and mental health and interpersonal and social skills are taught.
4. Experiential learning opportunities are made available.
5. Opportunities with community groups to further their knowledge and understanding of mental health problems are identified.

STANDARD V

The activities of daily living are utilized in a goal directed way in work with clients.

Rationale. A major portion of one's daily life is spent in some form of activity related to health and well-being. An individual's developmental and intellectual level, emotional state and physical limitations may be reflected in these activities. Therefore, nursing has a unique opportunity to assess and intervene in these processes in order to encourage constructive changes in the client's behavior so that each person may realize his full potential for growth.

Assessment Factors

1. An appraisal is made of the client's capacities to participate in activities of daily living based on needs, strengths and levels of functioning.
2. Clients are encouraged toward independence and self-direction by various skills such as motivating, limit setting, persuading, guiding and comforting.
3. Each person's rights are appreciated and respected.
4. Methods of communicating are devised which assure consistency in approach.

STANDARD VI

Knowledge of somatic therapies and related clinical skills are utilized in working with clients.

Rationale. Various treatment modalities may be needed by clients during the course of illness. Pertinent clinical observations and judgments are made concerning the effect of drugs and other treatments used in the therapeutic program.

Assessment Factors

1. Pertinent reactions to somatic therapies are observed and interpreted in terms of the underlying principles of each therapy.
2. A patient's responses are observed and reported.
3. The effectiveness of somatic therapies is judged and subsequent recommendations for changes in the treatment plan are made.
4. The safety and emotional support of clients receiving therapies is provided.
5. Opportunities are provided for clients and families to discuss, question and explore their feelings and concerns about past, current or projected use of somatic therapies.

STANDARD VII

The environment is structured to establish and maintain a therapeutic milieu.

Rationale. Any environment is composed of both human and nonhuman resources which may work for or against the person's well-being. The nurse works with people in a variety of environmental settings, e.g. hospital, home, etc. The milieu is structured and/or altered so that it serves the client's best interests as an inherent part of the overall therapeutic plan.

Assessment Factors

1. The effects of environmental forces on individuals are observed, analyzed and interpreted.
2. Psychological, physiological, social, economic and cultural concepts are understood and utilized in developing and maintaining a therapeutic milieu.
3. Communications within the environment are congruent with therapeutic goals.
4. All available resources in the environment are utilized when appropriate in the therapeutic efforts.
5. Nursing participation and its effectiveness in establishing and maintaining a therapeutic milieu are evaluated.

STANDARD VIII

Nursing participates with interdisciplinary teams in assessing, planning, implementing and evaluating programs and other mental health activities.

Rationale. In addition to the nurse, the number and variety of people working with clients in the mental health field today make it imperative that efforts be coordinated to provide the best total program. Communication, planning, problem-solving and evaluation are required of all those who work with a particular client or program.

Assessment Factors

1. Specific knowledge, skills and activities are identified and articulated so these may be coordinated with the contributions of others working with a client or a program.
2. The value of nursing and team member contributions are recognized and respected.
3. Consultation with other team members is utilized as needed.
4. Nursing participates in the formulating of overall goals, plans and decisions.
5. Skills are developed in small group process for maximum team effectiveness.

STANDARD IX

Psychotherapeutic interventions are used to assist clients to achieve their maximum development.

Rationale. People with mental health problems fashion many of their patterns of living and relating to others on a psychopathologic basis. In order to help clients achieve better adaptation and improved health, a nurse assists them to identify that which is useful and that which is not useful in their modes of living and relating. Alternatives available to them are identified.

Assessment Factors

1. Useful patterns and themes in the client's interactions with others are re-enforced.

2. Clients are assisted to identify, test out and evaluate more constructive alternatives to unsatisfactory patterns of living.
3. Principles of communication, problem-solving, interviewing and crisis intervention are employed in carrying through psychotherapeutic intervention.
4. Knowledge of psychopathology and its healthy adaptive counterparts are used in planning and implementing programs of care.
5. Limits are set on behavior that is destructive to self or others with the ultimate goal of assisting clients to develop their own internal controls and more constructive ways of dealing with feelings.
6. Crisis intervention is used to reduce panic of disturbed patients.
7. Long-term psychotherapeutic relationships with clients are undertaken.
8. Colleagues are utilized in evaluating the progress of the psychotherapeutic relationships and in formulating modification of intervention techniques.
9. Nursing participation in the therapeutic relationship is evaluated and modified as necessary.

STANDARD X

The practice of individual, group or family psychotherapy requires appropriate preparation and recognition of accountability for the practice.

Rationale. Acceptance of the role of therapist entails primary responsibility for the treatment of clients and entrance into a contractual agreement. This contract includes a commitment to see a client through the problem he presents or, if this becomes impossible, to assist him in finding other appropriate assistance. It also includes an explicit definition of the relationship, the respective roles of each person in the relationship, and what can realistically be expected of each person.

Assessment Factors

1. The potential of the nurse to function as a primary therapist is evaluated.
2. The accountability for practicing psychotherapy is recognized and accepted.
3. Knowledge of growth and development, psychopathology, psychosocial systems and small group and family dynamics is utilized in the therapeutic process.
4. The terms of the contract between the nurse and the client, including the structure of time, place, fees, etc., that may be involved, are made explicitly clear.
5. Supervision or consultation is sought whenever indicated and other learning opportunities are used to further develop knowledge and skills.
6. The effectiveness of the work with an individual, family or group is routinely assessed.

STANDARD XI

Nursing participates with other members of the community in planning and implementing mental health services that include the broad continuum of promotion of mental health, prevention of mental illness, treatment and rehabilitation.

Rationale. In our contemporary society, the high incidence of mental illness and mental retardation requires increased effort to devise more effective treatment and prevention programs. There is a need for nursing to participate in programs that strengthen the existing health potential of all members of society. In this effort cooperation and collaboration by all community agencies becomes imperative. Such concepts as early intervention and continuity of care are essential in planning to meet the mental health needs of the community. The nurse uses organizational, advisory or consultative skills to facilitate the development and implementation of mental health services.

Assessment Factors

1. Knowledge of community and group dynamics is used to understand the structure and function of the community system.
2. Current social issues that influence the nature of mental health problems in the community are recognized.
3. High risk population groups in the community are delineated and gaps in community services are identified.
4. Community members are encouraged to become active in assessing community mental health needs and planning programs to meet these needs.
5. The strength and capacities of individuals, families and the community are assessed in order to promote and increase the health potential of all.
6. Consultative skills are used to facilitate the development and implementation of mental health services.
7. The needs of the community are brought to the attention of appropriate individuals and groups, including legislative bodies and regional and state planning groups.
8. The mental health services of the agency are interpreted to others in the community. There is collaboration with the staff of other agencies to insure continuity of service for patients and families.
9. Community resources are used appropriately.
10. Nursing participates with other professional and nonprofessional members of the community in the planning, implementation and evaluation of mental health services.

STANDARD XII

Learning experiences are provided for other nursing care personnel through leadership, supervision and teaching.

Rationale. As leader of the nursing team, the nurse is responsible for the team's activities, and must be able to teach, supervise and evaluate the performance of nursing care personnel. The focus is on the continuing development of each member of the team.

Assessment Factors

1. Leadership roles and responsibilities are accepted.
2. Team members are encouraged to identify strengths and abilities. A climate is provided for the continuing self-development of each member.
3. A role model in giving direct nursing care is provided for the team.

4. The supervisory role is used as a tool for improving nursing care.
5. The client's needs, as well as the abilities of each member of the nursing team, are evaluated and assignments are based on these evaluations.

STANDARD XIII

Responsibility is assumed for continuing educational and professional development and contributions are made to the professional growth of others.

Rationale. The scientific, cultural and social changes characterizing our contemporary society require the nurse to be committed to the ongoing pursuit of knowledge which will enhance professional growth.

Assessment Factors

1. There is evidence of study of one's nursing practice to increase both understanding and skill.
2. There is evidence of participation in in-service meetings and educational programs either as an attendee or as a teacher.
3. There is evidence of attendance at conventions, institutes, workshops, symposia and other professionally oriented meetings and/or other ways to increase formal education.
4. There is evidence of systematic efforts to increase understanding of psychodynamics, psychopathology and avenues of psychotherapeutic intervention.
5. There is evidence of cognizance of developments in relevant fields and utilization of this knowledge.
6. There is evidence of assisting others to identify areas of educational needs.
7. There is evidence of sharing appropriate clinical observations and interpretations with professionals and other groups.

STANDARD XIV

Contributions to nursing and the mental health field are made through innovations in theory and practice and participation in research.

Rationale. Each professional has responsibility for the continuing development and refinement of knowledge in the mental health field through research and experimentation with new and creative approaches to practice.

Assessment Factors

1. Studies are developed, implemented and evaluated.
2. Responsible standards of research are used in investigative endeavors.
3. Nursing practice is approached with an inquiring and open mind.
4. The pertinent and responsible research of others is supported.
5. Expert consultation and/or supervision is sought as required. Judgment is used in assessing abilities as well as limitations to engage in research.
6. The ability to discriminate those findings which are pertinent to the advancement of nursing practice is demonstrated.
7. Innovations in theory, practice and research findings are made available through presentations and/or publications.

APPENDIX

D

GUIDELINES FOR WRITING PROCESS RECORDINGS

A process recording is one tool used in psychosocial nursing to help the student examine the interaction with the patient. The written recording contains precise notes on what transpired during the patient–student interaction.

PURPOSE

1. To provide a means of observing the reciprocal and circular nature of one-to-one interactions; that is, two individuals responding to and eliciting responses from one another.
2. To provide a means for the student to identify and understand the meanings of behavior, thoughts, and feelings, her own as well as the patient's.
3. To provide a tool for systematically recording and analyzing verbal and nonverbal interactions occurring in a one-to-one relationship.
4. To provide a means by which students can examine and evaluate nursing intervention and validate perceptions and interpretations.
5. To provide a means for developing skills in handling raw data gathered during a one-to-one interaction; these skills include collecting, ordering, analyzing, and synthesizing the data.
6. To provide a tool for applying theoretic concepts to practice.
7. To provide a means for planning purposeful intervention.
8. To increase observational skills.

FORMAT

The format in Table D.1 is suggested, but it may be varied as needed. The knowledge gained from a process recording depends on the amount of effort invested. Tape recording or videotaping each session aids in writing process recordings. In addition, we suggest keeping your process

These guidelines were developed by Reg Arthur Williams and Denise Conlin-Fort.

recordings. It is very enlightening to look at your interactions with patients later in your nursing career.

For further discussion of process recording, refer to: Travelbee J: Interventions in Psychiatric Nursing. Philadelphia, FA Davis, 1969, pp 117–137.

Table D.1. FORMAT FOR PROCESS RECORDING

Date: Time:
Number of interactions:
Location:
Brief description of the presenting problem(s):
Objectives for this interaction:

CONVERSATION	NONVERBAL COMMUNICATION AND PERCEPTIONS	NURSE'S FEELINGS AND THOUGHTS	ANALYSIS
The verbal exchange that transpires between the nurse and the patient. N: "________" P: "________"	The patient's nonverbal behavior; descriptive information about the environment and the patient available through the senses (what you see, smell, taste, touch, and hear)	Your emotional and intellectual responses to what is occurring	Theoretic concepts and reasons for utilizing interventions that increase your understanding of the patient's behavior; evaluate effective and ineffective therapeutic skills used in the interaction

Summarize the themes of the patient's concerns during this interaction. What are the plans for the next interaction?

APPENDIX

E

GUIDELINES FOR VISITING COMMUNITY AGENCIES

Students should select and visit community agencies in which mental health professionals from a variety of disciplines offer a range of services to the community. Services are aimed at the prevention as well as the treatment of mental illness. The range of available community services will reflect the scope of full comprehensive care.

Comprehensive service, as defined by the Community Mental Health Centers Act of 1963, includes ten major areas.

I. Five essential services, necessary for communities to qualify for federal funds:
   1. Inpatient services
   2. Outpatient services
   3. Partial hospitalization services:
      a. Day care
      b. Night care
      c. Weekend hospitalization
   4. Emergency service provided 24 hours per day within at least one of the three services above
   5. Consultation and education to community agencies and professional personnel

II. Full comprehensive service must also include:
   6. Diagnostic and evaluative service distinct from diagnostic and evaluative procedures inherent in other services
   7. Precare and aftercare services:
      a. Halfway house
      b. Vocational placement
      c. Foster home care
      d. Nursing home placement
      e. Home visiting
   8. Rehabilitation service:
      a. Vocational

These guidelines were developed by Denise Conlin-Fort.

   b. Recreational
   c. Resocialization
9. Training:
   a. In-service education for professionals and lay groups
   b. Field placements for students of various educational institutions
10. Research and evaluation

SUGGESTED APPROACH

1. With the assistance of the instructor, the student selects agencies she would like to visit. Selections should be based on personal interest and on the extent to which the agencies reflect current patterns in delivering mental health care service to the public.
2. The agency is contacted by the student.
3. An appropriate resource is identified, and specific details of the visit are arranged.
4. Include in your plans the purpose of your visit: date, time, length of visit.
5. Ascertain who at the agency will orient you to the facility. If no one person is available, plan how you will use your time at the agency to meet your objectives.
6. In evaluating the agency, the following are important aspects to consider:
   a. Objectives
   b. Name of agency
   c. Name and position of person orienting you to the facility
   d. Brief history of how the resource developed
   e. Types of services available
   f. Population served
   g. Mode of treatment employed
   h. Average length of contact patient will have with the agency
   i. Means by which an individual is referred or comes to the agency
   j. Who is eligible to receive services of the agency
   k. Cost of services
   l. Financial assistance available to defray cost of services
   m. Approximate number of staff employed
   n. Types of professionals and nonprofessional workers represented
   o. Brief description of how you perceive the roles of the various mental health care workers and how each contributes to the delivery of services
   p. Impression of the resource and how the services provided relate to the prevention and treatment of mental illness
   q. If possible, describe briefly how the community might view the agency in terms of the types of services available. What needs might members of the community identify that can be met by the agency? What is your impression of the way the agency and staff respond to expressed or felt needs of the community?

INDEX

A

F

G

M

N

R

S

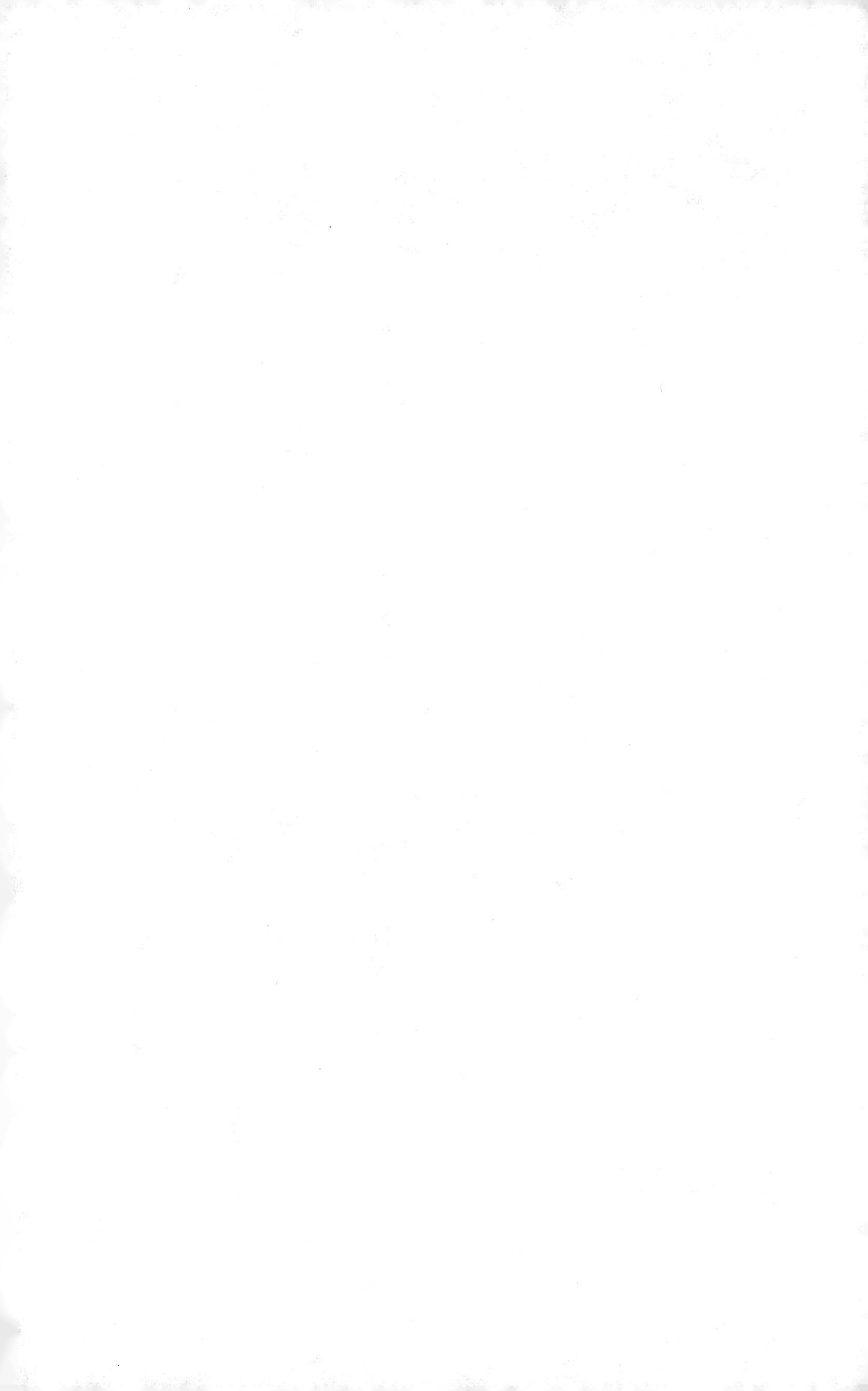